AF327014

Sleep Medicine

Clinical Practice

SLEEP - PHYSIOLOGY, FUNCTIONS, DREAMING AND DISORDERS

SLEEP - PHYSIOLOGY, FUNCTIONS, DREAMING AND DISORDERS

SLEEP MEDICINE

CLINICAL PRACTICE

ANTONIO DEL CASALE
ROBERTO BRUGNOLI
AND
PAOLO GIRARDI
EDITORS

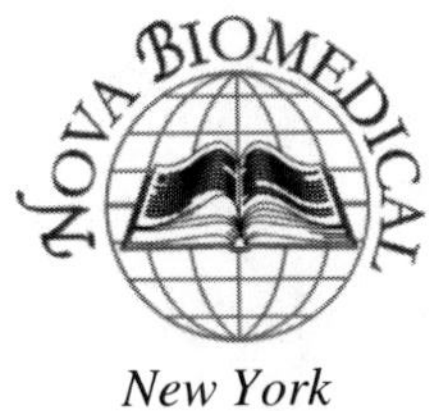

New York

Library of Congress Cataloging-in-Publication Data

ISBN: 978-1-62808-515-0

Library of Congress Control Number: 2013944374

Published by Nova Science Publishers, Inc. † New York

Contents

Preface vii
Roberto Tatarelli

Introduction ix
Paolo Girardi

Part I. Sleep Disorders: New Research and Clinical Evidence 1

Chapter I Fundamentals of Human Chronobiology 3
Daniele Serata, Chiara Rapinesi, Antonio Del Casale,
Georgios Demetrios Kotzalidis, Roberto Brugnoli
and Paolo Girardi

Chapter II Circadian Rhythm Sleep Disorders 17
Chiara Brugnoli, Antonio Del Casale,
Daniele Serata, Chiara Rapinesi
and Roberto Brugnoli

Chapter III Insomnia and Hypersomnias 27
Luigi Ferini-Strambi and Sara Marelli

Chapter IV Parasomnias 61
Daniele Serata, Chiara Rapinesi,
Antonio Del Casale and Roberto Tatarelli

Chapter V Sleep-Related Breathing and Movement Disorders 75
Luigi Ferini-Strambi, Sara Marelli and Andrea Galbiati

Chapter VI Risk Factors in Obstructive Sleep Apnea Syndrome:
Cohort Analysis 123
F. Chéliout-Héraut, M. Faye, F. Djouadi,
N. Zrek and F. Bour

Chapter VII Sleep Bruxism and Gastroesophageal Reflux
as a Peripheral Risk Factor 135
Shouichi Miyawaki, Takakazu Yagi, Kunihiro Nagayama,
Haruhito Ohmure, Kyoko Kanematsu and Yoko Sakoguchi

Part II. Sleep Disturbance in Psychiatric Disorders — 151

Chapter VIII — Sleep Disturbances and Related Psychopathologies — 153
Antonio Del Casale, Paolo Girardi,
Chiara Rapinesi, Daniele Serata,
Roberto Tatarelli and Gabriele Sani

Chapter IX — Sleep Disturbances in Anxiety Disorders — 163
Chiara Rapinesi, Antonio Del Casale,
Daniele Serata and Giovanni Manfredi

Chapter X — Sleep Disturbance in Mood Disorders — 181
Lidia Petrone, Stefano Porcelli
and Alessandro Serretti

Chapter XI — Sleep Disturbance in Schizophrenia — 217
Roberto Brugnoli, Simone Pallottino
and Paolo Girardi

Chapter XII — Substance-Related Sleep Disorders — 231
Alessandro E. Vento and Paolo Girardi

Part III. Diagnostic Techniques — 247

Chapter XIII — EEG and Polysomnography in Sleep Disorders — 249
Carla Buttinelli, Michela Ferraldeschi,
Miriam Tasillo and Manuela Giuliani

Chapter XIV — Neuroimaging in Sleep Medicine — 275
Antonio Del Casale, Valentina Corigliano,
Chiara Rapinesi, Daniele Serata,
Anna Comparelli and Stefano Ferracuti

Part IV. Psychoeducation and Pharmacotherapies — 303

Chapter XV — Psychoeducation in Sleep Medicine — 305
Paolo Girardi, Antonio Del Casale,
Chiara Brugnoli, Lavinia De Chiara,
Daniele Serata, Chiara Rapinesi
and Gloria Angeletti

Chapter XVI — Pharmacotherapies in Sleep Medicine — 319
Luigi Ferini-Strambi
and Sara Marelli

Index — 351

Preface

***Roberto Tatarelli*[*]**
Full professor of Psychiatry, "Sapienza" University
"Sant'Andrea" Hospital, Rome, Italy

The study of phenomena that occur during sleep has always aroused a great interest in various fields of human knowledge, both in religion and in philosophy, as well as in science. Hippocrates and Aristotle conducted different studies and observations on sleep and dreams, focusing on the changes that affect the state of consciousness between the waking and sleeping states. Freud even started from the observations and interpretation of dreams in the foundation of the psychoanalytic method. After the introduction of the electroencephalogram (EEG) by Hans Berger (1929), the beginning of modern sleep medicine began.

Currently, the scientific literature in this field is very vast, gathering different aspects of many medical specialties, mainly including psychiatry, neurology, pneumology, cardiology, internal medicine, and others. Precisely because of this broad extension, it is not completely explorable by clinicians and is not always adequate for their needs.

This book aims to be a point of reference for the basic principles of clinical practice in the field of sleep medicine. Its main objective is to provide a useful tool for both study and consultation, using a variety of figures and tables in each chapter.

This book deals with various aspects of sleep medicine: circadian rhythm neurophysiology, neurophysiopathology of sleep disorders, and multifaceted relationships between psychiatric disorders and sleep disturbances. Both electroencephalographic and the latest neuroimaging aspects are discussed. One major point concerns available psycho-educational treatments and pharmacotherapies of sleep disorders. In summary, several ideas and topics on sleep medicine are deeply discussed in an original manner.

---

[*] roberto.tatarelli@uniroma1.it.

Introduction

Paolo Girardi[*]

NESMOS Department (Neurosciences, Mental Health, and Sensory Organs)
Sapienza University of Rome, School of Medicine and Psychology
"Sant'Andrea" Hospital, Rome, Italy

A great interest in the nature of sleep and dreams thoroughly covers chronicled human history. Hindu Brihad-Aranyaka Upanishad gave much attention to sleep, dream and awareness of dreams [1], and Old and New Testaments of the Bible have often described dreams and their interpretation [2]. Edwin Smith, Ebers and Kahun medical papyri from ancient Egyptian described insomnia and the use of the opium, which very likely was the first hypnotic medication [3]. In Greek mythology, the god $Y\pi\nu o\varsigma$ was the personification of sleep, habitually represented holding poppies [4].

Hippocrates often referred to disordered sleep and dreams: he suggested that phenomena occurring during sleep and dream could be used for diagnosing somatic complaints [5]. He also stressed the importance of a well-established circadian rhythm in patients with organic diseases, particularly in those suffering from epilepsy. These patients should "spend the day awake and the night asleep. If this habit be disturbed, it is not so good… worse of all when he sleeps neither night nor day" [6]. Hippocrates, Aristotle and Galen considered the dream as a state of consciousness in which sensations are amplified, explaining in this way the realization of some "premonitory dreams".

After the classical era, the scientific interest in sleep and dreams was revived in the early 20th century, during which Sigmund Freud in The Interpretation of Dreams [7] theorized the unconscious nature of dreams. With Freud, dreams are a creation of one's individual psyche, and any dream can be interpreted by understanding definite underlying thoughts. These theories are the basis of all Freudian psychoanalytic thought.

Afterward, the field of Sleep Medicine was introduced in the 1970's. A milestone was the development of the electroencephalogram (EEG) in 1929 by the German psychiatrist Hans Berger. EEG allowed monitoring and studying brain activity, even during sleep [8]. Berger showed the varying EEG patterns correlated with wakefulness and sleep. Through EEG study

---

[*] Email: paolo.girardi@uniroma1.it.

it was well established that the brain is in a synchronized pattern of neuronal activation during sleep, and is not idle.

The father of American sleep research is largely considered Nathaniel Kleitman, who started in the 1920s at the University of Chicago, and studied sleep, wakefulness, and circadian rhythm. In 1951, Eugene Aserinsky, a doctoral student of Kleitman, observed the phenomenon of rapid eye movements, first in sleeping infants and soon after in adults [9]. As a result, Kleitman and William Dement established the cyclical nature of EEG recordings during sleep. Each cycle occurred at intervals between 90 and 100 minutes. They observed the association between REM sleep and dreaming. During REM sleep, brain wave patterns resembled light sleep. They classified sleep as either non-REM or REM [10].

To function adequately in a 24-hour cycle, the human central nervous system must synchronize with the external time. The central pacemaker that regulates circadian rhythms is the suprachiasmatic nucleus (SCN) situated in the anterior hypothalamus [11]. Light is the strongest stimulant for the SCN, which gets direct afferents from melanopsin-containing ganglion cells of the retina [12, 13]. During light exposure, the SCN inhibits the synthesis and release of melatonin by the pineal gland. Conversely, during the night (or in prolonged conditions of absence of light), the SCN clock stimulates the pineal gland to synthesize and releasing melatonin [14].

Optimal sleep is reached when sleep time aligns with endogenous circadian rhythm and wake propensity. The regulation of circadian rhythm and maintenance of optimal sleep are complex physiological processes that may undergo pathological disruption in several cases, including dyssomnias, parasomnias, sleep disorders associated with medical and/or psychiatric disorders, and other cases. At present, the International Classification of Sleep Disorders (ICSD-2) is the most used classification system, consisting in "a primary diagnostic, epidemiological and coding resource for clinicians and researchers in the field of sleep and sleep medicine" [15].

In this book we will discuss and present the most recent evidence on major sleep disorders.

We will first analyze all dyssomnias and parasomnias studied by sleep medicine. Subsequently, we expose sleep disturbances that may occur in the course of a mental disorder. In these contexts it is very important to emphasize two fundamental concepts. First, in patients with sleep disturbance due to an organic condition, restoring a stable circadian rhythm and obtaining an adequate number of hours of sleep through available treatments almost always improves the underlying organic disease. Second, sleep disorders and circadian rhythm disruption are, on the one hand, epiphenomena of an underlying mental disorder, and on the other constitute an authentic engine of illness, thus creating a vicious cycle of disease that becomes increasingly serious. In these cases, treating sleep disorders and circadian rhythm alterations significantly contributes to improving the mental health of the patient.

We will also give space to recent and interesting evidence obtained through polysomnography and neuroimaging studies.

Finally, regarding the treatment of sleep disorders, particular emphasis will be given to both current pharmacotherapies and psychoeducational and cognitive-behavioral therapies. Treating sleep disorders and re-establishing a good circadian rhythm constitute a primary goal for the physician in the treatment of patients suffering from a primary sleep disorder, and for patients who suffer from a sleep disturbance that is related to an underlying organic pathology or mental disorder.

References

[1]   Olivelle P. The Early Upanisads: annotated text and translation. New York: Oxford University Press, 1998.

[2]   The Catholic Study Bible. 2nd edition. Donald Senior, ed. New York: Oxford University Press, 2006.

[3]   Silverburg R. The Dawn of Medicine. Putnam Publishing, New York, 1975.

[4]   Smith W. A Dictionary of Greek and Roman biography and mythology. By various writers. Smith, William, Sir, ed. 1813-1893. Boston, MA: Little, Brown and co., 1867.

[5]   Jones WHS. Hippocrates On Dreams. Loeb Classical Library Vol IV, Harvard University Press, Cambridge, MA, 1923.

[6]   Lloyd GER. Hippocrates, the Sacred Disease, Aphorisms, and Prognosis. In: Lloyd GER, editor. Hippocratic writings. Boston: Penguin; 1983.

[7]   Freud S. The Interpretation of Dreams, third edition. Translated by Brill AA. New York: The Macmillan Company; 1913.

[8]   Berger H. Ueber das Elektoenkephalogram des Menschen. *J. Pschol. Neurol.* 1930;40:160-179.

[9]   Aserinsky E, Kleitman N. Regularly occurring periods of eye motility, and concomitant activity during sleep. *Science.* 1953;118:273-274.

[10] Dement W, Kleitman N. Cyclic variations in EEG during sleep and their relation to eye movements, body motility, and dreaming. *Electroenceph Clin. Neurophysiol.* 1957;9:673-690.

[11] Moore RY, Eichler VB. Loss of a circadian adrenal corticosterone rhythm following suprachiasmatic lesions in the rat. *Brain Res.* 1972;42(1):201-6.

[12] Bellingham J, Foster RG. Opsins and mammalian photoentrainment. *Cell Tissue Res.* 2002;309(1):57-71.

[13] Paul KN, Saafir TB, Tosini G. The role of retinal photoreceptors in the regulation of circadian rhythms. *Rev. Endocr. Metab. Disord.* 2009 Dec;10(4):271-8

[14] Pevet P, Challet E. Melatonin: both master clock output and internal time-giver in the circadian clocks network. J Physiol Paris. 2011;105(4-6):170-82.

[15] The International Classification of Sleep Disorders: Diagnostic and Coding Manual, ICSD-2. 2nd edn. Westchester, IL: American Academy of Sleep Medicine, 2005.

Part I.
Sleep Disorders:
New Research and Clinical Evidence

In: Sleep Medicine
Editors: A. Del Casale, R. Brugnoli and P. Girardi

ISBN: 978-1-62808-515-0
© 2013 Nova Science Publishers, Inc.

Chapter I

Fundamentals of Human Chronobiology

Daniele Serata, Chiara Rapinesi, Antonio Del Casale,*
Georgios Demetrios Kotzalidis, Roberto Brugnoli
and Paolo Girardi
Sapienza University, Rome
NESMOS (Neuroscience, Mental Health and Sensory Organs)
Department School of Medicine and Psychology

Abstract

Chronobiology is the study of biological temporal rhythms, including the circadian, weekly, seasonal, and annual rhythms. The term "circadian" comes from the Latin words "*circa*", meaning "around", and "*dies [-ēi]*", meaning "day". A circadian rhythm can be defined as any biological process that manifests an endogenous entrainable oscillation of about 24 hours. Circadian rhythm affects physiology, behavior, cognition, and the sleep-wake cycle in mammalians and humans. The master clock located in the suprachiasmatic nuclei (SCN) of the hypothalamus has a central role in circadian rhythm preservation. The human circadian time-keeping system is characterized by a composite architecture, with the central brain's SCN pacemaker and subsidiary clocks in nearly every cell. The sleep-wake cycle is a complex and dynamic phenomenon involving numerous cerebral structures, neuronal network, and neurotransmitters. Sleep is generally divided into non-rapid eye movement (NREM) sleep and rapid eye movement (REM) sleep. NREM and REM phases occur in the course of the sleep with cyclicity. Each phase has typical characteristics, including variations in brain wave patterns, eye movement type, and muscle tone. This chapter provides a general overview of the human circadian-generating systems and sleep physiology.

Keywords: Circadian rhythm, sleep physiology, NREM, REM

---

* Corresponding author: Dr. Daniele Serata"Sapienza" University, Rome.Email: seratadaniele@gmail.com.

Human Circadian Rhythm

The Circadian Clock

All biological activities in humans are characterized by cycles of varied lengths. The period of approximately one day is called "circadian". Circadian rhythm is homeostatically regulated. The main time-giver (*zeitgeber*) is solar light. In the absence of external time-givers, circadian rhythm has a period that differs from 24 hours [1].

The brain area of the endogenous circadian *zeitgeber* is the suprachiasmatic nucleus (SCN), which is located bilaterally in the hypothalamus, just above the optic chiasm. SCN contains the mechanism entertaining relations with the daily light-dark cycle, and has a major role in the regulation of the 24-hour rhythm.

From the retina through the retinohypothalamic tract, light-mediated input stimulates N-methyl-D-aspartate glutamatergic receptors in the SCN [2]. Here, circadian rhythms are maintained intracellularly by interlocking positive and negative feedback control of transcription and translation of three period genes (Per1-3), two cryptochrome genes (Cry1,2), and the "Clock" and "Bmal1" (brain and muscle ARNT-like 1) genes [2,3]. These feedbacks create molecular signals that produce a cascade that ends in changes of neural membrane potential. Circadian rhythms in the whole body are mainly coordinated in synchrony by the SCN [4], but clock genes are also expressed in extra-SCN brain regions and in peripheral tissues (fibroblasts).

Outside the SCN, other organs and areas have a role in maintaining circadian rhythm, including the retina, olfactory bulbs, piriform cortex, hippocampus, striatum, and the cerebellum express clock genes. These structures are also called "secondary clocks" [5]. Although their rule is not fully understood, they have a major role for timing behavioral and physiological tasks to underlie precise daily activities, including vigilance and sleep, motivation, learning, vision, and olfaction [6]. The circadian clock also drives several other physiological mechanisms, mainly body temperature, humoral signals, endocrine activities (including, for example, the hypothalamic-pituitary-adrenal axis), and feeding-related cues [7]. Different polysynaptic connections drive signals from the SCN. The major circadian relay from the adjacent sub-paraventricular zone runs dorsally and caudally into the dorsomedial hypothalamus; it can been considered as a crescent-shaped continuum of the medial hypothalamus [8]. Within the hypothalamus, projections to the paraventricular nucleus, preoptic area, pineal gland, and medio-basal nuclei make it possible to regulate daily rhythms of hormone secretion, including adrenocorticotropins, gonadotropins, melatonin, and other metabolic hormones [9]. The SCN can regulate both the ascending arousal system and sleep-regulatory centers, which themselves have reciprocal connections for the regulation of circadian rhythm (Figure 1).

The Ascending Arousal System

Wakefulness depends on the functioning of the ascending reticular activating system projecting to brain cortices. This system consists of: 1. cholinergic neurons in the pedunculopontine and laterodorsal tegmental nuclei; 2. noradrenergic neurons of the locus coeruleus; 3. serotonergic neurons in the dorsal raphe nucleus; 4. dopaminergic neurons of the ventral periaqueductal gray matter; 5. histaminergic neurons of the tuberomammillary nucleus. In general, neurons in all of these areas are more active during wakefulness than during sleep.

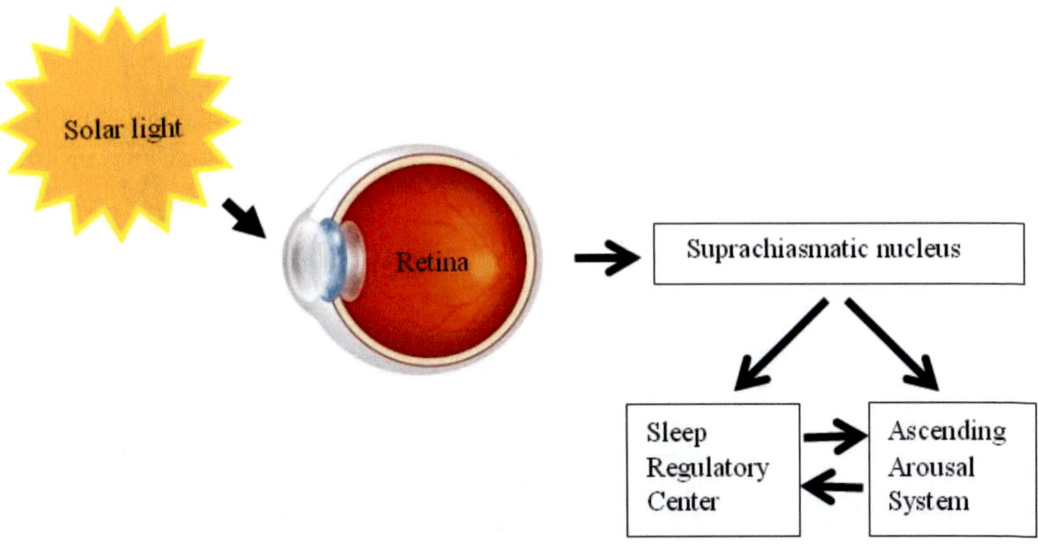

Figure 1. Simplipied regulatory circuits involved in wake and sleep.

In particular, the ascending arousal system is structured in two main pathways. The first pathway dorsally innervates the thalamus, and activates the relay neurons and reticular nuclei, which are essential for thalamo-cortical transmission. The pedunculopontine and laterodorsal tegmental nuclei, which are two major cholinergic structures in the brainstem and basal forebrain, innerve the main thalamic nuclei and are most active during wakefulness and rapid eye movement (REM) sleep, discharging more slowly during non-REM (NREM) sleep [8,10].

Thus, the dorsal tegmentum pathway is composed by cholinergic neurons active during wake and REM sleep (wake/REM-on). Also, acetylcholine release in the thalamus is high during wake and REM sleep. The cholinergic neurons from the laterodorsal tegmentum compactly innervate the medial, intralaminar, and other thalamic nuclei, the lateral hypothalamus, and the midbrain. During wake and REM sleep, they depolarize thalamic relay neurons, thus activating thalamo-cortical signaling with consequential fast cortical rhythms. During NREM sleep they are inactive. Other basal forebrain cholinergic neurons, whose discharge-rate is higher during wake and REM and lower during NREM sleep, project to the cortex, hippocampus, and amygdala.

The second pathway is ventral and mainly innerves the lateral hypothalamus and basal forebrain. It comprises a number of monoaminergic cells (noradrenergic neurons of the locus coeruleus, serotonergic neurons of the dorsal and median raphe nuclei, dopaminergic neurons of the ventral periaqueductal gray matter, and histaminergic neurons of the tuberomammillary nucleus). It receives input from the orexin and melanin-concentrating hormone neurons of the lateral hypothalamic area, as well as from GABAergic or acetylcholine neurons of the basal forebrain.

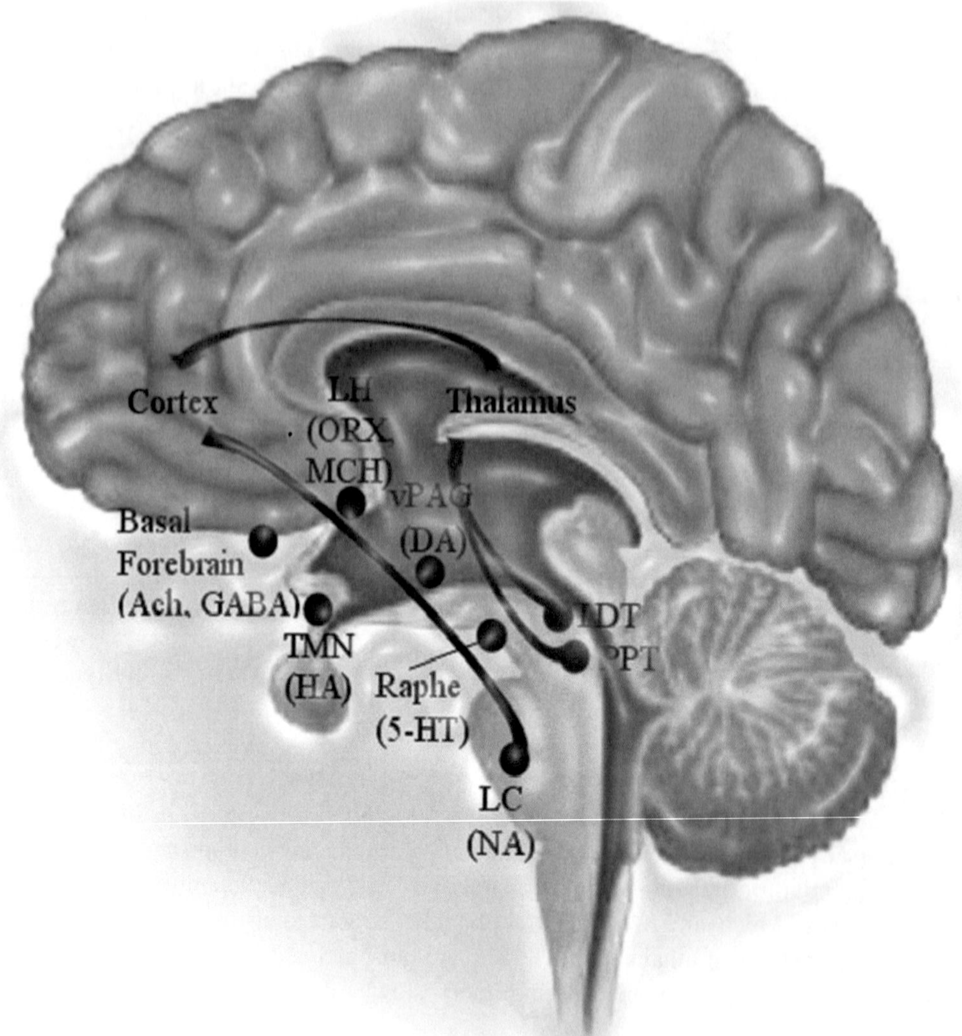

Figure legend: 5-HT: serotonin; Ach: Acetylcholine; DA: dopamine; GABA: gamma-aminobutiric acid; HA: histamine; LC: locus coeruleus; LDT: laterodorsal tegmentum; LH: lateral hypothalamus.

Figure 2. The ascending arousal system.

These two pathways forming the ascending arousal system operate to promote cortical arousal and to realize and maintain the waking state. Conversely, during the sleep state they are inhibited by neurons of the ventrolateral preoptic (VLPO) nucleus [11] (Figure 2).

The Sleep Regulatory System

The VLPO nucleus plays a crucial function, which is to deactivate the arousal system with the subsequent onset of the sleep state [12]. VLPO neurons are primarily active during sleep and release the inhibitory transmitters gamma-aminobutyric acid (GABA) and galanin. Loss of these neurons causes intense insomnia and sleep fragmentation [13].

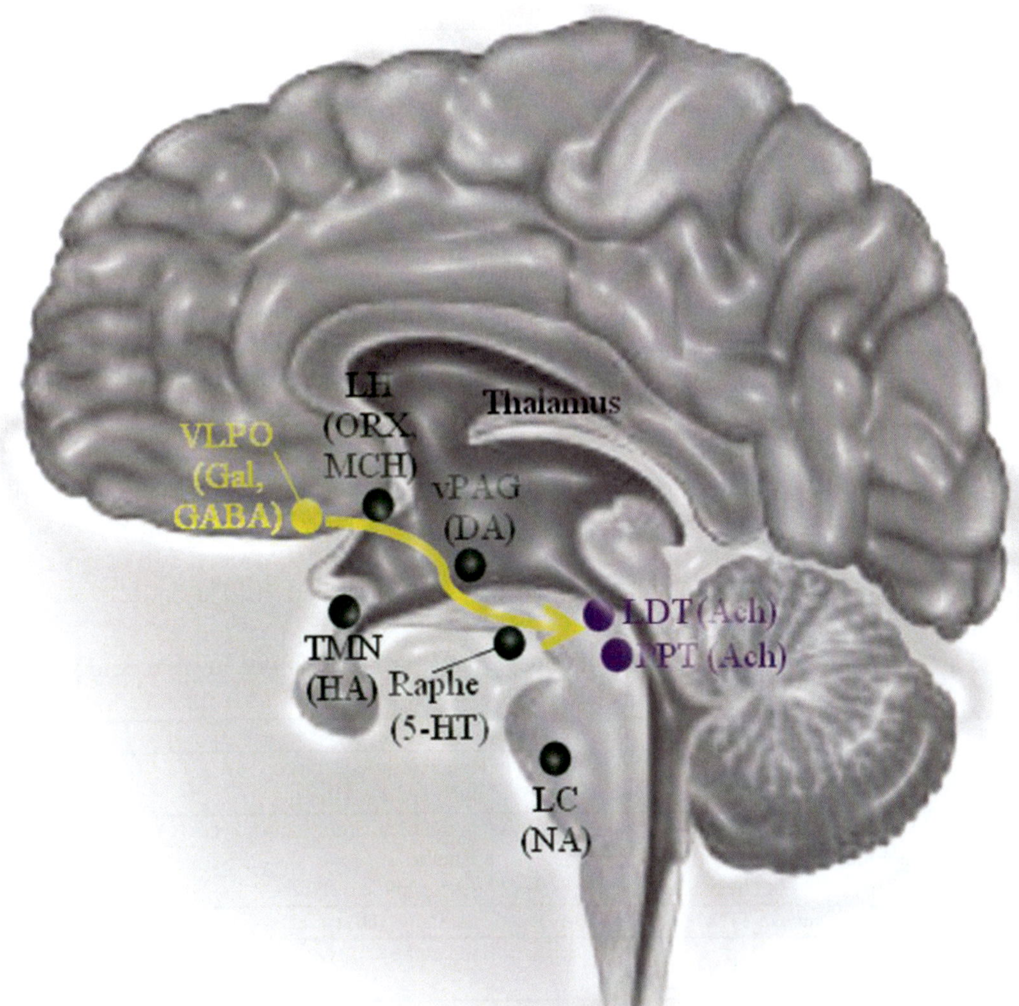

Figure legend. 5-HT: serotonin; Ach: Acetylcholine; DA: dopamine; GABA: gamma-aminobutiric acid; Gal: galanine; HA: histamine; LDT: laterodorsal tegmentum; LC: locus coeruleus; LH: lateral hypothalamus; MCH: melanin-concentrating hormone; NA: noradrenaline; ORX: orexin; PPT: pedunculopontine tegmentum; TMN: tuberomammillary nucleus; VLPO: ventrolateral preoptic nucleus; vPAG: ventral periaqueductal gray matter.

Figure 3. The sleep-regulatory system.

Two principal populations of neurons are located in the VLPO. The first is a cluster of neurons placed in its core (VLPOc) that projects most heavily to the tuberomammillary nucleus. The second population, more diffusely located, is included in the so-called extended VLPO (eVLPO), and mainly projects to the locus coeruleus and to dorsal and median raphe nuclei. The interactions between the eVLPO and the components of the arousal systems are mutually inhibitory.

In addition to GABA and galanin, neuropeptide S, another recently discovered neuromodulator, is co-expressed in glutamate-producing neurons situated for the most part in the pre-coeruleus region (an area located rostrally to the locus coeruleus), which projects to extensive brain areas, including sleep-wake regulatory regions such as the midline thalamic nuclei, lateral hypothalamus, and preoptic area. Intracerebroventricular administration of neuropeptide S increased locomotor activity and decreased sleep in rats [14].

Brain Areas and Associated Neurotransmitters Regulating the Circadian Rhythm

Beginning in the early 1930s, some key brain areas critically involved in maintaining the circadian rhythm were identified [15]. The anterior and posterior hypothalamus and the rostral midbrain were coupled with several other areas and associated neurotransmitters, including acetylcholine, serotonin, dopamine, GABA, and histamine (HA). Other neuromodulators like hypocretin 1 (Hcrt1) and 2 (Hcrt2), galanin, and neuropeptide S are also involved in circadian rhythm regulation.

The nerve cells of the neural networks that are involved in the regulation of the circadian rhythm are often characterized by a specific activity during each phase [16]. For example, some neurons are principally active during wake, other during REM only, still others during REM and wake, or during NREM only, or during both NREM and REM sleep.

Table 1. Brain areas and associated neurotransmitters involved in wake and sleep

Brain Areas	Neurotransmitters
Hypothalamic Areas (Lateral and Posterior)	Hypocretin 1 (Hcrt1) Hypocretin 2 (Hcrt2)
Ventrolateral Preoptic Area	Gamma-aminobutyric acid (GABA) Galanin Neuropeptide S (NPS)
Tuberomammillary Nucleus (TMN)	Histamine (HA)
Brainstem Regions Substantia Nigra & Ventral Tegmental Area	Dopamine
Reticular Formation Lateral Dorsal and Peduncolopontine Tegmentum (LDT/PPT)	Acetylcholine

Regarding the hypothalamic areas, the above mentioned lateral and posterior hypothalamus play a central role, being the main areas currently known as the source of the awake-promoting neuropeptides Hcrt1 and Hcrt2 [17]. These neuropeptides primarily stabilize transitions between wake and sleep. It is noteworthy that patients with narcolepsy with or without cataplexy have of loss of hypocretin neurons [18,19]. These neurons have a strong excitatory effect on cholinergic neurons of the basal forebrain that contribute to cortical arousal, but have no effect on GABAergic sleep-promoting neurons within the VLPO area. They have several excitatory projections to the dorsal raphe nucleus (Hrct1 and Hcrt2 receptors), locus coeruleus (Hcrt1 receptors), and tuberomammillary nucleus (Hcrt2 receptors). These regions in turn send inhibitory projections to hypocretin neurons.

The tuberomammillary nucleus is an important subnucleus of the posterior third of the hypothalamus. It receives stimulatory input from the lateral hypothalamus, and its activity is high during wake and absent during REM. It largely consists of histaminergic neurons that project to the cerebral cortex, amygdala, substantia nigra, dorsal raphe nucleus, locus coeruleus, and nucleus of the solitary tract. Histamine acting on neural H1 receptors produces wakefulness, while antihistamines (H1 receptor blockers) cause drowsiness or sleep. Its projections to the cerebral cortex directly amplify the cortical activations and arousal, while its output to the acetylcholinergic neurons of the basal forebrain and dorsal pons work similarly, but indirectly, by increasing the release of acetylcholine in the cerebral cortex [17].

The dopaminergic neurons are mainly sited in the substantia nigra and ventral tegmental area. For a long time it was thought that these neurons do not change their activation across sleep states, but recently some research has identified other dopaminergic neurons located in ventral periaqueductal gray matter, which are active during wakefulness but not during the sleep state. These periaqueductal cells send efferent to several major components of the circadian regulatory system, including the midline and intralaminar thalamus, VLPO, locus coeruleus, and medial-prefrontal cortex; they also project to cholinergic neurons of the basal forebrain, orexin/hypocretin cells in the lateral hypothalamic, and cholinergic cells of the pontine laterodorsal tegmental nuclei. These same dopaminergic neurons receive afferents from almost all the same areas, including the medial prefrontal cortex, VLPO, lateral hypothalamus, laterodorsal tegmental nuclei, and locus coeruleus [20].

Sleep Architecture

Sleep is a state of reduced awareness and responsiveness. The sleeping brain is relatively more responsive to internal than external stimuli, and the unconsciousness sleep state is characterized by dynamic processes that involve several brain areas and physiological systems. Sleep architecture refers to the basic structural organization of normal sleep. Sleep occurs in cycles, each usually composed of a period of NREM sleep followed by REM stage ("R" sleep) that cyclically alternate with each other. Sleep staging is based on electroencephalographic (EEG), electro-oculographic (EOG), and electromyographic (EMG) criteria. Knowing how to recognize certain EEG characteristics is essential for sleep staging.

EEG activity is described by frequency in cycles per second (hertz = Hz), amplitude (microvolts [μV]), and shape. The EEG frequency ranges from delta (<4 Hz), theta (4-7 Hz), alpha (8-13 Hz), and beta (>13 Hz) activities. The region (frontopolar, frontal, central, and occipital) of highest activity (amplitude) and the wave EEG activity patterns are important features. There are some particular patterns in EEG during sleep.

Sharp waves are narrow waves of 70 to 200 msec in duration, while *spikes* have a shorter duration of 20 to 70 msec. The so-called *alpha rhythm* consists of most prominent activity in occipital derivations, which is attenuated by eye opening and increased by eye closure. It is possible to use the term "alpha activity" to describe any EEG activity with a frequency in the alpha range (8-13 Hz). Bursts of alpha waves can also occur during stage R, typically at a frequency from 1 to 2 Hz slower than during wakefulness. *Sleep spindles* (*SSs*) are bursts of activity that arise from the thalamic reticular nucleus, with a frequency range from 11 to 16 Hz (usually 12-14) and a duration of 0.5 sec or greater (usually 0.5-1.5 sec) [21]. A *K complex* is a high-amplitude biphasic wave composed of an initial negative sharp wave (deflection up) followed by a slow wave, typically in frontal derivation. *Vertex sharp waves* are narrow-duration waves (<500 msec) prominent in central-vertex derivation during the transition between the sleep stages N1 and N2. The triangular-shaped *saw-tooth waves* generally occur during REM sleep (from 2 to 6 Hz) in the central derivations. The *slow wave activity* is composed by waves with a frequency range of 0.5 to 2 Hz (necessary from 2 to 0.5 sec duration) and a peak-to-peak amplitude greater than 75 µV in frontal derivations.

The recording of eye movements is made possible by the potential difference across the eyeball with the positive (+) front/cornea and the negative (–) back/retina. Eye movements are detected by EOG voltage changes associated with eye movement. Slow eye movements can be recorded with closed eyes, while awake, or during the first stage of NREM sleep. Rapid eye movements can be seen during eyes open wakefulness or stage "R" sleep.

Another important parameter is EMG. Monitoring chin EMG activity is important for identifying stage "R" (REM sleep). In this stage, the chin EMG is relatively reduced: the amplitude is equal to or lower than the lowest EMG amplitude in NREM sleep. The reduction in the chin EMG amplitude during REM sleep reflects global skeletal-muscle hypotonia.

NREM Sleep-Stage "N"

The previous classification of sleep stage distinguished the NREM sleep into 4 stages [22], which represent a continuum of relative depth sleep (table 2).

- Stage 1. Occurs at sleep onset and is characterized by standard muscle tone, eye movement, and wave patterns with low-voltage EEG (mixed frequency) waves, which are defined as "theta" waves, and constitute the predominant wave pattern of light sleep. This first emerges in infants at about 5 months of age. The amplitude of theta waves reaches its peak at 2-4 years and slowly declines through life. Stage 1 sleep lasts only a few minutes and can be easily interrupted, without awareness of having slept.
- Stage 2. Begins when K-complexes and sleep spindles (lasting at least 0.5 sec) appear on a background of theta waves. The K-complexes are the most evident characteristic of Stage 2 and can also be elicited by auditory stimuli. Sleep spindles are high-frequency bursts of electrical activity, ranging from 12 to 16 Hz. During stage 2 muscle tone persists and eye movements are usually slow or absent, although they may re-emerge for small intervals.
- Stage 3. The onset is defined when the EEG pattern comprises a percentage of 20-50% high-amplitude, low frequency (2 Hz) "delta" waves. Sleep spindles and K-complexes can still be identified in this stage.
- Stage 4: In this stage the EEG pattern has more than 50% high-amplitude, low-frequency waves. Muscle tone and eye movements are significantly diminished or not present during Stages 3 and 4.

The most recent classification of slow-wave sleep from the American Academy of Sleep Medicine (AASM) divides this NREM sleep into three stages: N1, N2, and N3, in which the previously defined sleep stages 3 and 4 were combined [22,23]. Low-amplitude mixed-frequency EEG waves with predominantly 4 to 7 Hz activity characterize the stage N1. Alpha EEG waves that occur during wakefulness are replaced during the N1 sleep stage by waves characterized by low amplitude and mixed frequency (4-7 Hz).

Table 2. The previous classification of Non-REM sleep

NREM Stage 75-80%	Duration (min) %	EEG pattern	Frequency (Hz)	Amplitude (mV)	Particular waves	Muscular tone (EMG)	Eyes movement (EOG)
1	1-7 min 2-5%	theta waves >50%	4-7 Hz	50-75 mV	sleep spindles	present	present
2	10-25 min 45-55%	theta waves, sigma waves	4-7 Hz 12-14 Hz	50-75 mV 5-50 mV	K complex, sleep spindles	present	slow or absent
3	2-10 min 3-8%	delta waves 20-50%	0,5-4 Hz	75 mV	K complex, sleep spindles	diminished or absent	diminished or absent
4	20-40 min 10-15%	delta waves 50%	0,5-4 Hz	75 mV	K complex, sleep spindles	diminished or absent	diminished or absent

Table 3. The recent classification of slow-wave sleep from the American Academy of Sleep Medicine (AASM) (Iber et al., 2007)

Non-REM sleep	Particular waves	Features
N1	LAMF waves vertex sharp waves	LAMF waves for >50% of the epoch
N2	KCs, SSs	LAMF EEG rhythm is present in epochs that contain, or are preceded by, K complexes or SSs
N3	SWA	20%-50% high-amplitude (> 75 microvolt), low-frequency (2Hz) delta waves

Legend: EEG: electroencephalographic; KCs: K complexes; LAMF: low-amplitude mixed-frequency; SSs: Sleep spindles; SWA: slow wave activity.

These waves occupy at least 50% of the epoch. The beginning of stage N1 can also be defined when alpha waves are not completely evident, but the presence of 4-7 Hz waves with slowing of background activity by at least 1 Hz compared with wakefulness, slow eye movements, or vertex sharp waves can be recorded. The N1 stage is characterized by the lack of SSs and K-complexes. Vertex sharp waves may also appear at the transition from stage N1 to N2.

Stage N2 starts with non-arousal EEG K-complexes or SSs during either the first half of the same stage or the last half of the previous epoch, with the lack of criteria for stage N3. Stage N2 continues if low-amplitude, mixed-frequency EEG rhythm is present in epochs that contain – or are preceded by – K-complexes or SSs.

Stage N3 is characterized by slow wave activity, with patterns that are equal to or greater than 20% of an epoch (≥6 sec). An EEG pattern of 20%-50% high-amplitude (>75 μV) and low-frequency (2 Hz) delta waves characterizes this stage. Slow wave activity is also distinguished in the EOG derivations, but slow and rapid eye movements are not present. The chin EMG is unpredictable, but typically less than during wake.

REM Sleep-Stage "R"

REM sleep is called "stage R" in the latest nomenclature [22,23]. In this stage, low-amplitude mixed-frequency activity generally characterizes the EEG (similar to stage N1).

Alpha activity is frequently more prominent than in stage N1, and has a frequency of 1-2 Hz lower than during wakefulness.

Stage R has three main features: 1. low-amplitude EEG (without K complexes or sleep spindles); 2. rapid eye movements; and 3. generalized skeletal-muscle hypotonia (detectable by low chin EMG). REM sleep is also characterized by several other physiological variations, including lower or absent deep tendon reflexes, irregular frequency and tidal volume of breath, penile tumescence, and amplified cardiac rhythm variability.

In general, EEG recordings show that REM sleep most closely resembles the waking state. Stage R ends when: 1. there is a transition to wakefulness or to sleep stage N3; 2. there is a transition to sleep stage N2 (appearance of K complexes or sleep spindles in the first half of the epoch); 3. an arousal occurs followed by slow eye movements; 4. a major body movement occurs, followed by slow eye movements; 5. chin EMG increases above the REM level for the majority of the epoch.

Control of Stage "R"

Several models have been proposed for the control of REM. In one model, the activity of REM-on neurons in the lateral dorsal tegmental/pedunculopontine tegmental nuclei is high, whereas activations in monoaminergic centers, including the tuberomammillary nucleus, dorsal raphe nucleus and locus coeruleus, are low. Different populations of REM-on cells located in the lateral pontine and pedunculopontine tegmentum stimulate effector cells in the medial pontine reticular formation (mPRF). These neurons in the mPRF are cholinoceptive. Infusion of cholinergic agonists into this area provokes the manifestations of REM sleep. Ponto-geniculo-occipital (PGO) waves and rapid eye movements correlate with the activity of specific areas in the mPRF that provide ascending projections. The pontine inhibitory area contains nuclei that are responsible for muscle atonia. The neurotransmitters GABA and glycine hypopolarize motor neurons resulting in REM sleep muscular atonia. Simultaneously, some neurons located in the medial medulla, with inhibitory projections to the LC, reduce the normal augmentation of muscle activity provided by the locus coeruleus [24].

Another purposed model is the so-called brainstem "flip-flop" switch [25], consisting of mutually inhibitory REM-off and REM-on areas in the mesopontine tegmentum. Each area contains GABAergic neurons that deeply innervate each other. The ventrolateral periaqueductal gray matter and lateral pontine tegmentum include the REM-off area, while the sublaterodorsal nucleus and precoeruleus area include the REM-on area. Both the REM-on and REM-off areas are jointly interconnected and inhibit each other.

REM-on glutamatergic neurons in the precoeruleus and medial parabrachial areas project to the medial septum–basal forebrain and activate the hippocampus (theta rhythm of REM sleep) and neocortex. REM-on glutamatergic neurons in the sublateraldorsal nucleus project to glycinergic/GABAergic interneurons in the spinal cord that, in turn, project to anterior horn cell motor neurons inducing muscle atonia.

The REM-off area can be inhibited by cholinergic neurons located in the peduncolopontine tegmentum and laterodorsal tegmentum, and by GABAergic and galanin neurons of the hypothalamic ventrolateral preoptic nucleus. Hypocretin (orexin) neurons provide stimulatory input to the REM-off neurons.

Physiological Changes During Sleep

Physiological changes during sleep involve many structures and systems, including the somatic and autonomic nervous system, the respiratory and cardiovascular systems, the endocrine and renal functions, and body temperature regulating system. These changes occur during both NREM and REM sleep (Table 4).

During NREM sleep, the autonomic nervous system shows an increase in parasympathetic tone and a decrease in sympathetic activity. REM sleep is associated with further increase of parasympathetic tone and intermittent increases in sympathetic activity.

NREM sleep is characterized by a burst of sympathetic-nerve activity related to the brief blood pressure and heart rate increases that follows K-complexes. Both sympathetic and hemodynamic changes may have a role in triggering ischemic events in patients affected by vascular disease during REM sleep [26].

Ventilation and respiratory flow manifests changes during sleep, becoming progressively faster and more unpredictable, particularly during REM sleep [27]. NREM sleep is associated with hypoventilation, which also characterizes REM sleep due to reduced muscle tone of the pharynx [28], reduced rib cage movement, and increased upper airway resistance related to defeat of the intercostals and upper airway muscular tone [29]. The cough reflex is also suppressed during both REM and NREM sleep. The hypoxic ventilatory response is lower in NREM sleep than during the waking state, and further decreases during REM sleep.

The circulatory system shows blood pressure and heart rate changes that are mainly determined by autonomic nervous system activity. Brief increases in blood pressure and heart rate occur with K-complexes, arousals, and outsized body movements [30,31]. The reported increased risk of myocardial infarction in the morning has been related to sharp increases in blood pressure and heart rate that accompany awakening [32].

Total blood flow and global metabolism in REM sleep is similar to wakefulness, while during NREM sleep these parameters are reduced in their average values. An exception is found in the limbic system (which is involved with emotions), and visual association areas, which both show metabolism and blood flow increases during REM sleep compared to wakefulness [33,34].

Regarding the renal system, decreased excretion of electrolytes during sleep and urine concentration and reduction have been reported [35].

Endocrine parameters such as growth hormone and thyroid hormone concentrations and melatonin secretion show changes during sleep. The first few hours subsequent to sleep onset temporally related to the first episode of slow-wave sleep are characterized by a peak in growth hormone secretion [36]. GH secretion and delta EEG wave activity have a temporal and quantitative relationship between themselves. Thyroid hormone secretion takes place in the late evening. The light-dark cycle affects melatonin secretion, which induces sleepiness by reducing an alerting effect from the SCN [29]. Global endocrine changes influence glucose regulation, insulin resistance, and corticotropic activity.

Circadian regulation also involves body temperature that is generally higher during the day than at night. During sleep, body temperature shows a gradual decline: heat production decreases and heat loss increases. During REM sleep, body temperature is not regulated, shivering and sweating are absent, and the temperature gradually approaches that of the surrounding environment. All these changes, together with EEG slow-wave activity, promote sleep onset and maintenance [37,38].

Table 4. Physiological changes during Non-REM and REM sleep

Physiological process	Non-REM	REM
Autonomic nervous system	Sympathetic nerve activity decreases and parasympathetic tone increases from wakefulness	Sympathetic nerve activity increases significantly from wakefulness
Circulatory system	Heart rate slows from wakefulness; blood pressure decreases from wakefulness	Heart rate increases compared to Non-REM; Blood pressure increases (up to 30%) from Non-REM
Respiratory system	Reduced hypoxic ventilatory response, respiration rate decreases from wakefulness, airway resistance increases from wakefulness	Increases and varies from Non-REM, reduced rib cage movement and increased upper airway resistance, coughing suppressed
Cerebral blood flow	Reduction in blood flow and metabolism	Total blood flow and metabolism is comparable to wakefulness and there is a relative increase in the limbic system and in visual association areas
Body temperature	Is regulated at lower set point than wakefulness, there a decrease in heat production and an increase in heat loss.	Is not regulated; no shivering or sweating; temperature drifts toward that of the local environment.

References

[1] Schulz P, Steimer T. Neurobiology of circadian systems. CNS Drugs 2009;23:3-13.

[2] Gillette MU, Tischkau SA. Suprachiasmatic nucleus: the brain's circadian clock. *Recent Prog. Horm. Res.* 1999;54:33-58; discussion 58-9.

[3] Albrecht U. Invited review: regulation of mammalian circadian clock genes. *J. App. Physiol.* 2002;92(3):1348-55.

[4] Ko CH, Takahashi JS. Molecular components of the mammalian circadian clock. *Hum. Mol. Genet.* 2006;15:271-7.

[5] Namihira M, Honma S, Abe H, Tanahashi Y, Ikeda M, Honma K. Daily variation and light responsiveness of mammalian clock gene, Clock and BMAL1, transcripts in the pineal body and different areas of brain in rats. *Neurosci. Lett.* 1999;267:69-72.

[6] Mendoza J, Challet E. Brain clocks: from the suprachiasmatic nuclei to a cerebral network. *Neuroscientist* 2009;15(5):477-88.

[7] Mohawk JA, Green CB, Takahashi JS. Central and peripheral circadian clocks in mammals. *Annu. Rev. Neurosci.* 2012;35:445-62.

[8] Saper CB, Scammell TE, Lu J. Hypothalamic regulation of sleep and circadian rhythms. *Nature* 2005;437(7063):1257-63.

[9] Kalsbeek A, Palm IF, La Fleur SE, Scheer FA, Perreau-Lenz S, Ruiter M, Kreier F, Cailotto C, Buijs RM. SCN outputs and the hypothalamic balance of life. *J. Biol. Rhythms* 2006;21(6):458-69.

[10] Hallanger AE, Levey AI, Lee HJ, Rye DB, Wainer BH. The origins of cholinergic and other subcortical afferents to the thalamus in the rat. *J. Comp. Neurol.* 1987;262(1):105-24.

[11] Schwartz JR, Roth T. Neurophysiology of sleep and wakefulness: basic science and clinical implications. *Curr. Neuropharmacol.* 2008;6(4):367-78.

[12] Sherin JE, Shiromani PJ, McCarley RW, Saper CB. Activation of ventrolateral preoptic neurons during sleep. *Science* 1996;271:216-219.

[13] Lu J, Greco MA, Shiromani P, Saper CB. Effect of lesions of the ventrolateral preoptic nucleus on NREM and REM sleep. *J. Neurosci.* 2000;20:3830-3842.

[14] Brown RE, Basheer R, McKenna JT, Strecker RE, McCarley RW. Control of sleep and wakefulness. Physiol Rev 2012;92:1087-187.

[15] Von Economo C. Sleep as a problem of localization. *J. Nerv. Ment. Dis.* 1930;71:249-259.

[16] Espana RA, Scammell TE. Sleep neurobiology for the clinician. *Sleep* 2004;27:811-820.

[17] De Lecea L, Kilduff TS, Peyron C, Gao X, Foye PE, Danielson PE, Fukuhara C, Battenberg EL, Gautvik VT, Bartlett FS 2nd, Frankel WN, van den Pol AN, Bloom FE, Gautvik KM, Sutcliffe JG. The hypocretins: hypothalamus-specific peptides with neuroexcitatory activity. *Proc. Natl. Acad. Sci. U S A* 1998;95(1):322-7.

[18] Nishino S, Ripley B, Overeem S, Lammers GJ, Mignot E. Hypocretin (Orexin) deficiency in human narcolepsy. *Lancet* 2003;355:39-40.

[19] Thannickal TC, Nienhuis R, Siegel JM: Localized loss of hypocretin (orexin) cells in narcolepsy without cataplexy. *Sleep* 2009;32:993-998.

[20] Lu J, Jhou TC, Saper CB. Identification of wake-active dopaminergic neurons in the ventral periaqueductal gray matter. *J. Neurosci.* 2006;26:193-202.

[21] McCormick L, Nielsen T, Nicolas A, Ptito M, Montplaisir J. Topographical distribution of spindles and K-complexes in normal subjects. *Sleep* 1997;20(11):939-41.

[22] American Academy of Sleep Medicine. International classification of sleep disorders, 2nd ed: Diagnostic and coding manual. American Academy of Sleep Medicine, Westchester, IL: 2005. Rechtschaffen A, Kales A. *A manual of standardized terminology, techniques and scoring system for sleep stages of human subjects.* Washington, DC: Public Health Service, US: Government Printing Office; 1968.

[23] Iber C, Ancoli-Israel S, Chesson A, Quan SF for the American Academy of Sleep Medicine. *The AASM Manual for the Scoring of Sleep and Associated Events: Rules, Terminology and Technical Specifications.* Westchester: American Academy of Sleep Medicine; 2007.

[24] McCarley RW. Mechanisms and models of REM sleep control. *Arch. Ital. Biol.* 2004;142:429-67.

[25] Lu J, Sherman D, Devor M, Saper CB: A putative flip- flop switch for control of REM sleep. *Nature* 2006;441:589-94.

[26] Somers VK, Dyken ME, Mark AL, Abboud FM. Sympathetic-nerve activity during sleep in normal subjects. *N. Engl. J. Med.* 1993;328(5):303-7.

[27] Simon PM, Landry SH, Leifer JC. Respiratory control during sleep. In: Lee-Chiong TK, Sateia MJ, Carskadon MA, editors. *Sleep Medicine.* Philadelphia: Hanley and Belfus; 2002. pp. 41-51.

[28] Krieger J. Respiratory physiology: Breathing in normal subjects. In: Kryger M, Roth T, Dement WC, editors. *Principles and Practice of Sleep Medicine.* 4th ed. Philadelphia: Elsevier Saunders; 2000. pp. 229-241.

[29] Parker KP, Dunbar SB. Cardiac nursing. In: Woods SL, Froelicher ESS, Motzer SU, Bridges E, editors. *Sleep. 5th ed.* Philadelphia: Lippincott Williams and Wilkins; 2005. pp. 197-219.

[30] Blasi A, Jo J, Valladares E, Morgan BJ, Skatrud JB, Khoo MC. Cardiovascular variability after arousal from sleep: time-varying spectral analysis. *J. Appl. Physiol.* 2003;95(4):1394-404.

[31] Tank J, Diedrich A, Hale N, Niaz FE, Furlan R, Robertson RM, Mosqueda-Garcia R. Relationship between blood pressure, sleep K-complexes, and muscle sympathetic nerve activity in humans. *Am. J. Physiol. Regul. Integr. Comp. Physiol.* 2003;285(1):R208-14.

[32] Floras JS, Jones JV, Johnston JA, Brooks DE, Hassan MO, Sleight P. Arousal and the circadian rhythm of blood pressure. *Clin. Sci. Mol. Med. Suppl.* 1978;4:395s-397s.

[33] Madsen PL, Schmidt JF, Wildschiødtz G, Friberg L, Holm S, Vorstrup S, Lassen NA. Cerebral O2 metabolism and cerebral blood flow in humans during deep and rapid-eye-movement sleep. *J. Appl. Physiol.* 1991;70(6):2597-601.

[34] Madsen PL, Holm S, Vorstrup S, Friberg L, Lassen NA, Wildschiødtz G. Human regional cerebral blood flow during rapid-eye-movement sleep. *J. Cereb. Blood Flow Metab.* 1991;11(3):502-7.

[35] Buxton OM, Spiegel K, Van Cauter E. Modulation of endocrine function and metabolism by sleep and sleep loss. In: Lee-Chiong TL, Sateia MJ, Carskadon MA, editors. *Sleep Medicine.* Philadelphia: Hanley & Belfus; 2002. pp. 59-69.

[36] Takahashi Y, Kipnis DM, Daughaday WH. Growth hormone secretion during sleep. *J. Clin. Invest.* 1969;47:2079-90.

[37] Szymusiak R. Sleep Research Society. SRS Basics of Sleep Guide. Westchester, IL: Sleep Research Society; 2005. *Thermoregulation and sleep*; pp. 119-126.

[38] Szymusiak R, Gvilia I, McGinty D: Hypothalamic control of sleep. *Sleep Med.* 2007;8:291-301.

In: Sleep Medicine
Editors: A. Del Casale, R. Brugnoli and P. Girardi

ISBN: 978-1-62808-515-0
© 2013 Nova Science Publishers, Inc.

Chapter II

Circadian Rhythm Sleep Disorders

Chiara Brugnoli, **Antonio Del Casale, Daniele Serata,***
Chiara Rapinesi and Roberto Brugnoli
Sapienza University, Rome
NESMOS (Neuroscience, Mental Health and Sensory Organs) Department
School of Medicine and Psychology

Abstract

Circadian rhythm sleep disorders, according to the ICSD-2, comprise a list of complaints sharing a common pathophysiological basis of misalignment between internal circadian rhythms and the desired or required time for sleep. The sleep disturbance produces sleep and wake periods that occur at inappropriate times, resulting in a complaint of insomnia or excessive sleepiness for patients. Diagnostic criteria include social or occupational impairment, and a diagnosis of CRSDs is appropriate only in the absence of other primary sleep disorders. The CRSDs recognized by ICSD-2 are: 1) Delayed sleep phase syndrome; 2) Advanced sleep-phase syndrome; 3) Non-24 hours sleep-wake syndrome; 4) Jet lag syndrome; 5) Shift work disorder; 6) Irregular sleep-wake pattern; 7) Circadian rhythm sleep disorder due to medical condition; 8) Circadian rhythm sleep disorder due to drug or substance; 9) Circadian rhythm sleep disorder, not otherwise specified [1].

Introduction

The definition "Circadian rhythm sleep disorders" comprises a list of nine disorders grouped by a common underlying chronophysiologic basis. According to the international classification of sleep disorders, second edition (ICSD-2), these disorders are due to a

---

* Corresponding author: Dr. Chiara Brugnoli "Sapienza" University, Rome. Email: chiarabrugnoli@gmail.com.

misalignment between the patient's sleep pattern and the sleep pattern that is desired, with involvement of the timing and duration of sleep [1].

The alteration of the circadian timing system leads to insomnia or excessive sleepiness, causing sleep to occur at inappropriate times, as well as wake periods, with the complaint of the patient.

The pathogenesis of these disorders often includes a misalignment between the endogenous circadian rhythm and environmental factors, or an internal disruption in the circadian timekeeping system, involving both exogenous and endogenous factors in the alteration [2].

Endogenous factors include the regulation of the intrinsic human circadian period, called τ (tau). This period is normally slightly longer than 24 hours and is under the major control of the suprachiasmatic nucleus (SCN) of the hypothalamus. The SCN regulates the sleep-wake cycle, core body temperature and secretion of melatonin and cortisol integrating external factors, such as light-dark cycles, social activities and food intake, and the intrinsic oscillation of SCN cells (τ).

Environmental stimuli are essential to adapt the intrinsic circadian period to the 24-hour light-dark cycle, since they can induce a daily advance in the circadian rhythm, which otherwise would last 24.2 hours each day [3]. Light is one of the most powerful environmental inputs for the synchronization of the SCN to the light-dark cycle, acting via the retino-hypothalamic tract (RHT), which connects photosensitive retinal ganglion cells to the SCN [4].

Circadian rhythm sleep disorders are characterized by a persistent or recurrent pattern of sleep disturbances due to alteration in these circadian endogenous and exogenous timekeeping systems (ICSD-2) [1]. According to the ICSD-2, the condition must be associated with impairment including social or occupational functioning, and diagnosis of CRSDs should not be made if the complaints underlie another sleep disorder, such as insomnia or narcolepsy [1]. We will here deal with the circadian rhythm sleep disorders in their principal clinical, epidemiological, and therapeutic aspects (Table 1).

Delayed Sleep Phase Syndrome

Delayed Sleep Phase Syndrome (DSPS) is a disorder in which the major sleep episode is delayed with respective to the desired bedtime. This causes a consequent difficulty in awakening at the required time in the morning.

This is the most frequent Circadian Rhythm Sleep Disorder with an incidence of 0.15% in the adult population [5].

Affected people usually report they cannot get to sleep until 2 a.m. At 6 a.m., there is great difficulty in waking up in time for social or occupational activities, and daytime sleepiness is present, especially in the morning hours. When not obliged to maintain a certain schedule, these patients usually sleep for a normal duration, although at a delayed phase relatively to local time [6,7].

The syndrome usually develops in early childhood or adolescence, with a predominance in the young boys. The duration of DSPS symptomatology varies from one month to decades, with a potential occupational, scholastic and social dysfunction. Chronic sedative or alcohol use or abuse accompanies some cases as a complicating feature [1].

Table 1. Circadian Rhythm Sleep Disorders

Circadian Rhythm Sleep Disorders	Description	Treatment
Delayed Sleep Phase Syndrome (DSPS)	The major sleep episode is delayed relatively to the desired sleep and wake up times, with sleep-onset insomnia and inability to get awake at the chosen time	Timed Light therapy; Timed melatonin; Chronotherapy
Advanced Sleep Phase Syndrome (ASPS)	The major sleep episode is advanced in relation to the desired clocktime, with evening sleepiness and early awakenings	Timed Light therapy; Timed melatonin; Chronotherapy
Non-24 hours Sleep-Wake Syndrome	Chronic pattern with one or two hours of progressive daily delay in sleep-onset and wake times	Timed melatonin in blind individuals. Timed melatonin, Chronotherapy and timed Light exposure in sighted individuals
Jet Lag Syndrome	Temporary condition of insomnia, excessive sleepiness, reduced alertness and somatic symptoms associated with a rapid travel across multiple time zones	Appropriate light exposure, Timed Melatonin, Hypnotics, Stimulants according to the direction of the flight (Eastward vs Westward travels)
Shift Work Disorder	Insomnia or excessive sleepiness related with a work schedule that occurs during the habitual hours of sleep or on irregular hours	Planned Sleep Schedule (Naps); Timed light exposure; Stimulants; Hypnotics
Irregular sleep-wake pattern	Alternated and disorganized episodes of sleeping and waking behaviors throughout the day	Timed Light exposure; Planned Sleep Schedule; Timed Melatonin for younger mentally impaired individuals
Circadian Rhythm Sleep Disorder due to Medical Condition	Insomnia or excessive daytime sleepiness directly related to medical condition	Timed Light exposure; Sleep Hygiene; Hypnotics
Circadian Rhythm Sleep Disorder due to Drug or Substance	Insomnia or excessive daytime sleepiness due to the use of drugs or substances	Avoid the entailed medication; Timed Light exposure; Sleep Hygiene
Circadian Rhythm sleep disorder Not Otherwise Specified (NOS)	Insomnia or excessive daytime sleepiness in a pattern that doesn't meet criteria for other circadian rhythm disorders	Timed Light exposure, Sleep Hygiene

The pathophysiology of this disorder can be attributed to a longer τ (the free running period of circadian rhythms in absence of external cues), a misaligned phase relationship between endogenous clock and sleep-wake cycles, and an altered sleep homeostasis; more often, patients with DSPS are thought to have a weak ability to phase advance their circadian systems in response to normal environmental cues, and they suffer because they try to live on a normal schedule but their biological clocks are not in phase with that schedule.

Polysomnographic recordings show a prolonged sleep latency. Sleep architecture and amount are otherwise normal for age. Sleep log and actigraphy monitoring can help in diagnosis.

These subjects are usually perplexed about the failure of their efforts to advance the timing of sleep onset: they try going to bed early, having a family member get them up in the morning, using sleeping pills or performing relaxation techniques, but no treatment seems to be permanently successful.

AASM standards of practice parameters recommend as effective treatments for DSPS light therapy with concurrent administration of exogenous melatonin (Guideline), and chronotherapy as an useful option [1]. A strict schedule and good sleep hygiene are essential in maintaining any beneficial effects of treatment.

Advanced Sleep Phase Syndrome

Advanced Sleep Phase Syndrome (ASPS) is a condition in which patients cannot remain awake until a desired clocktime, feeling very sleepy before 8 p.m.; at the same time, they wake up very early in the morning, usually before 2 or 3 a.m. These subjects suffer from a chronic inability to posticipate the onset of the major sleep episode or extend sleep later into the morning hours, resulting in a complaint for not being able to engage in evening activities due to the need to retire much earlier than the social norm [8]. Unlike other sleep maintenance disorders, the early morning awakening occurs after a normal period of undisrupted sleep, and daytime activities are not affected by somnolence.

Polysomnographic features during the patient's habitual sleep period include a normal sleep onset, sleep latency, and sleep duration relative to age. Daytime alertness is also normal [1]. Sleep logs and actigraphy demonstrates and advance in the habitual sleep time. This disorder is apparently rare and theoretically associated with aging. Men and women are equally affected.

Patients with ASPS are presumed to have a deficient phase-delay capability and melatonin and core body temperature levels that cycle hours earlier than an average person. A familial ASPS has been described as an autosomal dominant genetic disease with a mutation in the circadian clock gene PER2 [9]. This results in a shorter period of the physiological intrinsic circadian period τ.

Affected people can suffer for negative personal or social consequences. Attempts to work on night shifts or take part of social events may result in drowsiness, difficulty staying awake or embarrassing episodes of falling asleep. These symptoms have to be present for at least three months to complete the diagnosis. Treatment options for AASM practice parameters comprise evening light therapy and avoidance of early morning light. Timed melatonin is also listed as indicated for the treatment of ASPS.

Non-24 Hours Sleep-Wake Syndrome

This disorder is described by a daily delay in sleep onset and wake times amounted to 1 or 2 hours each day. The delay is due to abnormal synchronization between the 24-hour light-dark cycle and endogenous circadian rhythms. These patients seem to have a sleep-wake pattern that could be considered normal for individuals living without environmental time cues (the intrinsic circadian rhythm lasts approximately 25 hours), such as non-affected people in time-isolation experiments. The sleep phase of these subjects periodically changes, sometimes being in phase between their internal biological rhythm and social conventions, and sometimes being totally desynchronized with the world's sleep and wake times [1].

When the circadian phase is concurrent with a normal sleep-wake period, patients can be asymptomatic, but as the delay rolls by, complaints will consist in difficulty in initiating sleep at night or sleepiness during the day, depending on sleep phases. Sleep diary and the use of an actigraph can demonstrate a progressive phase delay in the sleep pattern of these subjects.

Unlike patients with DSPS, these subjects do not achieve a normal sleep pattern out of work and school duties.

This disorder appears to be rare in the general population, but is often described in totally blind patients. Rarely this syndrome is present in sighted people [10], and is usually accompanied in these latter cases by a schizoid or avoidant personality disorder, or mental retardation.

In blind subjects, the pathophysiology comprises the absence of visual environmental information about the light-dark cycle. These cues are crucial for the 24-hour time information, acting on the retino-hypothalamic tract on the suprachiasmatic nucleus of the hypothalamus, and their lack allows for the intrinsic phase delay to be manifested. In sighted people, the causes of this disorder should include above all personality factors.

Individuals affected by non-24 hours sleep-wake syndrome are partially or totally unable to work or function on a conventional daily schedule, as the disorder often presents as chronic and intractable. Treatment options in blind individuals include the administration of melatonin before the desired bedtime. In sighted patients, daytime sun exposure, a regular sleep-wake schedule and timed melatonin may represent a valid option, although treatment recommendations are less clear for these subjects.

Jet Lag Syndrome

Jet lag is characterized by a misalignment between endogenous circadian rhythms and local time caused by rapid travel across multiple time zones. This disorder is described by excessive difficulties in initiating or maintaining sleep, sleepiness, decrease in subjective daytime alertness and somatic symptoms after a rapid travel across at least two time zones [1]. The inability to adjust the internal clock rapidly to long-distance air travel can also bring emotional distress and gastrointestinal disturbances. The severity and duration of the symptoms is variable, depending on the number of time zone crossed, sleep loss during travel, and individual susceptibility.

The sleep-wake disturbances generally abate after 2-3 days in the arrival location, although it is estimated that it takes about one day per hour of time zone change to adjust. Westwards travel is better tolerated because the body is phase advanced compared with local time.

Elderly people appear to be more likely to develop these symptoms compared to those under age 30; however, the disorder usually represents an occasional, self-limiting inconvenience.

The treatment of jet lag comprises general sleep hygiene measures, timed light exposure and timed melatonin.

Timed light exposure is of primary importance in shifting circadian clock: a strategic avoidance or exposure to light can help travellers accommodate their circadian rhythm in an efficient way [11,12]. In particular, some specific tips can be administered depending on the direction of the flight: Eastern travels require a phase advance (because the subject is phase delayed) and in this case patients will benefit from avoiding light exposure on arrival. On the other hand, in Westward flights the patient is phase advanced relative to local time and requires a phase delay, and will benefit from a light outdoor exposure on arrival.

Timed melatonin was found to improve the quality of sleep and alleviate daytime symptoms of jet lag [13]. The utility of standard hypnotics is still not well established [2].

Shift Work Disorder

Shift work disorder consists of symptoms of excessive sleepiness or insomnia related with a work period (usually night works) that occurs during the habitual sleep phase. This is a common problem in industrialized countries, where a substantial proportion of the population works in an occupation requiring shift work, and sometimes night shift work.

The sleep complaint usually entails a reduction of one to four hours in sleep length duration after a night shift, often accompanied with sleepiness during shifts and impaired mental ability due to reduced alertness.

The consequences can affect work duties with reduced performance capability as well as social life due to the necessity to employ a large part of free time to recover sleep. Actigraphy and sleep logs can be helpful in demonstrating an altered sleep-wake pattern corresponding that of the shift work disorder. The condition usually persists for the duration of the work-shift period. Its pathophysiology is related to the conflict between the requirement to work during the night and physiological nocturnal sleepiness, together with sleepiness due to the lack of sleep. Risk factors include advanced age and female sex.

The recommended treatments for this disorder include timed bright light exposure, planned sleep schedule (naps) and stimulants such as caffeine and modafinil. Exposition of bright light during night shifts induces an effective circadian adaptation [14]. Data about the administration of timed melatonin are inconsistent, and one study found that the use of melatonin was not effective if there was a concurrent exposition of bright light during night shift works [15].

Strategic, short napping before or in the first period of the shift was found to be beneficial [16]; the employment of stimulants, especially modafinil, provided significant improvement in alertness and performance [17]. Caffeine is still effective, but not addressed specifically to patients with shift work disorder [2].

Irregular Sleep-Wake Pattern

This disorder is characterized by alternated and disorganized episodes of sleeping and waking behavior throughout the day. Elderly patients with dementia or subjects living in an institutional setting are more susceptible to this sleep-wake pattern [18]. Total sleep time in the 24 hours is usually normal for age, but there are no single sleep periods of normal length, and the chance to find these patients asleep is unpredictable during the day and night. The consequence of this disorganization is excessive sleepiness and napping during daytime, and difficulty in initiating or maintaining the sleep during the night [1]. These subjects, especially those institutionalized or with brain dysfunction, refer wake times as sleepy and may experience subjective cognitive impairment.

Sleep logs kept by patients can highlight the lack of an established circadian pattern of sleep onset and wake time. Factors precipitating an irregular sleep-wake pattern include diffuse brain dysfunction with a diminished response to environmental agents such as light, an irregular daytime routine, and limited exposure to exercise and social activities.

Its pathophysiology can include an involvement of the endogenous circadian system in subjects with diffuse brain affection, or a voluntary started and perpetuated pattern by neurologically intact patients. The condition tends to be chronic, with a minimum duration of three months.

Recommended treatments comprise timed light exposure, a planned sleep schedule, and daytime activities. Melatonin was not found to be effective in these patients [19], especially those elderly with dementia, while younger mentally impaired individuals found some benefit [20].

Circadian Rhythm Sleep Disorder Due to Medical Condition

This disorder comprises several circadian sleep disturbances directly originated by a medical condition. Patients complain of insomnia or excessive sleepiness, with a sleep pattern that seems to be out of alignment with normal sleep times.

An underlying medical condition provoking the alteration of the circadian time-keeping system is a necessary condition for this diagnosis [1]. Medical diseases that can be related with a misalignment of circadian rhythms are heterogeneous, and include dementia, since the circadian rhythms system decreases and becomes weaker; movement disorders such as Parkinson's disease, in which there is sleep fragmentation, insomnia, and daytime sleepiness; blindness for the lack of an important zeitgeber, the light; hepatic encephalopathy with sleep disturbance related to toxins filtered in the bloodstream.

Diagnosis can be aided by sleep logs and actigraphy.

Treatments for circadian rhythm sleep disorder due to a medical condition include sleep hygiene and light exposure, as well as an administration of hypnotic medication. A change of treatment of the underlying medical condition can be useful if medications improve the circadian sleep disorder component (for example, certain Parkinson's medications increase insomnia or daytime sleep attacks).

Circadian Rhythm Sleep Disorder Due to Drug or Substance

Similarly to CRSD due to a medical condition, this disorder can be diagnosed if the altered sleep pattern is directly caused by a drug or substance. Drugs and substances can produce various types of abnormal sleep timing patterns, depending on the substance, the subjective reaction to a specific medication and the strength of personal circadian rhythms.

There are a multitude of prescription drugs, herbs and vitamins, illicit drugs or substances that can cause sleepiness or wakefulness at the wrong times.

Diagnosis is usually made using a sleep diary or an actigraph; treatment is directed to stopping or reducing the use of the entailed substance. Light exposure and correct sleep hygiene are also recommended [1].

Circadian Rhythm Sleep Disorder, Not Otherwise Specified

In this disorder, criteria for a circadian rhythm sleep disorder are satisfied, with a misalignment in patient's sleep times; however, the pattern cannot meet the criteria for any other circadian sleep disorder. Diagnosis can be made using a sleep diary or an actigraphy. The treatment aims at helping patients recover a long sleep time during the night and a long wake time during the day. Timed light exposition and sleep hygiene can be helpful [1].

References

[1] American Academy of Sleep Medicine: ICSD-2 *International Classification of Sleep Disorders*, 2nd ed. Diagnostic and Coding Manual. Westchester, IL: American Academy of Sleep Medicine, 2005.

[2] Sack RL, Auckley D, Auger RR, et al: American Academy of Sleep Medicine. Circadian rhythm sleep disorders: part I, basic principles, shift work and jet lag disorders. An American Academy of Sleep Medicine review. *Sleep* 2007;30:1460-83.

[3] Czeisler CA, Duffy JF, Shanahan TL, et al: Stability, precision, and nearly 24 hour period of the human circadian pacemaker. *Sleep* 1999;284:2177-81.

[4] Lowrey PL, Takahashi JS: Mammalian circadian biology: elucidating genome-wide levels of temporal organization. Annu Rev *Genomics Hum. Genet.* 2004;5:407-41.

[5] Schrader H, Bovim G, Sand T. The prevalence of delayed advanced sleep phase syndromes. *J. Sleep Res.* 1993;2(1):51-5.

[6] Wyatt JK. Delayed sleep phase syndrome: pathophysiology and treatment options. *Sleep* 2004;27:1195-203.

[7] Wyatt JK. Circadian rhythm sleep disorders. *Pediatr. Clin. North Am.* 2011;58(3):621-35.

[8] Auger RR: Advanced related sleep complaints and advanced sleep phase disorder. *Sleep Med. Clin.* 2009;4:219-27.

[9] Hamet P, Tremblay J. Genetics of the sleep-wake cycle and its disorders. Metabolism. 2006;55(10 Suppl 2):S7-12.

[10] Hayakawa T, Uchiyama M, Kamei Y, et al: Clinical analysis of sighted patients with non-24 hour sleep-wake syndrome. *Sleep* 2005;28:945-52.

[11] Daan S, Lewy AJ: Scheduled exposure to daylight: a potential strategy to reduce "jet lag" following transmeridian flight. *Psychopharmacol. Bull.* 1984;20:566-8.

[12] Sack RL. Clinical practice. *Jet lag. N. Engl. J. Med.* 2010;362(5):440-7.

[13] Boivin DB, James FO: Circadian adaptation to night-shift work by judicious light and darkness exposure. *J. Biol. Rhythms.* 2002;17(6):556-67.

[14] Suhner A, Schlagenhauf P, Höfer I, Johnson R, Tschopp A, Steffen R: Effectiveness and tolerability of melatonin and zolpidem for the alleviation of jet lag. *Aviat. Space Environ. Med.* 2001;72:638-46.

[15] Crowley SJ, Lee C, Tseng CY, Fogg LF, Eastman CI: Combinations of bright light, scheduled dark, sunglasses, and melatonin to facilitate circadian entrainment to night shift work. *J. Biol. Rhythms* 2003;18:513-23.

[16] Sallinen M, Härmä M, Akerstedt T, Rosa R, Lillqvist O: Promoting alertness with a short nap during a night shift. *J. Sleep Res.* 1998;7:240-7.

[17] Czeisler CA, Walsh JK, Roth T, et al: US Modafinil in Shift Work Sleep Disorder Study Group. Modafinil for excessive sleepiness associated with shift-work sleep disorder. *N. Engl. J. Med.* 2005;353:476-86.

[18] Zee PC, Vitiello MV: Circadian rhythm disorder: irregular sleep wake rhythm. *Sleep Med. Clin.* 2009;4:213-18.

[19] Singer C, Trachtenberg RE, Kaye J, et al: A multicenter, placebo controlled trial of melatonin for sleep disturbance in Alzheimer's disease. *Sleep* 2003;26:893-901.

[20] Pillar G, Shahar E, Peled N, et al: Melatonin improves sleep wake patterns in psychomotor retarded children. *Pediatr. Neurol.* 2000;23:225-28.

In: Sleep Medicine
Editors: A. Del Casale, R. Brugnoli and P. Girardi

ISBN: 978-1-62808-515-0
© 2013 Nova Science Publishers, Inc.

Chapter III

Insomnia and Hypersomnias

Luigi Ferini-Strambi* and Sara Marelli
Department of Clinical Neurosciences, Sleep Disorders Center,
Università Vita-Salute San Raffaele, Milan, Italy

Abstract

Insomnia is a common clinical problem that often exists as a chronic condition. Usually the etiology is multifactorial and it is frequently comorbid with psychiatric and medical disorders or in association with underlying sleep disorders. A wide spectrum of psychologic and physiologic factors has been identified as possible vulnerabilities for primary insomnia. Dominant models include psychophysiologic and hyperarousal processes.

A diagnosis of insomnia must confirm both the existence of nocturnal symptoms and a clinically significant impact during the patient's waking state. Nocturnal symptoms include difficulty initiating or maintaining sleep, early awakening, and interrupted or nonrestorative sleep. Daytime symptoms include distress about poor nocturnal sleep and impairment in any role function or other aspects of overall well-being. The assessment of insomnia begins with an initial diagnostic interview. During the initial interview the clinician must obtain sufficient information to correctly diagnose the insomnia subtype and contributing factors. Following the interview, objective measures of sleep can be used to rule out other sleep disorders when clinically indicated, laboratory tests may be ordered to rule out suspected comorbid medical conditions, and subjective self-report measures can be used to supplement information gathered in the initial interview.

Excessive daytime somnolence (EDS) is a prevalent problem in medical practice and in society in general. EDS can be caused by various conditions, including circadian rhythm disorders, obstructive sleep apnea (OSA), or other causes of disturbed nocturnal sleep. Several different types of hypersomnia of central origin, such as narcolepsy (with and without cataplexy), recurrent hypersomnia, idiopathic hypersomnia, behaviorally induced insufficient sleep syndrome, narcolepsy/hypersomnia due to medical condition, hypersomnia due to drug and substance, and nonorganic hypersomnia have been

---

* Email: ferinistrambi.luigi@hsr.it.

described and classified. Various methods have been developed to assess EDS (although each of them has limitations), and one of the objective polytrophic measures for sleep tendency and REM sleep abnormalities (i.e., MSLT) has been included in the diagnostic criteria for EDS of central origin.

Although much progress has been made in discovering the pathophysiology of narcolepsy in humans (i.e., hypocretin ligand deficiency), much more remains to be understood and far less is known about other primary conditions of EDS.

Insomnia

Diagnostic Definition of Insomnia

Insomnia has a range of clinical manifestations and involves a multitude of physical and psychological factors. The traditional diagnostic descriptions of insomnia have often included a designation as to whether the condition is "primary" or "secondary." These terms have historically been intended to indicate that insomnia is either a symptom or a function of another medical or psychiatric condition or has arisen of its own accord without subordinate relationship to another disorder. The diagnostic definitions of insomnia have changed in the last decades.

The modern approach to diagnosis and classification of insomnia started with the publication of the initial nosology of the Association of Sleep Disorders Centers (ASDA), released in 1979 [1]. This manual groups disorders that are primarily associated with insomnia (disorders of initiating and maintaining sleep) into a single major category with eight subheadings (e.g., "psychophysiological" or "associated with psychiatric/ substances/ breathing disturbance"). In the first edition of the International Classification of Sleep Disorders (ICSD) [2], the major insomnia categories were clumped into intrinsic or extrinsic dyssomnias and secondary disorders. The recent publication of ICSD-2 [3] reverted to a distinct category for major insomnia diagnoses, although it should be noted that insomnia may appear as a symptom of numerous other disorders classified under their own distinct heading. In the ICSD-2, a diagnosis of insomnia must confirm both the existence of nocturnal symptoms and a clinically significant impact during the patient's waking state. Nocturnal symptoms include difficulty initiating or maintaining sleep, early awakening, and interrupted or nonrestorative sleep. Daytime symptoms include distress about poor nocturnal sleep and impairment in any role function or other aspects of overall well-being.

The Diagnostic and Statistical Manual of Mental Disorders, fourth edition (DSM-IV) of the American Psychiatric Association published in 1994 included a major heading for sleep disorders [4]. The approach to classification paralleled ICSD, first edition in its use of dyssomnias as a major heading, though was understandably far more parsimonious in its level of detail. The edition of the DSM-IV TR adopted an approach that is consistent with the ICSD-2.

An important goal of DSM-V sleep nosology will be to improve recognition of sleep disorders by mental health and general medical clinicians, to improve appropriate referrals to a sleep specialist, and to improve the approach to treatment of sleep disorders that are comorbid with other health conditions. The major changes under consideration include: (1) eliminating the diagnosis of "primary insomnia" in favor of "insomnia disorder," with concurrent specification of clinically comorbid conditions (both medical and psychiatric). Making this change will allow also to (2) eliminate "sleep disorder related to another mental disorder" and "sleep disorder due to a general medical condition," in favor of "insomnia disorder" (or "hypersomnia disorder") with concurrent specification of clinically comorbid conditions. These changes move away from the causal attribution inherent in DSM-IV and simply specify clinically relevant comorbidities. As such they are consistent with the data and recommendations of the 2005 National Institutes of Health (NIH) State of the Science position on classification of insomnia disorders. The 2005 NIH State of the Science Conference on Chronic Insomnia recommends that the term "comorbid insomnia" replace that of secondary insomnia [5]. The principal reason for this recommendation would seem to lie in the fact that, regardless of its origins, chronic insomnia appears to be characterized by certain specific psychological and physiological characteristics that, in many cases at least, give rise to a condition that is relatively autonomous, that does not necessarily resolve with treatment of the primary medical or psychiatric condition, and that does respond effectively to therapies aimed at the more specific aspects of the insomnia process itself.

The criteria underscore that the patient has a sleep disorder (either insomnia or hypersomnia) that warrants independent clinical attention, in addition to mental/psychiatric or medical disorders also present.

Incidence and Prevalence of Insomnia

Insomnia is a common public health problem, affecting virtually all ages and socioeconomic strata. Most epidemiological studies place the prevalence of occasional or intermittent insomnia at about 30% to 40% of the general population and that of chronic insomnia at roughly 10% to 15% [6-11].

However, several considerations apply. It has become clear that the prevalence data are significantly influenced by the operational definition of insomnia that is employed in these studies. For example, Ohayon and Roth have pointed out that investigations utilizing only a single identifier such as "difficulty getting to sleep" or "difficulty staying asleep" as a marker for insomnia are likely to overestimate the prevalence of the disorder [12]. Duration as a qualifier (greater than one month duration) has relatively little impact since most of the sample meets this criterion. However, the presence of other factors such as dissatisfaction, dread of going to bed, or the presence of hyperarousal (e.g., excessive mental activity in bed) proves critical in defining clinically relevant insomnia. In addition, earlier epidemiological studies of insomnia failed to include a criterion of daytime consequences, a factor that further narrows and defines the population. That said, the large European study that incorporated the criteria described above still demonstrated an insomnia prevalence of 11%, although only two-thirds (6.8%) received a sleep disorder diagnosis, while the remainder received mental disorder diagnoses [12]. The important lesson to be derived from these data is that insomnia is a complex condition that is characterized not only by a complaint about sleep but also by an individual's assessment of and response to this complaint, as well as the consequences of the condition.

Few studies have investigated the prevalence of insomnia using operational definitions such as those set forth in the ICSD and DSM-IV, specifying what proportion of respondents satisfied the criteria to reach a diagnosis of insomnia disorder. Ohayon and Reynolds [13] performed a cross-sectional study involving 25,579 individuals aged 15 years and over representative of the general population of France, the United Kingdom, Germany, Italy, Portugal, Spain and Finland. The participants were interviewed on sleep habits and disorders managed by the Sleep-EVAL expert system using DSM-IV and ICSD classifications. At the complaint level, too short sleep (20.2%), light sleep (16.6%), and global sleep dissatisfaction (8.2%) were reported by 37% of the subjects. At the symptom level (difficulty initiating or maintaining sleep and non-restorative sleep at least 3 nights per week), 34.5% of the sample reported at least one of them. At the criterion level, (symptoms + daytime consequences), 9.8% of the total sample reported having them. At the diagnostic level, 6.6% satisfied the DSM-IV requirement for positive and differential diagnosis. However, many respondents failed to meet diagnostic criteria for duration, frequency and severity in the two classifications, suggesting that multidimensional measures are needed.

It is obvious that the prevalence of insomnia is substantially higher among certain populations. Women manifest insomnia more often than men at a ratio of about 2:1 [14-17].

This higher prevalence may not be entirely a function of higher incidence but rather of a lower remission rate, at least in the elderly. Moreover, higher rates of mood and anxiety disorders in women may also lead to chronic insomnia, although our current understanding raises the possibility that the converse is also true. Rates of chronic insomnia are clearly higher in clinic populations, including both psychiatric and medical clinics, and exceed 50% in some studies [9, 18, 19]. Sleep disturbance is a particular concern for the elderly, and epidemiological data are consistent with this. Depending on the definition and severity ratings, studies suggest an insomnia prevalence rate of anywhere from about 25% to over 40% [20, 21]. It has been reported that the incidence of insomnia is higher in older adults than younger adults, but is most often associated with other age-related conditions, rather than age per se.

Sleep difficulties are significantly associated with medical and psychiatric comorbidities and the presence of multiple medical conditions has been found to be detrimental to sleep quality. Insomnia is often disregarded by health care practitioners. The reasons for this are not clear but may represent, in part, a perception of this condition as less significant than other medical problems that may come to their attention. However, in surveys comparing health-related quality of life in a variety of chronic health conditions, insomnia sufferers demonstrate impairments that are on the same order as congestive heart failure and major depressive disorder [22-24] performed a cross-sectional study in three general practices in Auckland, New Zealand.

Consecutive patients from the waiting room were asked to complete a nine-page questionnaire on possible causes of insomnia. In total, 1517 patients were approached and 955 completed the nine-page questionnaire (63%). Of the 41% who reported difficulty with sleeping, primary insomnia occurred in 12% of the population (95% confidence interval = 9% to 15%); 50% had depression, 48% had anxiety and 43% had general (physical) health problems. Obstructive sleep apnoea occurred in 9% and delayed sleep phase disorder in 2%.

The results of several epidemiological studies suggest that clinicians must consider insomnia as significant risk factor for development of new psychiatric disorders including depression, anxiety disorders, and substance abuse. Moreover, chronic insomnia may adversely affect the course and outcome of other medical disorders, either through impaired treatment adherence, promotion of complicating psychiatric disorders, or direct impact on physiological function (e.g., lowering of pain threshold).

Pathophysiology

The experience of insomnia may result from numerous influences, including both psychologic and physiologic processes. The etiology of insomnia episodes is often multifactorial and the relative effects of different influences may vary over time. Key factors initiating an episode may no longer contribute to the persistence of insomnia as new other factors exert greater influence on the maintenance on the insomnia symptoms [25].

An individual's vulnerabilities for developing insomnia can involve genetic and cultural factors, personality characteristics, personal history, and assorted habits and routines. Comorbid disorders and other physical conditions (e.g., pregnancy and menopause), medication and other substance use, and environmental disturbances all may initiate insomnia episodes that then may be sustained by these elements or become complicated further by emergent perpetuating factors. Among these new processes, promoting the continuance of an insomnia episode may be the evolution of a psychologically conditioned excessive arousal associated with attempts to sleep; maladaptive sleep-related behaviours, attitudes, and beliefs; and physiologic abnormalities associated with an experience of excessive arousal.

Triggers of transient insomnia episodes, typically lasting up to a few days or weeks, are generally easily identifiable. Chronic insomnia, persisting for one month or longer, is more likely to be heterogeneous in etiology. For conceptual convenience, chronic insomnia may be classed as either primary or comorbid. Primary insomnia is presumed to exist independent of other disorders, while comorbid insomnia is thought to evolve with some contribution from co-occurring conditions. However, insomnia patients with and without other disorders may share fundamental vulnerabilities [26].

Several theoretical models of the etiology and evolution of primary insomnia have been elaborated [27]. Generally, these highlight either psychologic or physiologic underlying processes, and attempt to account for the full spectrum of nighttime and daytime insomnia symptoms. A common denominator among the recent models is an appreciation of primary insomnia not just as a nighttime sleep disturbance with daytime consequences, but rather as a 24-hour disorder that deleteriously affects the experiences of both sleep and wakefulness [28].

Insomnia etiology models have focused on personality features, behavioural associations, and cognitive experiences. It has been reported that persistent insomnia more likely occurs in people who internalized psychologic disturbances [29]. Worry and rumination with associated emotional and physiologic arousal have been core elements in the initiation and persistence of insomnia in the cognitive models. In advocating a stimulus-control treatment for insomnia, Bootzin emphasized the role of behavioural routines in sustaining insomnia [30]. The importance of arousing and conditioned psychologic processes is inherent in Spielman's model of predisposing, precipitating, and perpetuating factors influencing the development of insomnia [25]. A general cognitive model of chronic insomnia begins with an acute event associated with rumination and worry that leads to cognitive and physiologic arousal and development of the subsequent symptoms associated with insomnia [27]. The focus on nighttime sleeplessness and perceived daytime consequences, along with the evolution of psychologic conditioning, reinforces and perpetuates the insomnia in a self-propagating manner.

Some authors have proposed a neurocognitive insomnia model noting that people with chronic insomnia are not awake because they are worrying, but rather that they are worrying because they are awake [27].

The neurocognitive model is based on the behavioural perspective that insomnia occurs acutely in association with predisposing and precipitating factors (for example psychosocial stressors), and chronically in association with perpetuating factors (for example extension of time in bed). The behavioural perspective is extended by explicitly allowing the possibility that conditioned arousal may act as a perpetuating factor. Arousal is expressed in terms of somatic, cognitive and cortical activation. Hence, the bed and the sleep environment and its circumstances become stimuli for arousal instead of "de-arousal". It is hypothesized that the cortical arousal (experienced subjectively as increased cognitive activity and measurable on an electroencephalographic level by increased fast frequencies of the sleep EEG) occurs as a result of classical conditioning and promotes abnormal levels of sensory and information processing, and of long-term memory formation. These phenomena are directly linked to sleep continuity disturbances and/or sleep state misperception. Specifically, enhanced sensory processing around sleep onset and during sleep is thought to render the insomniac subject especially vulnerable to perturbation by environmental (or other) stimuli, and these events can directly interfere with sleep initiation and/or maintenance. Enhanced information processing during sleep may distort the distinction between sleep and wakefulness and might thus account for the tendency of many insomniac patients to judge sleep (objectively measured) as wakefulness. Enhanced memory formation for the events around sleep onset and arousals during sleep may interfere with the subjective experience of sound and uninterrupted sleep. An increased ability to encode and retrieve information in insomnia would be expected to correlate with altered assessments about sleep latency, wakefulness after sleep onset and sleep duration.

An early study investigating physiologic correlates of insomnia noted increased activation in poor sleepers before sleep onset and during sleep, as evidenced by increased heart rate, basal skin resistance, core body temperature, and phasic vasoconstriction [31]. Some authors [32] have explored the relationship of sleep characteristics, indicators of hyperarousal, objective daytime sleepiness, and subjective daytime symptoms in a series of experiments. Among these have been studies with yoke-controlled normals with sleep limited to the insomnia subject patterns and investigations producing insomnia symptoms in normal sleepers given high-dose caffeine for one week. They have concluded that elevated arousal produces both poor sleep and related symptoms in insomnia patients.

Among the physiologic parameters studied in controlled insomnia research studies have been metabolic rate, heart-rate variability, electromyographic activity, hypothalamic pituitary axis (HPA) activity, immune function and cytokine levels, thermoregulation, and EEG patterns. Abnormalities of the stress-response system have been the focus of several hyperarousal insomnia models and have stimulated the design of numerous clinical investigations.

Vgontzas and colleagues examined the relationships of cortisol and cytokines with characteristics of sleep and waking in populations of sleep-disordered individuals, including chronic insomnia subjects [33]. The authors found a shift of tumor necrosis factor (TNF) and interleukin (IL)-6 secretions from nighttime to daytime in the chronic insomnia group and hypothesized that this might explain daytime fatigue and performance decrements. Their findings of 24-hour cortisol hypersecretion in insomnia subjects could help explain nighttime difficulty falling asleep.

Sleep onset normally is associated with substantial thermoregulatory changes. It has been argued that insomnia may be associated with abnormalities in these processes.

Thermoregulatory research has shown that subjects with sleep-onset insomnia had impaired heat loss capacity in peripheral regions in association with sleep onset [34].

EEG studies have demonstrated increased beta and gamma range activity in insomnia subjects [35]. Alterations in sleep EEG microstructure as represented in cyclic alternating pattern (CAP) rate correlate with poor sleep [36]. A study employing event-related potentials that indicate the processing of auditory information during sleep in insomnia subjects demonstrated an enhancement in attention and a decrease in inhibitory processes that normally facilitate sleep onset [37].

In contrast to neuroendocrine and neurophysiological studies, which allow only indirect conclusions about the function and activity of the human brain, neuroimaging methods such as single photon emission computed tomography (SPECT), positron emission tomography (PET) and magnetic resonance imaging (MRI) allow a more direct approach to brain structure and function.

A SPECT study [38] imaging conducted around the sleep onset interval in patients with primary insomnia and in good-sleeper subjects showed that patients with insomnia exhibited a consistent pattern of hypoperfusion across eight preselected regions of interest, with the most marked effect being observed in the basal ganglia. The frontal, medial, occipital and parietal cortices also showed significant decreases in blood flow compared to good sleepers. Interestingly, after successful behavioural therapy abnormal values in insomniacs returned to baseline [39].

A PET study [40] acquired data from patients with chronic insomnia and controls from an interval during wakefulness and during consolidated non-REM sleep. This study for the first time gave direct evidence for the hypothesis of central nervous hyperarousal in insomnia. Insomniac patients showed increased global glucose metabolism during wakefulness and non-REM sleep. Additionally, it was found that patients with insomnia exhibited smaller declines in relative glucose metabolism from wakefulness to sleep in wake-promoting regions including ascending reticular activating systems, the hypothalamus and thalamus. Similar effects were also observed in areas associated with cognition and emotion, including the amygdala, hippocampus, insular cortex and the anterior cingulate and prefrontal cortices. The same authors [41], by using PET again, described a correlation between increased brain metabolism in the pontine tegmentum, thalamocortical networks in a frontal, anterior temporal and anterior cingulated distribution and the quantity of nocturnal wake times in patients with primary insomnia.

The apparent contradictions between the SPECT and PET studies may be due to several factors. First of all, the PET studies allowed a 20-min 'window' of measured brain activity as opposed to 2 min in the SPECT studies. It is so far unknown whether the assumed hyperarousal is a dynamic process with periods of instability, switching from reduced to increased brain metabolism, or whether we have to deal with a stable process throughout the entire night. Given the cyclic nature of the sleep process itself, with its well-known oscillations between slow wave and REM sleep, and other dynamic changes with even shorter period lengths during sleep, it seems reasonable to assume that the hypothetical hyperarousal too fluctuates, which might explain why neuroimaging methods with different sampling times may produce divergent results.

Riemann and colleagues [42] performed MRI study during the wake state during daytime) and found a reduction in hippocampal volumes in chronic insomniacs compared to healthy control sleepers. This finding is in good agreement with animal studies on the effects of sleep loss and sleep deprivation on neurogenesis in the hippocampus. It remains to be determined whether these alterations in hippocampal structures are directly related to the insomnia (i.e. a consequence of chronic sleep loss) or to the associated increased cortisol excretion, or whether they precede the development of insomnia.

The first functional MRI (fMRI) study in a sample of patients with primary insomnia used a category and a letter fluency task as stimulation paradigms [43] during the wake state in the MRI scanner. This study revealed a hypoactivation of the medial and inferior prefrontal cortical areas in primary insomnia (in the absence of behavioural differences) compared to good sleeper controls. Rescanning after successful cognitive–behavioral therapy revealed a normalization of these patterns of activation in the patients with insomnia. The authors interpret their data as evidence for a differential recruitment of other brain regions for successful task completion in the insomniac patients, whom they consider 'high achievers' on a behavioral level (as demonstrated by improved performance on rather simple tasks but decreased performance on more complex tasks relative to controls).

Using proton magnetic resonance spectroscopy to determine brain GABA levels *in vivo* in patients with primary insomnia, Winkelmann and colleagues [44] demonstrated a global reduction in GABA in the brains of patients compared to good sleepers. Since GABA is the most prevalent inhibitory neurotransmitter in the CNS, these results support the assumption that in primary insomnia the central nervous balance between inhibition and excitation is compromised.

Diagnostic Tools for Insomnia

The assessment of insomnia begins with an initial diagnostic interview. During the initial interview, it is fundamental to obtain sufficient information to correctly diagnose the insomnia subtype and contributing factors. Following the interview, objective measures of sleep may be used to rule out other sleep disorders when clinically indicated, laboratory tests might be ordered to rule out suspected comorbid medical conditions, and subjective self-report measures can be used to supplement information gathered in the initial interview.

a)   History

The clinician must evaluate patients' current sleep patterns, the history of their sleeping problems, the current state of their homeostatic and circadian drives regulating normal sleep, factors that contribute to hyperarousal, and other factors that might interfere with the normal process of sleep. The latter include comorbid sleep, medical, or psychiatric disorders, substance use, current medications, and the patient's response to his or her insomnia, including behaviours originally initiated in an effort to improve sleep.

A careful analysis of the patient's current sleep-wake schedule attends to a multitude of nocturnal and daytime sleep parameters. Nocturnal parameters include latency to sleep onset, wake after sleep onset, and the discrepancy between the desired and actual wake-up time. Parameters that allow evaluation of the regularity and circadian placement of sleep episodes include bedtime, lights out, final wake-up time, and time out of bed. Daytime sleep parameters include the timing, frequency, and length of naps, as well as the perceived ability to fall asleep during the day, given the opportunity. It is also important to collect information about the patient's sleep environment, including noise and comfort levels in the bedroom.

Since many patients tend to generalize their sleep problem on the basis of their worst night, it is important to identify a concrete time frame for discussing the sleep pattern.

Usually the most recent typical week works well. It is also helpful to acknowledge the variability of sleep-wake schedules by encouraging patients to report day-to-day variability of their sleep-wake pattern. Daily sleep diaries completed prior to the initial interview can further promote the efficiency and accuracy of this portion of the interview.

It is fundamental that the initial diagnostic interview include an evaluation of comorbid conditions, whether sleep-related or more general medical or psychiatric problems. Both the conditions and their treatments can contribute to insomnia. Thus, the interview should include a review of systems most commonly associated with disturbed sleep, a physical examination, and additional laboratory tests when indicted (e.g., thyroid function and prostate-specific antigen). Detailed information about medications and over-the-counter remedies taken to improve sleep quality is important. A comprehensive list of a patient's medications for other conditions is also essential. The most relevant medications to attend to in the context of assessment of insomnia are those that produce hyperarousal, such as stimulants, steroids, b-agonist medications, and some psychotropic medications. Medications in the latter class, such as antidepressant drugs, can cause insomnia or hypersomnolence and may exacerbate restless legs and periodic limb movements during sleep.

Concerning the comorbid conditions, the following are the most common medical conditions associated with insomnia: hyperthyroidism, chronic pain associated with rheumatologic disorders, pulmonary diseases (most notably obstructive pulmonary disease typically treated with steroids), cardiac disorders (particularly when treated with b-agonist medications), gastrointestinal reflux, and auto-immune conditions treated with steroids. In addition, the potential impact of gender-specific factors must be considered. These include menstrual phase effects on sleep in young women, menopausal symptoms in middle-aged women, and prostate disease in older men.

Psychiatric disorders, particularly depressive disorders, account for up to 40% of cases of chronic insomnia encountered in sleep centers. Because depressed patients may focus on sleep complaints, most notably sleep continuity disturbances and early awakening, to the exclusion of other mood disorder symptoms, a routine evaluation of depressive disorders is important. Because anxiety disorders are associated with disturbances to the sleep system, the clinician or researcher should seek information regarding heightened general anxiety and perceived stress. Assessing comorbid psychiatric disorders and their relationship to the fluctuation in insomnia symptoms can help with differential diagnosis and treatment planning. In particular, this can aid in deciding when to refer for treatment of the comorbid psychiatric disorder.

b)   Subjective Assessment Tools

The sleep diary (or sleep log) is the primary tool for providing data on a night-to-night basis. In addition to characterizing the frequency and severity of the nighttime problem, the sleep diary can provide useful information on the variability of the patient's sleep-wake habit, circadian tendencies, patterns of medication use, and nap behaviours. While sleep diaries may provide prospective data on the sleep problem, questionnaires provide retrospective data on global indices of insomnia severity and take into account both nocturnal and daytime symptoms. Among several sleep questionnaires that provide retrospective data on global indices of insomnia severity, the following two are largely used: the Insomnia Severity Index (ISI) and the Pittsburgh Sleep Quality Index (PSQI). Both are well validated, easy to administer and often used in research as well as clinic settings.

The ISI [45, 46] is a seven-item scale that measures the degree of severity on three nighttime symptoms (difficulty falling asleep, difficulty staying asleep, problem waking too early) and daytime consequences, distress, and dissatisfaction. Each item is rated on a five-point scale and the total score provides an index of severity of the insomnia. The instruction is to "rate the current (i.e., last 2 weeks) severity of your insomnia problem(s)." Guidelines for interpreting the total score are as follows: 0-7 (no significant insomnia), 8-14 (sub-threshold insomnia), 15-21 (moderate insomnia), 22-28 (severe insomnia). [45] In addition, a score > 14 has been found to be the optimum cut-off for insomnia as a disorder [45]. It should be highlighted that the ISI is exclusively focused on insomnia symptoms and does not provide information on sleep pattern and frequency of disturbed sleep.

The PSQI is a 19-item scale that measures general sleep disturbances over a one-month interval [47]. The PSQI provides a global severity of sleep disturbance based on questions about sleep patterns, frequency of sleep onset, and maintenance difficulties, as well frequency of a range of other sleep disturbances (e.g., snoring, feeling too hot or too cold, dreams, and pain), medication use, and a range of daytime consequences. Each item is ranked on a 0-3 scale. Scoring the PSQI consists of deriving scores for the following seven components: subjective sleep quality, sleep latency, sleep duration, sleep efficiency, sleep disturbance, use of sleep medication, and daytime dysfunction, from which a global score is derived. A score >5 represents clinically meaningful insomnia. More specifically, this cut-off score indicates moderate sleep problems in at least three sleep components or severe sleep problems in at least two areas.

c)   Objective Assessment Tools

In clinical settings, objective measures of sleep are used for differential diagnosis of other sleep disorders and when paradoxical insomnia is suspected.

Polysomnography (PSG) is routinely used for the diagnosis of several sleep disorders, but it is not routinely indicated for the diagnosis of insomnia [48]. Nevertheless, PSG can help rule out a sleep-disordered-breathing (SDB) when clinical symptoms are present and could be useful when insomnia does not respond to an adequate course of treatment. Night-to-night variability and the "first-night" effect (i.e., poor sleep associated with adapting to the laboratory setting and recording equipment) are greater for measures of sleep continuity relevant to insomnia than for indices of SDB and periodic leg movements. Contemporary home-based PSG studies, which are typically unattended, allow the collection of a full montage of sleep data. Unlike laboratory PSG studies, the first-night effect of home-based PSG is generally absent, suggesting that home PSG provides more reliable data on sleep continuity of insomniacs [49].

Another possible ambulatory monitoring is actigraphy. Actigraphs are wristwatch-sized devices containing a motion sensor that records and stores information on gross motor activity. Typical epoch length for insomnia studies is one minute, and most devices also include an event marker that can indicate events of interest, such as the onset and offset of the intended sleep period. Some models have additional features, such as light sensors or programmable alarm prompts, so that the user may mark subjective ratings of interest. Unlike PSG, which evaluates sleep based on multiple channels of information (EEG, electromyography and electrooculography), actigraphy determines sleep-wake states based solely on wrist movement. Consequently, sleep and wake states during the intended sleep period can be estimated but actigraphs do not provide information about sleep stages.

Correlations between actigraphy and PSG-derived sleep parameters vary depending on the specific actigraphy model and specific scoring algorithm. When used in primary insomnia, actigraphy appears to have acceptable agreement with PSG on measures such as number of awakenings, total time spent awake after sleep onset, total sleep time, and sleep efficiency, but not latency to sleep onset [50]. The main advantage of actigraphy is its suitability for recording sleep-wake data continuously for long periods of time in the patient's habitual sleep environment. It is recommended that actigraphs be used along with sleep diaries to confirm timing of lights out and the end of the sleep period and to allow rejecting of artefacts. It is also recommended that actigraphs be used for at least three consecutive 24-hour periods [51].

Subtypes of Insomnia

As previously reported, over the years a number of categorizations and definitions of insomnia have been devised for clinical and research purposes. Inconsistency in definition inevitably has led to inconsistency in the methods used to measure and to diagnose insomnia. In the last years, there have been calls for greater precision and consistency in the categorizations and diagnoses of insomnia. According to the ICSD-2, eleven subtypes of insomnia may be distinguished. We now report the more frequently observed in the clinical practice.

a) Adjustment Insomnia

Adjustment insomnia has a number of alternate names (acute insomnia, transient insomnia, short-term insomnia, stress-related insomnia, transient psychophysiological insomnia, adjustment disorder). It is by definition a transient or short-term insomnia related to an identifiable stressor. Adjustment insomnia occurs more commonly in older adults and women. Evidence suggests that in a given year 15% to 20% of adults experience some adjustment insomnia.

Although sleep disturbance is the primary symptom of adjustment insomnia, this sleep disorder is frequently associated with waking psychological symptoms of arousal such as anxiety, worry, and ruminative thoughts. Anxiety-related physical symptoms such as muscle tension, gastrointestinal upset, and headaches are also often present as well as daytime symptoms of fatigue, impaired concentration, and irritability.

Adjustment insomnia is, by its short duration, the presence of a known precipitant, and absence of a learned or association component. The onset is usually acute with a less than three-month time course. The time course of the resolution of the insomnia depends on the speed at which the stressor resolves or the individual adapts to a chronic stressor. If the sleep problem lasts longer than a few months, alternate diagnoses should be considered.

b) Psychophysiological Insomnia

Psychophysiological insomnia has a number of alternate names: primary insomnia, learned insomnia, conditioned insomnia, and chronic insomnia among others.

Psychophysiological insomnia is rare among children and most frequent in women. This condition is a very common form of insomnia affecting 1% to 2% of the general population and 12% to 15% of those who seek treatment at sleep centers.

Psychophysiological insomnia is characterized by physical and/or psychological arousal that interferes with sleep. Attention to and worry about their ability or inability to sleep are characteristic of patients with this disorder and are the primary foci for cognitive behavioural treatments for insomnia. Hyperarousal has been found to be a 24-hour-a-day phenomenon in patients with psychophysiological insomnia. They have been found to be more alert in the daytime than would be expected according to their sleep complaints, and they are more alert at night than asymptomatic control subjects. Although hyperarousal is the distinguishing feature of psychophysiological insomnia, it should be noted that heightened arousal is not exclusive to this form of insomnia. Another component of psychophysiological insomnia has been conceptualized as a "learned" or "conditioned" element found to be well treated by stimulus control treatment. A defining characteristic of conditioned insomnia is its association with place. Stimulus control is predicated on blocking the learned association between the bed and sleeplessness.

The onset of psychophysiological insomnia may be insidious or acute. In its insidious forms, adult patients often report having had symptoms in adolescence or young adulthood. As mentioned above, adjustment insomnia if unresolved can lead to psychophysiological insomnia. Psychophysiological insomnia, in turn, if not treated can be enduring. Thus, duration could be seen as a major distinction between adjustment and psychophysiological insomnia. Potential complications of psychophysiological insomnia include the appearance of a first episode or recurrence of major depression and/or the abuse of over-the-counter or prescription sleep-promoting medications.

c)   Paradoxical Insomnia

In this type of insomnia (otherwise known as sleep state misperception, pseudo-insomnia, or sleep hypochondriasis), subjective sleep complaints are not supported by objective findings nor is there the level of daytime impairment that would be expected given the severity of complaints (e.g., little or no sleep) about nighttime sleep.

Paradoxical insomnia seems to be most common among young and middle aged adults. The condition can persist for months or years without change in symptoms or presentation. The prevalence of paradoxical insomnia in the general population is unknown. Among clinical populations the prevalence is less than 5%.

Overestimation of sleep latency or extreme underestimation of time spent asleep as compared with objective sleep recordings are the core characteristics of this disorder. The objective/ subjective discrepancy is greater than in other insomnias.

There has been considerable discussion as to the nature of this complaint. It is possible that the discrepancy between subjective and objective measures in this type of insomnia is due to the inability of objective measures to detect whatever is causing the individual to perceive his/her sleep as disturbed or inadequate.

d)   Idiopathic Insomnia

The core characteristic of idiopathic insomnia is a long-standing complaint of insomnia initiated in infancy or childhood and persisting through adulthood. The prevalence is approximately 0.7% of adolescents and 1% of very young adults. Among sleep clinic patients, the prevalence is less than 10%. There are no data reported regarding the sex distribution of this disorder.

The typical complaint is a lifelong difficulty with sleep. Sleep difficulties can be sleep initiation, repeated awakenings, or short sleep duration. Insomnia is persistent with few extended periods of remission. A notable feature is the absence of specific precipitants of the condition. Baseline sleep associated with this condition, however, can worsen in the presence of factors that typically precipitate insomnia such as psychosocial stressors or medical conditions.

This condition is associated with risk of major depression or substance abuse that may develop from patients' attempts to ameliorate their sleep problem.

Hypersomnias

Diagnostic Definition of Hypersomnia

Somnolence is a complex state, determined by multiple factors such as quantity and quality of prior sleep, circadian time, drugs, attention, motivation, environmental stimuli, and various medical, neurological, and psychiatric conditions. Somnolence is clearly welcomed when sleep is desired, however at other times becomes an unwanted symptom. Pathological or inappropriate somnolence is clinically termed hypersomnia or excessive daytime sleepiness (EDS). Subjects with hypersomnia are unable to stay alert and awake during the major waking episodes of the day resulting in unintended lapses into sleep. Sleepiness can vary in severity. In some cases, sleepiness is associated with large increases in the total daily amount of sleep without feeling of restoration. In other cases, sleepiness may be alleviated temporarily by naps but recurs shortly thereafter. In most cases, excessive sleepiness is a chronic symptom. It must occur for at least three months prior to diagnosis.

EDS has been associated to several causes. They can be categorized into the following types:

1) Insufficient or nonrestorative sleep
   a) Sleep restriction
   b) Sleep fragmentation
2) Hypersomnias of central origin
   a) Central nervous system (CNS) pathology/dysfunction
   b) Hypersomnia due to medical/neurological disorder
   c) Hypersomnia due to drugs
   d) Hypersomnia due to mood disorders
3) Alterations in the circadian rhythm
4) Sleepiness due to multiple factors

Concerning sleep restriction, it is well known that total and partial sleep deprivation in normal subjects produces EDS [52, 53]. Total sleep deprivation does not usually represent a diagnostic problem since it is easy to detect. Partial sleep restriction can be more difficult to recognize either because the patient may underestimate it [54] or because it may coexist with other known causes of sleepiness.

Behaviourally induced insufficient sleep should be suspected when the patient (i) has an unusually high sleep efficiency, (ii) reports about two hours more sleep on each weekend day more than each weekday, or (iii) when the appearance of sleepiness is preceded by a change in the sleep patterns of the patient, particularly a reduction in the usual number of hours of sleep.

Sleep restriction can occur in patients because of medical disorders causing pain, limited mobility, nicturia, dyspnea, etc. and may be a cause of daytime sleepiness. EDS due to sleep restriction can also coexist with other causes of sleepiness, such as sleep disordered breathing, narcolepsy, etc., complicating not only the diagnosis, but also the treatment of the condition. Interestingly, in some disorders like insomnia or restless leg syndrome there is no such clear relationship between degree of sleep reduction or fragmentation and daytime sleepiness.

In routine clinical practice there is only one condition that can be associated with such a high level of sleep fragmentation and it is obstructive sleep apnea (OSA). In fact, sleep fragmentation has been shown to be more relevant in producing EDS than the oxyhemoglobin desaturation occurring in OSA [55]. However, other authors found that apnea/hypoxemia is the most important explanations for EDS in OSA [56].

The ICSD-2[3] recognizes a vast differential of etiologies of hypersomnolence: those types of hypersomnolence due to sleep-related breathing disorders, circadian rhythm sleep disorders, or other causes of disturbed sleep, and those with a cause of central origin. The main groups of central origin hypersomnias include narcolepsy, recurrent hypersomnia (including Kleine–Levin syndrome and menstrual-related hypersomnia), idiopathic hypersomnia, behaviourally induced insufficient sleep syndrome, hypersomnia due to medical conditions or drugs, nonorganic hypersomnia, and unspecified physiological hypersomnia.

Pathophysiology

Sleepiness and hypersomnia are terms used in a variety of ways. Sleepiness describes at least three different aspects: 1) the physiological need state for sleep, also called sleep propensity; 2) the subjective perception of the need for sleep; 3) and the behavioural signs (yawning, closing of the eyelids, motor slowing, lapses in attention, etc.) that a subject displays when approaching sleep. Not every sleepy patient will show parallel changes in the above three aspects. Hypersomnia is also used indistinctively to describe EDS, prolonged sleep duration, or both. Using hypersomnia as synonym of EDS may not be always accurate. Not everybody experiencing sleepiness will fall asleep, particularly if sleepiness is not severe, and on the other hand, people who need ten or more hours of nocturnal sleep (and could be considered as suffering from hypersomnia) may not have EDS at all if they get enough nocturnal sleep.

At least two different approaches have been used to understand how sleep and sleepiness occurs: studies of sleep regulation and studies of the neural circuitry underlying sleep-wake states.

The studies of sleep regulation indicate that the tendency to fall asleep is not a fixed value, since it oscillates continuously due to the interaction of several factors or processes. Some of them act relatively slowly (hours) and others function in a more short-term basis. The two slow-acting ones are the homeostatic process, which accumulates sleep propensity during waking and dissipates it with sleep, and the circadian process, a clock-like mechanism which tends to limit the appearance of sleep to a time of day where it is more ecologically appropriate [57, 58]. In a conventional 24-hour schedule, sleepiness is highest in the middle of the night with a second peak in the afternoon, whereas alertness is highest in the evening.

However, the model does not explain how the homeostatic need for sleep is generated and which are the neural substrate and biochemical basis of this regulation. Moreover, the knowledge of the circadian system circuitry, centered in the suprachiasmatic nuclei (SCN) of the hypothalamus [59], is impressive, however it is unclear if the SCN function by promoting exclusively an arousal drive that opposes the need for sleep, by producing both arousing and sleep-promoting signals depending on the time of day, or simply by acting as a gate which opens when accumulated sleep exceeds a given threshold and closes whenever accumulated sleep falls below another threshold. The neural substrate of the gate and its thresholds is not known.

In the study of sleep regulation, researchers generally use protocols that specifically avoid influences from social interaction, work or food schedules, physical activity, etc. in order to unmask the effects of the homeostatic and circadian processes. The focus on these two processes may lead to assume that they are the only factors determining the tendency to fall asleep. However, there are other arousing (or sleep-promoting) contextual factors that can influence the appearance of sleepiness and sleep and may be clinically relevant.

For example, sleep is difficult in the presence of fear, anxiety, or severe pain. Ambient noise, change in temperature, posture, motor activity and motivation are other factors present in real life that clearly modify the impact of sleep loss in acute sleep deprivation studies [53] and likely influence the presence of sleepiness in healthy subjects [60] and in patients with sleep disorders. Watching alone a boring TV program favours sleep whereas the presence of other people in the room delays it [61]. Moreover, contextual factors may vary from one moment to the next and the same situation may not have equal effect on different subjects.

In summary, homeostatic, circadian, contextual and individual factors interact in generating sleep propensity of a subject. The high complexity of these interactions in the real world is what makes the measurement of sleepiness so difficult.

The neural mechanisms maintaining sleep and wakefulness are relatively well known. Wakefulness is maintained by a complex network of multiple, parallel systems [62] whose components originate in the cholinergic pontine nuclei, the noradrenergic locus coeruleus, the serotonergic raphe nuclei in the pons/midbrain junction, the histaminergic tuberomandibular and hypocretinergic (orexinergic) nuclei in the posterior hypothalamus, the cholinergic basal forebrain, and the glutamatergic thalamocortical systems and probably a dopaminergic ventral periaqueductal gray area in the midbrain [63].

Cortical areas are activated by widespread projections from these nuclei through different thalamic and extrathalamic pathways and probably cooperate in maintaining arousal [64]. Most of these systems are maximally active during wakefulness and are likely responsible for this behavioural state and its electroencephalographic (EEG) correlate. However, the relative importance of each of these systems in producing the arousal level of an individual is not well known since isolated dysfunction of these systems is really difficult to identify in humans. In cataplexy, a clinical situation, deactivation of serotoninergic and noradrenergic systems and poor functioning of the hypocretin/orexin systems is not incompatible with alertness, suggesting that the histaminergic system (with perhaps the contribution of the cholinergic, glutamatergic and dopaminergic systems) is able to maintain arousal, at least for the relatively short duration of the cataplectic attack [65]. Out of the episodes of cataplexy, narcoleptics may also have periods of normal alertness, suggesting that other arousal systems can produce wakefulness without the help of the hypocretinergic system, although they cannot maintain it for long periods. Moreover, the SCN have an important role in maintaining arousal because, after their selective destruction, the other arousal systems are unable to sustain relatively long periods of wakefulness [66, 67].

Sleep is associated with activation of the basal forebrain and the hypothalamic ventrolateral preoptic (VLPO) area together with deactivation of arousal systems, but it is not completely clear which goes first. The thalamus, the nucleus tractus solitarius in the lower medulla [62, 64] and various cortical areas (premotor, posterior supraorbital, and somesthetic) [68] are also other areas that when stimulated with repetitive low frequency electrical stimuli induce sleep. Although the preoptic area (ventrolateral and median preoptic) has a central role in sleep promotion and some of its neurons show a gradual increase in their firing rates before sleep onset [69], an intriguing fact is that the firing rate of VLPO area neurons during waking does not increase with sleep deprivation; it only increases when the animals actually sleep, suggesting that it is more related to the production of sleep than to the level of sleepiness [70].

Concerning the mechanisms governing the transition between sleep and wakefulness, sleep-promoting neurons in the VLPO and wake-promoting neurons (lateral hypothalamic orexin neurons) are mutually antagonistic (ie, inhibit each other) and form a "flip-flop switch," a type of circuit that results in rapid and complete transition in behavioural state. The flip-flop switch circuitry of the wake-sleep regulatory system produces the typical sleep pattern seen in healthy adults, with consolidated waking during the day and alternation between NREM and REM sleep at night. Breakdown in this circuitry both results in and explains the manifestations of a variety of sleep disorders including hypersomnia [71].

Diagnostic Tools for Hypersomnia

a) Daytime History and Physical Examination

Physiological daytime napping is common before the age of five years, so it is difficult to identify a pathologically sleepy preschool-age child. In a school-age child, however, habitually falling asleep in the classroom, while being driven in an automobile, at the dinner table, while watching television, or while reading should arouse suspicion of significant daytime sleepiness. A gradual increase in the consumption of caffeinated beverages or nicotine may be also observed. Adults with significant sleepiness may show involuntary napping in socially inappropriate situations like talking or eating. Their performance at work can also suffer.

Periods of hypersomnia lasting 10 to 14 days in teenagers in association with hyperphagia or hypersexual behaviour may suggest the Kleine–Levin syndrome [72]. Inadequate sleep hygiene, substance abuse, and drug-seeking behaviour may also mimic a primary disorder of vigilance like narcolepsy/idiopathic hypersomnia. A medication history for prescription and over-the counter agents is therefore critical. Low self-esteem, sadness, and social withdrawal may suggest underlying depression. It is also important to inquire what impact daytime sleepiness has had on the quality of life.

The history should assess bedtime, sleep onset time, sensorimotor disturbance suggestive of restless legs syndrome, bedtime rituals, habitual snoring, mouth breathing, periods of observed apnea, nocturnal awakenings and associated abnormal motor behaviour, and how alert the person feels upon awakening in the morning.

The height, weight, body mass index (BMI), occipitofrontal head circumference, and blood pressure of our patient with hypersomnia must be recorded. Obstructive sleep apnea (OSA) may be associated with high BMI. The patient should be assessed for craniofacial abnormalities like micrognathia, dental malocclusion, enlarged tongue size, and midface hypoplasia. A deviated nasal septum, swollen inferior turbinates, tonsillar hypertrophy, and mouth breathing may also be especially seen in children with OSA. Consultation with an otolaryngologist may be required to exclude adenoidal hypertrophy. Brainstem anomalies like the Chiari type II malformation can be associated with hoarseness of the voice, decreased gag reflex, and abnormal tendon reflexes. Neuromuscular disorders like myotonic dystrophy are associated with chronic obstructive hypoventilation due to a combination of oropharyngeal muscle weakness leading to airway collapse, combined with diminished respiratory muscle excursion. Home videos, when available, also provide valuable clues to nocturnal seizures, parasomnias and other abnormal motor activities that may cause sleep fragmentation.

b) Subjective Assessment Tools

Questionnaire surveys of sleepiness are useful in epidemiological research, but they may also serve as screening instruments in clinical practice. Because sleep is a multidimensional phenomenon, subjective, unidimensional measures like the Epworth sleepiness scale (ESS) and the Stanford Sleepiness Scale (SSS) correlate only weakly with objective measures of sleepiness.

The ESS is the most widely self-administered questionnaire in sleep clinical practice [73]. It has been validated in a variety of clinical disorders (Table 1) and proven to be reliable [74-77].

Table 1. The mean ESS item-scores

Subjects	Mean Epworth score	Reference
Young male students	5.6	Johns and Patterson (2000) (unpublished)
Older male students	6.6	"
Young female students	6.7	"
Older female students	5.7	"
Narcolepsy	19.6	Parkes et al. (1998)
Severe OSA patients	18.4	"
Controls (age 33-37 yrs)	5.7	Bloch et al. (1999)
Elderly females	6.6	Broman et al. (2000)

Eight questions estimate the patient's chance of dozing off on a zero to three scale during common activities such as while sitting and reading, watching television, sitting inactive in a public place, as a passenger in a car, lying down in the afternoon, sitting talking to somebody, after lunch, and while driving after stopping for a few minutes at a traffic light. The maximum score is 24, and values up to 10 are physiologic and that above 12 correlate with pathological daytime sleepiness. In the original description by Johns, the questionnaire was administered to 188 adults, including 30 healthy controls and 150 patients with sleep disorders consisting of primary snoring, OSA, narcolepsy, idiopathic hypersomnia, insomnia, and periodic limb movement disorder [73]. The controls showed a mean ESS score of 5.9+/-2.2, with no significant gender difference. All patients with narcolepsy and idiopathic hypersomnia had higher ESS scores (>10) than controls. Scores >16 were felt to reflect severe sleepiness. One drawback of the ESS is that patients frequently underestimate the severity of their own sleepiness. Others have difficulty distinguishing sleepiness from fatigue.

The SSS is a self-rating scale, in which patients are asked to choose from one to seven statements that best describe their level of sleepiness at a specific time of the day [78]. It reliably measures the effects of partial sleep deprivation, but there can be subjective underestimation of sleepiness, as for the ESS. The SSS, that has not been validated against other physiological measures, does not capture the true, multidimensional nature of sleepiness.

Karolinska Sleepiness Scale is another scale developed in 1990 by Akerstedt and Gillberg [79] and frequently applied in the occupational health field. It uses a nine-point scale that ranges from one being very alert to nine being very sleepy and trying hard to stay awake. Patients are asked to rate their sleepiness in the five minutes immediately prior to taking the test. A score of seven or more denotes pathological sleepiness.

c) Objective Assessment Tools

The diagnosis of sleep-disordered breathing, a frequent cause of daytime sleepiness, can be made by comprehensive sleep studies in a sleep laboratory, but also using measurement of oxygen desaturation at home or portable equipment for cardiorespiratory monitoring, according to pretest probabilities, individual experience and local preferences [80].

Overnight oximetry analysis is a simple screening tool for sleep-disordered breathing [81]. Oximetry data must be visually inspected and interpreted by clinicians knowledgeable in distinguishing artefact from the "saw-toothed" (cyclical) oscillations in the oxyhemoglobin saturation that are caused by apneas/hypopnea [82]. The sensitivity and specificity of oximetry in the diagnosis of OSA are dependent on its severity—in a study in subjects with suspected OSA, some authors found that for those with apnea-hypopnea index (AHI) > 25, the sensitivity was 100% and specificity was 95% [83]. When the AHI was >15, the sensitivity and specificity fell to 75% and 86%, respectively, and when the AHI was >5, the sensitivity and specificity dropped to 60% and 80%, respectively. A normal overnight oximetry essentially excludes moderate/severe OSA, but does not exclude mild OSA or upper airway resistance syndrome (UARS), nor does it rule out etiologies of sleepiness that are unrelated to sleep-disordered breathing.

Concerning portable monitoring, various systems are now available that seek to improve convenience and comfort by recording only a limited number of cardiorespiratory parameters, with some of these devices designed for home use without a technologist in attendance. Despite the technological advances in portable-monitor devices, there remains a lack of standardization in terms of signals recorded, sensors, signal processing, and data analysis. Large differences can exist between monitors, even those within the same classification. Greater standardization is required. The proper role for these portable monitors remains a matter of significant debate.

A Task Force of the American Academy of Sleep Medicine [84] makes the following recommendations: unattended portable monitoring (PM) for the diagnosis of OSA should be performed only in conjunction with a comprehensive sleep evaluation. Clinical sleep evaluations using PM must be supervised by a practitioner expert in sleep medicine. PM may be used as an alternative to polysomnography (PSG) for the diagnosis of OSA in patients with a high pretest probability of moderate to severe OSA. PM is not appropriate for the diagnosis of OSA in patients with significant comorbid medical conditions or in patients suspected of having comorbid sleep disorders. PM may be indicated for the diagnosis of OSA in patients for whom in-laboratory PSG is not possible by virtue of immobility, safety, or critical illness. At a minimum, PM must record airflow, respiratory effort, and blood oxygenation.

In the investigation of disorders leading to daytime sleepiness such as narcolepsy, idiopathic hypersomnia, and periodic hypersomnia (Kleine–Levin syndrome), the nocturnal in-laboratory PSG should be performed for the differential diagnosis. The PSG must be performed the night before the two traditional objective tests for the evaluation of sleepiness: the multiple sleep latency test (MSLT) [85] and the maintenance of wakefulness test (MWT) [86]. MSLT is the "gold standard" for the assessment of daytime sleepiness in adults and children [87]. The strengths of the test lie in its intuitive design (sleepy individuals are more likely to fall asleep than those who are not sleepy), its reliability, and the availability of normative data across various ages. It has also been validated in conditions such as sleep loss, sleep disruption, and hypnotic and alcohol use [88]. One major indication for the MSLT is suspected narcolepsy or idiopathic hypersomnia.

The MSLT is commenced 1.5 to 3 hours after the final morning awakening. The test consists of the provision of five nap opportunities at two hourly intervals, e.g., 0900 hours, 1100 hours, 1300 hours, 1500 hours, and 1700 hours. Central and occipital EEG (C3-O1, C4-O2), eye movements (right outer canthus to left outer canthus), and chin EMG need to be recorded. One of the eye movement sensors is placed slightly above the outer canthus, and the other slightly below the outer canthus. This arrangement facilitates capture of both horizontal and vertical eye movements. The time constant for the electrooculogram (EOG) should be long enough to allow for the recording of slow rolling eye movements that typically herald the onset of NREM sleep. At the designated hour, lights are turned off, the patient is advised to relax, close the eyes, and try to fall asleep while the electrophysiological parameters are being monitored. If no sleep occurs, the nap opportunity is terminated 20 minutes following "lights out," and the patient is designated as having a sleep latency of 20 minutes (the maximum). If the patient falls asleep, the test is continued for 15 minutes after sleep onset. Sleep is scored in 30-second epochs. The time interval between "lights out" and electroencephalographic sleep onset is designated the sleep latency. A mean of the sleep latency (MSL) is derived from averaging the sleep latency of the five nap opportunities. Reference values for the MSL at various ages, as well as reported values in several pathological conditions, are listed in Table 2 [89-91].

Table 2. MSL at MSLT in different sleep disorders

Sleep disorders	Mean sleep latency (time in minutes)
Narcolepsy	2.9 ± 2.7
Idiopathic Hypersomnia	8.7 ± 4.9
Insomnia	> 10
Normative controls decades	
20's	12.7 ± 7.0
30's	10.4 ± 3.7
40's	11.4 ± 5.1
50's	12.1 ± 1.1
60's	11.2 ± 5.2
80's	15.2 ± 6.1

A SOREMP (Sleep Onset REM Period) is defined as the occurrence of REM sleep within 15 minutes of sleep onset. About 80% of patients with narcolepsy show two or more SOREMPs during the MSLT. False positives may occur in patients with severe OSA who have suppression of nocturnal REM sleep with a consequent daytime REM sleep rebound. The diagnostic sensitivity of the MSLT for the diagnosis of narcolepsy has been estimated around 61%, while the diagnostic specificity when two or more SOREMPs are present is around 94%. If the presence of two or more SOREMPs is combined with a MSL <5 minutes, then the diagnostic specificity rises to 97%. A limitation of the MSLT is its "floor" effect— e.g., in pathologically sleepy subjects with MSL <5 minutes, it cannot help determine whether an individual with a MSL of 2 minutes is somehow different from an individual with MSL of 1 minute. The normal values for the MSLT were derived from the study of healthy, sleep-deprived subjects, thus, its application to subjects with sleep disorders also poses limitations—we do not know whether sleepiness resulting from sleep deprivation and that due to sleep disorders are qualitatively identical. The MSLT can control for environmental variables such as light, ambient temperature, and noise, but it cannot control for internal psychological factors like motivation and anxiety that might also impact sleep latency.

MWT is a mirror image opposite of the MSLT [87]. It is a test of daytime alertness and measures the ability to stay awake during the daytime in a darkened, quiet environment. Electrodes are applied for monitoring the EEG, eye movements, and chin EMG in a manner identical to the MSLT. The patient is provided four opportunities to stay awake in a darkened, quiet room at two hourly intervals, starting at 1.5 to 3 hours after the final morning awakening. The patient sits is advised to "sit still and remain awake for as long as possible." Each trial ends after 40 minutes if no sleep occurs or after three epochs of unequivocal sleep. As in the MSLT, patients undergoing the MWT show their shortest MSL around 1300 hours. The physiological MSL on the MWT is 30.4 _ 11.2 minutes. The upper limit of the 95% confidence interval is 40 minutes. Using 20-minute MWT trials, Mitler and colleagues [92] found that subjects with narcolepsy were able to stay awake only for an average of 6 minutes as compared with 19 minutes in normal control subjects. The MWT is useful in monitoring response to therapy in daytime sleepiness when the patient is being treated and in instances where one needs to ensure adequate daytime alertness for occupational reasons (airline pilots, truck drivers, etc.). The drawback is that normative data are limited. It is unclear whether the MWT correlates reliably with alertness in the real-life day-to-day setting.

Subtypes of Hypersomnia

a) Narcolepsy

Narcolepsy is a disorder in which the boundaries of wakefulness and normal sleep, most notably REM sleep, are blurred; features of sleep intrude into the state of wakefulness and vice versa [93].

It has been divided into various categories, including those with cataplexy, those without cataplexy, those due to a medical condition.

Narcolepsy was first thought to be a genetically determined autoimmune disorder when a link between narcolepsy and the human leukocyte antigen (HLA) DR2 and HLA DQ6 was identified in Japan in 1986 [94]. This association was confirmed in 96% of Caucasians diagnosed with narcolepsy, and later shown to be primarily due to DQB1*0602 across multiple ethnic groups [95]. Narcoleptics with cataplexy have been found to have DQB1*0602 positivity more often than those without cataplexy; moreover, a positive correlation between DQB1*0602 positivity and severity of cataplexy has been identified [95, 96]. In 2000, following on parallel discoveries in animal models [97], most cases of human narcolepsy with cataplexy were found to have low cerebrospinal fluid (CSF) hypocretin-1 [98].

A dramatically decreased number of hypocretin producing cells in the brain of narcoleptic patients has been reported in some post-mortem studies [99, 100].

Narcolepsy-cataplexy usually manifests during adolescences and often the onset is insidious. As the name implies, narcolepsy with cataplexy is a syndrome characterized by the presence of both excessive daytime somnolence and cataplexy. Although sleepiness can be welcome if an individual wants to sleep, it can be pathological when it results in a tendency to fall asleep at inappropriate times. Excessive daytime somnolence is often the first symptom to appear in narcolepsy with cataplexy and may be induced by a variety of different factors, including the quality and quantity of one's sleep, drugs, circadian components, environmental stimuli, motivation, and any number of psychiatric, medical, and neurological conditions [101].

Some narcoleptics have demonstrated unintentional periods of sleep during times of desired wakefulness, as during interactive conversation, during intercourse, and while eating. These irresistible periods of sleep are referred to as sleep attacks [101, 102]. Interestingly, patients may feel refreshed for a brief period of time after they take a short nap (approximately 10–15 minutes), but then feel sleepy again after a few hours. These individuals have an inability to stay awake or asleep for prolonged periods of time rather than a requirement of increased sleep amounts. The ICSD-2 requires a daily complaint of sleepiness for a minimum of three months. Essentially pathognomonic for narcolepsy-cataplexy, cataplexy is characterized by a bilateral loss of muscle tone triggered by strong emotions (laughter, anger, and surprise); it is usually brief in duration, on the order of a few seconds to several minutes [103]. It often presents within a couple of years from the onset of daytime sleepiness. In mild cases, there may simply be a loss of facial tone, head droop, slurred speech, or jaw drop. Severe attacks are marked by a collapse to the ground. Reflexes cannot be elicited during this event. Cardiac and respiratory muscles are spared; consciousness is maintained, and the patients retain complete memory of the event. Patients may try to avoid conditions that provoke cataplexy.

As narcoleptic patients fall asleep or awaken from sleep, they may experience sleep paralysis, which is an inability to move or speak [104]. It usually persists for 10 seconds to several minutes before resolving spontaneously. An external stimulus, like the touch or the voice of another person, may also halt the paralysis. Muscles of respiration and eye control are spared, but a sense of fright may be present. This phenomenon is present in approximately 40% to 80% of narcoleptics. Importantly, however, up to 40% to 50% of normal individuals have reported isolated episodes of sleep paralysis, although the symptom is typically mild and rare.

Vivid and realistic hallucinations at sleep onset (hypnagogic) or on awakening (hypnopompic) have been reported in 40% to 80% of narcoleptics [102]. The hallucinations are usually visual.

Automatic behaviour typically manifests in cases of severe sleepiness [102]. This phenomenon is characterized by an interruption of purposeful activity by a sleep attack or a microsleep episode such that performance is markedly impaired; the individual furthermore demonstrates no recollection of the event. One example is the case where a patient who is sleepy may continue to speak on the phone but in an inarticulate manner.

Narcoleptic patients with cataplexy are generally not true "hypersomniacs"; indeed patients do not typically sleep a larger amount over a 24-hour period when compared with normal individuals. Moreover, a large part of individuals with narcolepsy with cataplexy have disturbed nocturnal sleep with repeated awakenings and restlessness [101, 105]. Nocturnal PSG usually shows a sleep latency of less than 10 min, an increase in the amount of nonrapid eye movement (NREM) stage N1 sleep, and sleep fragmentation. About 25% to 50% of people with this disorder also demonstrate a SOREMP. Two or more SOREMPs and a mean latency to sleep of less than eight minutes are expected on an MSLT as criteria for the diagnosis of narcolepsy.

Several medical disorders have been shown to be a direct cause of narcolepsy. Those that have resulted in narcolepsy with cataplexy include neurosarcoidosis, hypothalamic tumors, multiple sclerosis (with plaques in the hypothalamus), autosomal-dominant cerebellar ataxia with deafness, Neimann–Pick type C disease, paraneoplastic syndromes with anti-Ma2 antibodies [106-108]. Other medical conditions, such as head trauma, multiple system atrophy, Parkinson's disease, myotonic dystrophy, and Prader–Willi syndrome have resulted in narcolepsy without cataplexy [109, 110].

Approximately 0.02% to 0.067% of the population in the United States and Western Europe are affected with narcolepsy with cataplexy. In Japan, the prevalence has been reported between 0.16% and 0.18%, and in Israel the prevalence of narcolepsy has been reported as 0.0002% [111]. Both sexes may be affected equally. The peak onset of symptoms occurs in adolescence with a second peak around the age of 40; about 10% of cases are diagnosed before 10 years old and 5% after 50 years old. Symptoms of narcolepsy are not progressive but usually persist for life.

In clinical samples, narcolepsy without cataplexy is thought to account for about 10% to 50% of the narcoleptic population. The exact population prevalence of narcolepsy without cataplexy is unknown.

In several case studies in the second half of the 20th century, psychiatric symptoms were reported to be present in narcolepsy. Of these, depressive mood has been most often described, in addition to personality and sexual disorders. Furthermore, the possible relation between narcolepsy and schizophrenia has received attention many times. Only recently, however, well-controlled studies using formal diagnostic instruments have been performed, in order to further define the psychiatric comorbidity of narcolepsy [112].

Symptoms of depression have been assessed repeatedly in patient series, and suggested to be highly prevalent [113-118]. In more recent years, the relation between depression and narcolepsy was assessed in different ways: as a "secondary outcome" in quality of life studies, using self report depression severity scales, and with more formal psychiatric diagnostic instruments. Using self report questionnaires, a high prevalence of depression was found in narcolepsy, for example with the Beck Depression Inventory [119-123]. In the quality of life studies of Vignatelli and colleagues, predictors for the different quality of life domains were calculated. The presence of depressive symptoms was the main stable independent predictor of health-related quality of life across a 5-year period [123], stressing the importance of paying attention to mood status in narcoleptic patients. Other authors used the Schedules for Clinical Assessment in Neuropsychiatry in a large cohort of narcolepsy patients and compared this to an age and sex-matched control group [124]. They chosed to adjust the diagnostic criteria of depression by excluding sleep symptoms and fatigue, but retaining concentration problems and weight changes. With these criteria, the authors did not find an overrepresentation of major depression. However, there clearly was a higher level of depressive symptoms that could not just be explained by the narcolepsy symptoms per se: depressive mood (30%), pathological guilt (22%), crying (25%), and anedonia (27%) were clearly and significantly overrepresented [124].

In contrast to depression, anxiety in narcolepsy received minor attention in the past [125-126]. However, more recently a strikingly high level of anxiety disorders, with 35% of patients receiving an anxiety disorder classification, compared to 3% in population controls has been found [124]. Narcolepsy patients reported more panic attacks (22%), as well as social phobias (20%). In part, these anxiety symptoms seem to be explained by a certain loss of control associated with the narcolepsy symptoms, for example when experiencing cataplectic attacks in public. Anxiety may also be triggered by daytime remembrance of hypnagogic hallucinations, which would explain the presence of more specific phobias such as fear of insects or situational fears, e.g., for water or pools [124].

Given that hypnagogic hallucinations form part of the core symptomatology of narcolepsy, it is not surprising that a possible overlap between narcolepsy and psychotic disorders such as schizophrenia has often been suspected or suggested. In one of the earlier studies, Sours found "frank schizophrenic reactions" in 10 out of 75 narcolepsy patients, although the criteria for this particular diagnosis were not reported [125]. Out of 20 patients, Roy et al. found one with a schizophreniform psychosis [114]. Later studies did not find psychotic or schizophrenic patients in the narcolepsy cohorts [115-116]. Some authors have discussed the differentiation of narcolepsy from schizophrenia as well as possible reciprocal relationships between the two [127-129]. Several options have been raised: the existence of a "psychotic form" of narcolepsy, coincident combinations of the two disorders, as well as stimulant-induced psychosis. The latter possibility was supported by the controlled study of Vourdas and colleagues: in this evaluation of 45 cases, 4 patients had a history of psychosis, all of which were most likely to be amphetamine-induced [130].

In a case-control study, any indication for an increased prevalence of schizophrenia or any other psychotic disorder in narcolepsy compared to population controls has been found [131]. In some patients, reality testing was compromised to a certain degree, and delusional memories were present in a few. These symptoms could be attributed to difficulties separating true memories from those constructed out of sleep-related hallucinations. The authors also compared the details of the hallucinatory experiences in the narcolepsy group to a cohort of schizophrenia patients, finding that there was a clear separation in the sensory pattern. Where schizophrenic hallucinations are typically auditory in origin, hallucinations in narcolepsy are much more "multimodal" in origin, combining visual, auditory, as well as tactile experiences.

b) Recurrent Hypersomnia

Kleine-Levin syndrome is a rare sleep disorder that mainly affects adolescents and is characterised by relapsing-remitting episodes of severe hypersomnia, cognitive impairment, apathy, derealisation, and psychiatric and behavioural disturbances [132]. It was first described in 1925 by Kleine [133] and later by Levin in 1936 [134]. The duration of each episode can vary from days to weeks. Episodes may occur rarely or multiple times per month and have no clear periodicity. The severity and duration of symptoms may decrease with successive episodes [135].

Cognitive abnormalities, such as a feeling of derealisation, are core to the symptomatology during episodes. Individuals afflicted with this disorder sleep 16 hours or more each day and may eat copious quantities on awakening. While they are awake, they may be hypersexual, withdrawn, dull, confused, and inattentive. Abnormal behaviour, such as aggression, irritability, or other odd behaviour, may be present, especially when the patient is abruptly awakened. In most cases, the disorder spontaneously remits within 2 to 10 years after onset. Between episodes, patients generally have normal sleep patterns, cognition, mood, and eating habits. During episodes, electroencephalography might show diffuse or local slow activity. Normal sleep cycling is present on PSG, and MSLTs demonstrate pathologic sleepiness without evidence of SOREMP. Functional imaging studies have revealed hypoactivity in thalamic and hypothalamic regions, and in the frontal and temporal lobes. It has been postulated that the disorder may be due to an abnormality of the limbic-hypothalamic pathway. On the basis of an association identified with the HLA DQB1*02, a viral or autoimmune etiology has been suggested.

Menstrual-related hypersomnia occurs within the first few months after menarche [136].

Repeated episodes of hypersomnia tend to persist for approximately one week and spontaneously resolve at the time of menses. Prolonged remission has been observed to occur with use of oral contraceptives, suggesting a hormone imbalance may be responsible for this disorder.

c) Idiopathic Hypersomnia with and without Long Sleep Time

The hallmark of idiopathic hypersomnia with and without long sleep time is constant, severe excessive daytime somnolence [137]. Those individuals with a long sleep time generally sleep around 12 to 14 hours per night (although a sleep time of greater than 10 hours is sufficient for this group) and may also nap for 3 to 4 hours through the day. Those without a long sleep time sleep may have a major sleep episode that is normal or slightly longer than that seen in normal individuals (but the duration is less than 10 hours); they may inadvertently nap during the day. Sleep fragmentation is not observed in either group. Waking up in the morning or at the end of naps is almost always laborious. Patients report sleep drunkenness, or confusion, on awakening [138]. An alarm clock alone is often insufficient to awaken these people. Peripheral vascular complaints, migraines, and orthostatic hypotension with syncope have been reported to occur in association with this disorder. Sleep paralysis and hypnagogic hallucinations may be sometimes observed.

Idiopathic hypersomnia is unusual in prepubertal children, and does not show predominance for either gender. Typically, patients with idiopathic hypersomnia with or without long sleep time present with symptoms before the age of 25 years. It appears to have a nonprogressive course; rare spontaneous remission has been noted [139]. Idiopathic hypersomnia with long sleep time may be hereditary, and an autosomal-dominant mode of inheritance has been suggested. It is important to differentiate idiopathic hypersomnia with long sleep time from depression with hypersomnia. Both groups of patients demonstrate normal amounts of NREM and REM sleep on PSG, although there may be a greater amount of slow wave sleep [140]. Other sleep disorders, such as periodic limb movement disorders and sleep-related breathing disorders, must either be ruled out or appropriately managed before a diagnosis of idiopathic hypersomnia with or without long sleep time may be properly established. An MSLT in either of these patients may demonstrate one or no SOREMPs. Whether or not long sleep time is present, patients with idiopathic hypersomnia have a short mean latency to sleep. In idiopathic hypersomnia without prolonged daily sleep amounts, an MSLT is mandatory for the diagnosis and must document a mean sleep latency below or equal to eight minutes. Patients with idiopathic hypersomnia have been studied via spectral analysis of their EEG during sleep. Such research has suggested a decreased sleep pressure, as measured during the first two nocturnal sleep cycles. All subjects studied so far have demonstrated normal levels of hypocretin-1 in the CSF [141, 142]. Billiard and Dauvilliers have performed neurochemical studies of CSF monoamine metabolites and found a decrease in noradrenergic metabolites [139]. Decreased CSF histamine levels have been identified in a group of idiopathic hypersomnia and narcolepsy patients with normal hypocretin levels [143].

d) Behaviourally Induced Insufficient Sleep

This disorder is present in people who repeatedly acquire suboptimal amounts of sleep to such an extent that their daytime alertness is affected [144]. Although these individuals have no difficulty with sleep onset or sleep maintenance, they continuously subject themselves to sleep deprivation. It is possible for them to manifest hypnagogic hallucinations or sleep paralysis. Secondarily, they may go on to develop poor concentration, fatigue, irritability, malaise, reduced motivation, and restlessness, which are all expected psychological and physiological hallmarks of sleep deprivation. Depression, social withdrawal, and stimulant abuse may be observed in these subjects. Though individuals of any age or gender may develop this problem, adolescents may be slightly more inclined to manifest symptoms as social reassures restrict their sleep; they may report that they sleep for extended periods of time at night on holidays or over the weekend [145-146]. It can be challenging to establish a diagnosis of behaviourally induced insufficient sleep syndrome in a patient who physiologically requires particularly large quantities of sleep. These subjects do not necessarily need to undergo a PSG or MSLT to establish their diagnosis. If they increase their total sleep time and note a subsequent resolution of their symptoms, then the diagnosis is clear. Individuals who have had polysomnographic monitoring demonstrate a high sleep efficiency (usually over 90%), a decreased latency to sleep, and a long sleep time. NREM and REM sleep occur in a normal distribution.

References

[1]   Association of Sleep Disorders Centers. Diagnostic classification of sleep and arousal disorders, first edition. *Sleep* 1979; 2(1):1-137.

[2]   American Sleep Disorders Association. *International Classification of Sleep Disorders.* Rochester, MN: American Sleep Disorders Association, 1990.

[3]   American Academy of Sleep Medicine. *International Classification of Sleep Disorders, 2nd ed. Diagnostic and Coding Manual.* Westchester, IL: American Academy of Sleep Medicine, 2005.

[4]   American Psychiatric Association. *Diagnostic and Statistical Manual of Mental Disorders* (DSM-IV). Washington DC: American Psychiatric Association, 1994.

[5] National Institutes of Health. National Institutes of Health State of the Science Conference statement on Manifestations and Management of Chronic Insomnia in Adults, June 13-15, 2005. *Sleep* 2005; 28(9):1049-57.

[6] Hohagen F, Kappler C, Schramm E, Rink K, Weyerer S, Riemann D et al. Prevalence of insomnia in elderly general practice attenders and the current treatment modalities. *Acta Psychiatr. Scand.* 1994; 90(2):102-8.

[7] Hatoum HT, Kania CM, Kong SX, Wong JM, Mendelson WB. Prevalence of insomnia: a survey of the enrollees at five managed care organizations. *Am. J. Manag. Care* 1998; 4(1):79-86.

[8] Ohayon MM. Prevalence of DSM-IV diagnostic criteria of insomnia: distinguishing insomnia related to mental disorders from sleep disorders. *J. Psychiatr. Res.* 1997; 31(3):333-46.

[9] Simon GE, VonKorff M. Prevalence, burden, and treatment of insomnia in primary care. *Am. J. Psychiatry* 1997; 154(10):1417-23.

[10] Kessler RC, Berglund PA, Coulouvrat C, Hajak G, Roth T, Shahly V, et al. Insomnia and the performance of US workers: results from the America insomnia survey. *Sleep* 2011 Sep 1;34(9):1161-71.

[11] Kraus SS, Rabin LA. Sleep America: managing the crisis of adult chronic insomnia and associated conditions. J Affect Disord 2012 May;138(3):192-212.

[12] Ohayon MM, Roth T. What are the contributing factors for insomnia in the general population? *J. Psychosom. Res* .2001; 51(6):745-55.

[13] Ohayon MM, Reynolds CF 3rd. Epidemiological and clinical relevance of insomnia diagnosis algorithms according to the DSM-IV and the International Classification of Sleep Disorders (ICSD). *Sleep Med.* 2009 Oct;10(9):952-60.

[14] Sateia MJ, Doghramji K, Hauri PJ, Morin CM. Evaluation of chronic insomnia. An American Academy of Sleep Medicine review. *Sleep* 2000; 23(2):243-308.

[15] Foley DJ, Monjan A, Simonsick EM, Wallace RB, Blazer DG. Incidence and remission of insomnia among elderly adults: an epidemiologic study of 6,800 persons over three years. *Sleep* 1999; 22(suppl 2):S366-S372.

[16] Ohayon MM, Bader G. Prevalence and correlates of insomnia in the Swedish population aged 19-75 years. *Sleep* Med 2010 Dec;11(10):980-6.

[17] Terzano MG, Parrino L, Cirignotta F, Ferini-Strambi L, Gigli G, Rudelli G, et al.; Studio Morfeo Committee. Studio Morfeo: insomnia in primary care, a survey conducted on the Italian population. *Sleep* Med 2004 Jan;5(1):67-75.

[18] Shochat T, Umphress J, Israel AG, Ancoli-Israel S. Insomnia in primary care patients. *Sleep* 1999; 22(suppl 2):S359-S365.

[19] Soehner AM, Harvey AG. Prevalence and functional consequences of severe insomnia symptoms in mood and anxiety disorders: results from a nationally representative sample. *Sleep*. 2012 Oct 1;35(10):1367-75.

[20] Maggi S, Langlois JA, Minicuci N, Grigoletto F, Pavan M, Foley DJ. Sleep complaints in community-dwelling older persons: prevalence, associated factors, and reported causes. *J. Am. Geriatr. Soc.* 1998; 46(2):161-8.

[21] Ancoli-Israel S. Sleep and its disorders in aging populations. *Sleep Med.* 2009 Sep.;10 Suppl 1:S7-11.

[22] Leger D, Scheuermaier K, Philip P, Paillard M, Guilleminault C. SF-36: evaluation of quality of life in severe and mild insomniacs compared with good sleepers. *Psychosom. Med.* 2001; 63(1):49-55.

[23] Katz DA, McHorney CA. The relationship between insomnia and health-related quality of life in patients with chronic illness. *J. Fam. Pract.* 2002; 51(3):229-35.

[24] Arroll B, Fernando A 3rd, Falloon K, Goodyear-Smith F, Samaranayake C, Warman G. Prevalence of causes of insomnia in primary care: across-sectional study. *Br. J. Gen. Pract.* 2012 Feb;62(595):e99-103.

[25] Spielman AJ, Caruso LS, Glovinsky PB. A behavioral perspective on insomnia treatment. *Psychiatr. Clin. North. Am.* 1987; 10:541-53.

[26] Drake CL, Roth T. Predisposition in the evolution of insomnia: evidence, potential mechanisms, and future directions. *Sleep Medicine Clinics* 2006; 1:333-49.

[27] Perlis ML, Smith MT, Pigeon WR. Etiology and pathophysiology of insomnia. In: Kryger MH, Roth T, Dement WC, eds. Principles and Practice of Sleep Medicine. 4th ed. Philadelphia, PA: *Elsevier*, 2005:714-25.

[28] Edinger JD, Bonnet MH, Bootzin RR, Doghramji K, Dorsey CM, Espie CA et al.; American Academy of SleepMedicine Work Group. Derivation of research diagnostic criteria for insomnia: report of an American Academy of Sleep Medicine work group. *Sleep* 2004; 27:1567-96.

[29] Kales A, Caldwell AB, Preston TA, Healey S, Kales JD. Personality patterns in insomnia. theoretical implications. *Arch. Gen. Psychiatry* 1976; 33:1128-34.

[30] Bootzin RR, Nicassio PM. Behavioral treatments for insomnia. In: Hersen M, Eisler RM, Miller PM, eds. *Progress in Behavior Modification*, Vol 6. New York: Academic Press, 1978:1-45.

[31] Monroe LJ. Psychological and physiological differences between good and poor sleepers. *J. Abnorm. Psychol.* 1967; 72:255-64.

[32] Bonnet MH, Arand DL. Hyperarousal and insomnia. *Sleep Med. Rev.* 1997; 1:97-108.

[33] Kapsimalis F, Basta M, Varouchakis G, Gourgoulianis K, Vgontzas A, Kryger M. Cytokines and pathological sleep. *Sleep* Med 2008;9:603-14.

[34] van den Heuvel C, Ferguson S, Dawson D. Attenuated thermoregulatory response to mild thermal challenge in subjects with sleep-onset insomnia. *Sleep* 2006; 29:1174-80.

[35] Perlis ML, Smith MT, Andrews PJ, Orff H, Giles DE. Beta/gamma EEG activity in patients with primary and secondary insomnia and good sleeper controls. *Sleep* 2001; 24:110-7.

[36] Parrino L, Ferrillo F, Smerieri A, Spaggiari MC, Palomba V, Rossi M et al. Is insomnia a neurophysiological disorder? The role of sleep EEG microstructure. *Brain Res. Bull.* 2004; 63:377-83.

[37] Yang CM, Lo HS. ERP evidence of enhanced excitatory and reduced inhibitory processes of auditorystimuli during sleep in patients with primary insomnia. *Sleep* 2007; 30:585-92.

[38] Smith MT, Perlis ML, Chengazi VU, Pennington J, Soeffing J, Ryan JM, et al. Neuroimaging of NREM sleep in primary insomnia: a Tc-99-HMPAO single photon emission computed tomography study. *Sleep.* 2002 May 1;25(3):325-35.

[39] Smith MT, Perlis ML, Chengazi VU, Soeffing J, McCann U. NREM sleep cerebral blood flow before and after behavior therapy for chronic primary insomnia: preliminary

single photon emission computed tomography (SPECT) data. *Sleep Med.* 2005 Jan;6(1):93-4.

[40] Nofzinger EA, Buysse DJ, Germain A, Price JC, Miewald JM, Kupfer DJ. Functional neuroimaging evidence for hyperarousal in insomnia. *Am J. Psychiatry.* 2004 Nov;161(11):2126-8.

[41] Nofzinger EA, Nissen C, Germain A, Moul D, Hall M, Price JC, et al. Regional cerebral metabolic correlates of WASO during NREM sleep in insomnia. *J. Clin. Sleep Med.* 2006 Jul 15;2(3):316-22.

[42] Riemann D, Voderholzer U, Spiegelhalder K, Hornyak M, Buysse DJ, Nissen C, et al. Chronic insomnia and MRI-measured hippocampal volumes: a pilot study. *Sleep.* 2007 Aug;30(8):955-8.

[43] Altena E, Van Der Werf YD, Sanz-Arigita EJ, Voorn TA, Rombouts SA, Kuijer JP, et al. Prefrontal hypoactivation and recovery in insomnia. *Sleep.* 2008 Sep;31(9):1271-6.

[44] Winkelman JW, Buxton OM, Jensen JE, Benson KL, O'Connor SP, Wang W, et al. Reduced brain GABA in primary insomnia: preliminary data from 4T proton magnetic resonance spectroscopy (1H-MRS). *Sleep.* 2008 Nov; 31(11):1499-506.

[45] Bastien CH, Vallieres A, Morin CM. Validation of the Insomnia Severity Index as an outcome measure for insomnia research. *Sleep Med.* 2001; 2(4):297-307.

[46] Morin C. Insomnia. New York: Guilford Press, 1993.

[47] Buysse DJ, Reynolds CF, Monk TH, Berman SR, Kupfer DJ. The Pittsburgh sleep quality index: a new instrument for psychiatric practice and research. *Psychiatry Res.* 1989; 28(2):193-213.

[48] Kushida CA, Littner MR, Morgenthaler T, Alessi CA, Bailey D, Coleman J Jr, et al. Practice parameters for the indications for polysomnography and related procedures: an update for 2005. *Sleep* 2005; 28(4):499-521.

[49] Edinger JD, Fins AI, Sullivan RJ Jr., Marsh GR, Dailey DS, Hope TV et al. Sleep in the laboratory and sleep at home: comparisons of older insomniacs and normal sleepers. *Sleep* 1997; 20(12):1119-26.

[50] Lichstein KL, Stone KC, Donaldson J, Nau SD, Soeffing JP, Murray D et al. Actigraphy validation with insomnia. *Sleep* 2006; 29(2): 232-39.

[51] Littner M, Kushida CA, Anderson WM, Bailey D, Berry RB, Davila DG et al. Practice parameters for the role of actigraphy in the study of sleep and circadian rhythms: an update for 2002. *Sleep* 2003; 26(3):337-41.

[52] Dinges DF, Rogers NL, Baynard MD. Chronic sleep deprivation. In: Kryger MH, Roth T, Dement WC, eds. Principles and Practice of Sleep Medicine. 4th ed. Philadelphia: *Elsevier Saunders*, 2005:50–67.

[53] Bonnet MH. Acute sleep deprivation. In: Kryger MH, Roth T, Dement WC, eds. Principles and Practice of Sleep Medicine. Philadelphia: *Elsevier Saunders*, 2005:51–66.

[54] Banks S, Dinges DF. Behavioral and physiologic consequences of sleep restriction. *J. Clin. Sleep Med.* 2007; 3(5):519–28.

[55] Seneviratne U, Puvanendran K. Excessive daytime sleepiness in obstructive sleep apnea: prevalence, severity, and predictors. *Sleep Med.* 2004 Jul;5(4):339-43.

[56] Lee SJ, Kang HW, Lee LH. The relationship between the Epworth Sleepiness Scale and polysomnographic parameters in obstructive sleep apnea patients. *Eur. Arch. Otorhinolaryngol.* 2012 Apr;269(4):1143-7.

[57] Borbe'ly AA. A two process model of sleep regulation. *Hum. Neurobiol.* 1982; 1(3):195–204.

[58] Tononi G, Cirelli C. Sleep function and synaptic homeostasis. *Sleep Med. Rev.* 2006; 10(1):49–62.

[59] Gooley JJ, Saper CB. Anatomy of the circadian system. In: Kryger MH, Roth T, Dement WC, eds. Principles and Practice of Sleep Medicine. 4th ed. Philadelphia: *Elsevier Saunders*, 2005:335–50.

[60] De Valck E, Cluydts R, Pirrera S. Effect of cognitive arousal on sleep latency, somatic and cortical arousal following partial sleep deprivation. *J. Sleep Res.* 2004; 13(4):295–304.

[61] Sharafkhaneh A, Hirshkowitz M. Contextual factors and perceived self-reported sleepiness: a preliminary report. *Sleep Med.* 2003; 4(4):327–31.

[62] Jones BE. From waking to sleeping: neuronal and chemical substrates. *Trends Pharmacol. Sci.* 2005; 26 (11):578–86.

[63] Lu J, Jhou TC, Saper CB. Identification of wake-active dopaminergic neurons in the ventral periaqueductal gray matter. *J. Neurosci.* 2006; 26(1):193–202.

[64] Siegel J. The Neural Control of Sleep and Waking. New York: Springer, 2002.

[65] John J, Wu MF, Boehmer LN, Siegel JM. Cataplexy-active neurons in the hypothalamus: implications for the role of histamine in sleep and waking behavior. *Neuron* 2004; 42(4):619–34.

[66] Edgar DE, Dement WC, Fuller CA. Effect of SCN lesions on sleep in squirrel monkeys: evidence for opponent processes in sleep-wake regulation. *J. Neurosci.* 1993; 13(3):1065–79.

[67] Dijk DJ, Lockley SW. Integration of human sleep-wake regulation and circadian rhythmicity. *J. Appl. Physiol.* 2002; 92(2):852–62.

[68] Pen~aloza-Rojas JH, Elterman M, Olmos N. Sleep induced by cortical stimulation. *Exp. Neurol.* 1964; 10:140–7.

[69] McGinty D, Szymusiak R. Sleep-promoting mechanisms in mammals. In: Kryger MH, Roth T, Dement WC, eds. *Principles and Practice of Sleep Medicine.* Philadelphia: Elsevier Saunders, 2005:169–84.

[70] Saper CB, Chou TC, Scammell TE. The sleep switch: hypothalamic control of sleep and wakefulness. *Trends Neurosci.* 2001; 24(12):726–31.

[71] Saper CB. The neurobiology of sleep. Continuum (Minneap Minn). 2013;19(1 Sleep Disorders):19-31.

[72] Arnulf I, Rico TJ, Mignot E. Diagnosis, disease course, and management of patients with Kleine-Levin syndrome. *Lancet Neurol.* 2012;11(10):918-28.

[73] Johns MW. A new method for measuring daytime sleepiness: the Epworth sleepiness scale. *Sleep* 1991; 14:540–5.

[74] Johns MW. Sensitivity and specificity of the multiple sleep latency test (MSLT), the manteinance of wakefulness test and the Epworth sleepiness scale: failure of MSLT as a gold standard. *J. Sleep Res.* 2000;9(1):5-11.

[75] Parkes JD, Chen SY, Clift SJ, Dahlitz MT, Dunn G. The clinical diagnosis of the narcoleptic syndrome. *J. Sleep Res.,* 1998, 7: 41-52.

[76] Bloch KE, Schoch OD, Zhang JN, Russi EW. German version of the Epworth sleepiness scale. *Respiration,* 1999, 66: 440-7.

[77] Broman JE, Bengtson H, Hetta J. Psychometric properties of a Swedish version of the Epworth sleepiness scale. *J. Sleep Res.,* 2000, 9 (Suppl. 1): 27.

[78] Hoddes EDW, Zarcone V. The development and use of the Stanford Sleepiness Scale. *Psychophysiology* 1972; 9:150.

[79] Akerstedt T, Gillberg M. Subjective and objective sleepiness in the active individual. *Int. J. Neurosci.* 1990; 52:29–37.

[80] Thurnheer R. Diagnostic approach to sleep-disordered breathing. *Expert Rev. Respir. Med.* 2011;5(4):573-89.

[81] Netzer N, Eliasson AH, Netzer C, Kristo DA. Overnight pulse oximetry for sleep disordered breathing in adults: a review. *Chest* 2001; 120:625–33.

[82] Batchelder KA, Mannheimer PD, Mecca RS, Ojile JM.. Pulse oximetry saturation patterns detect repetitive reductions in airflow. *J. Clin. Monit. Comput.* 2011;25(6):411-8.

[83] Cooper BG, Veale D, Griffiths CJ, et al. Values of nocturnal oxygen saturation as a screening test for sleep apnea. *Thorax* 1991; 46(8):586–8.

[84] Collop NA, Anderson WM, Boehlecke B, Claman D, Goldberg R, Gottlieb DJ, Hudgel D, Sateia M, Schwab R; Portable Monitoring Task Force of the American Academy of Sleep Medicine Clinical guidelines for the use of unattended portable monitors in the diagnosis of obstructive sleep apnea in adult patients. Portable Monitoring Task Force of the American Academy of Sleep Medicine. *J. Clin. Sleep Med.* 2007 ,15;3(7):737-47.

[85] Carskadon MA, Dement WC, Mitler MM, Roth T, Westbrook PR, Keenan S. Guidelines for the multiple sleep latency test (MSLT): a standard measure of sleepiness. *Sleep* 1986; 9:519–24.

[86] Mitler MM, Walsleben J, Sangal RB, Hirshkowitz M. Sleep latency on the maintenance of wakefulness test (MWT) for 530 patients with narcolepsy while free of psychoactive drugs. *Electroencephalogr. Clin. Neurophysiol.* 1998; 107(1):33–8.

[87] Littner MR, Kushida C, Wise M, Davila DG, Morgenthaler T, Lee-Chiong T, Hirshkowitz M, Daniel LL, Bailey D, Berry RB, Kapen S, Kramer M; Standards of Practice Committee of the American Academy of Sleep Medicine. Practice parameters for the clinical use of the multiple sleep latency test and the maintenance of wakefulness test. *Sleep* 2005; 1 28(1):113–21.

[88] Kotagal S, Goulding P. The laboratory assessment of daytime sleepiness. *J. Clin. Neurophysiol.* 1996; 13(3):208–18.

[89] Arand D, Bonnet M, Hurwitz T, Mitler M, Rosa R, Sangal RB. The clinical use of the MSLT and MWT. *Sleep.* 2005;28(1):123-44.

[90] Huang L, Zhou J, Li Z, Lei F, Tang X. Sleep perception and the multiple sleep latency test in patients with primary insomnia. *J. Sleep Res.* 2012;21(6):684-92.

[91] Wise MS. Objective measures of sleepiness and wakefulness: application to the real world? *J. Clin. Neurophysiol.* 2006;23(1):39-49.

[92] Mitler MM, Gujavarty KS, Browman CP. Maintenance of wakefulness test: a polysomnographic technique for evaluation and treatment efficacy in patients with excessive somnolence. *Electroencephalogr. Clin. Neurophysiol.* 1982; 53(6):658–61.

[93] Dauvilliers Y, Arnulf I, Mignot E. Narcolepsy with cataplexy. *Lancet* 2007 10;369(9560):499-511.

[94] Honda Y, Juji T, Matsuki K, et al. HLA-DR2 and Dw2 in narcolepsy and in other disorders of excessive somnolence without cataplexy. *Sleep* 1986; 9:133–42.

[95] Mignot E, Ling L, Rogers R, et al. Complex HLA-DR and DQ interactions confer risk for narcolepsy– cataplexy in three ethnic groups. Am J Hum Genet 2001; 68:686–99.

[96] Mignot E, Hayduk R, Black J, et al. HLA DQB1*0602 is associated with cataplexy in 509 narcoleptic patients. *Sleep* 1997; 20(11):1012–20.

[97] Chemelli RM, Willie JT, Sinton CM, et al. Narcolepsy in orexin knockout mice: molecular genetics of sleep regulation. Cell 1999; 98:437–51.

[98] Nishino S, Ripley B, Overeem S, et al. Hypocretin (orexin) deficiency in human narcolepsy. *Lancet* 2000; 355:39–40.

[99] Peyron C, Faraco J, Rogers W, et al. A mutation in a case of early onset narcolepsy and a generalized absence of hypocretin peptides in human narcoleptic brains. *Nat. Med.* 2000; 6:991–7.

[100] Thannickal TC, Moore RY, Nienhuis R, et al. Reduced number of hypocretin neurons in human narcolepsy. *Neuron* 2000; 27:469–44.

[101] Black J, Brooks SN, Nishino S. Narcolepsy and syndromes of primary excessive daytime somnolence. *Semin. Neurol.* 2004; 24:271–82.

[102] Overeem S, Mignot E, van Dijk, et al. Narcolepsy: clinical features, new pathophysiologic insights, and future perspectives. *J. Clin. Neurophysiol.* 2001; 18:78–105.

[103] Okun ML, Lin L, Pelin A, et al. Clinical aspects of narcolepsy–cataplexy across ethnic groups. *Sleep* 2002; 25:27–35.

[104] Koziorynska EI, Rodriguez AJ. Narcolepsy: clinical approach to etiology, diagnosis, and treatment. *Rev. Neurol. Dis.* 2011;8(3-4):e97-106.

[105] Dauvilliers Y, Billiard M, Montplaisir J. Clinical aspects and pathophysiology of narcolepsy. *Clin. Neurophysiol.* 2003; 114:2000–17.

[106] Arii J, Kanbayashi T, Tanabe Y, et al. A hypersomnolent girl with decreased CSF hypocretin level after removal of a hypothalamic tumor. *Neurology* 2001; 56:1775–6.

[107] Kanbayashi T, Abe M, Fujimoto S, et al. Hypocretin deficiency in Niemann–Pick type C with cataplexy. *Neuropediatrics* 2003; 34:52–3.

[108] Vankova J, Stepanova I, Jech R, et al. Sleep disturbances and hypocretin deficiency in Niemann–Pick disease type C. *Sleep* 2003; 26:427–30.

[109] Overeem S, van Hilten JJ, Ripley B, et al. Normal hypocretin-1 levels in Parkinson's disease patients with excessive daytime sleepiness. *Neurology* 2002; 58:498–9.

[110] Martinez-Rodriguez JE, Lin L, Iranzo A, et al. Decreased hypocretin-1 (orexin-A) levels in the cerebrospinal fluid of patients with myotonic dystrophy and excessive daytime sleepiness. *Sleep* 2003; 26:287–90.

[111] Dauvilliers Y, Arnulf I, Mignot E. Narcolepsy with cataplexy. *Lancet.* 2007, 10;369(9560):499-511.

[112] Fortuyn HA, Mulders PC, Renier WO, Buitelaar JK, Overeem S. Narcolepsy and psychiatry: an evolving association of increasing interest. *Sleep Med.* 2011;12(7):714-9.

[113] Sours J.A. Narcolepsy and other disturbances in the sleep-waking rhythm: a study of 115 cases with review of the literature. *J. Nerv. Ment. Dis.* 1963;137:525-42.

[114] Roy A. Psychiatric aspects of narcolepsy. *Br. J. Psychiatry.* 1976 Jun;128:562-5.

[115] Kales A, Soldatos CR, Bixler EO Caldwell A, Cadieux RJ, Verrecchio JM, Kales JD. Narcolepsy-cataplexy. II. Psychosocial consequences and associated psychopathology. *Arch. Neurol.* 1982;39(3):169-71.

[116] Krishnan RR, Volow MR, Miller PP, Carwile ST. Narcolepsy: preliminary retrospective study of psychiatric and psychosocial aspects. *Am. J. Psychiatry.* 1984;141(3):428-31.

[117] Baker TL, Guilleminault C, Nino-Murcia G, Dement WC. Comparative polysomnographic study of narcolepsy and idiopathic central nervous system hypersomnia. *Sleep.* 1986;9(1 Pt 2):232-42.

[118] Mosko S, Zetin M, Glen S, Garber D, DeAntonio M, Sassin J, McAnich J, Warren S. Self-reported depressive symptomatology, mood ratings, and treatment outcome in sleep disorders patients. *J. Clin. Psychol.* 1989;45(1):51-60.

[119] Dauvilliers Y, Paquereau J, Bastuji H, Drouot X, Weil JS, Viot-Blanc V. Psychological health in central hypersomnias: the French Harmony study. *J. Neurol. Neurosurg. Psychiatry.* 2009;80(6):636-41.

[120] Daniels E, King MA, Smith IE,. Shneerson JM. Health-related quality of life in narcolepsy. *J. Sleep Res.* 2001;10(1):75-81.

[121] Vandeputte M, de Weerd A. Sleep disorders and depressive feelings: a global survey with the Beck depression scale. *Sleep Med.* 2003;4(4):343-5.

[122] Vignatelli L, D'Alessandro R, Mosconi P, Ferini-Strambi L, Guidolin L, De Vincentiis A, Plazzi G; GINSEN (Gruppo Italiano Narcolessia-Studio Epidemiologico Nazionale). Health-related quality of life in Italian patients with narcolepsy: the SF-36 health survey. *Sleep Med.* 2004;5(5):467-75.

[123] Vignatelli L, Plazzi G, Peschechera F, Delaj L, D'Alessandro R. A 5-year prospective cohort study on health-related quality of life in patients with narcolepsy. *Sleep Med.* 2011;12(1):19-23.

[124] Fortuyn HA, Lappenschaar MA, Furer JW, Hodiamont PP, Rijnders CA, Renier WO, Buitelaar JK, Overeem S. Anxiety and mood disorders in narcolepsy: a case-control study. *Gen. Hosp. Psychiatry.* 2010;32(1):49-56.

[125] Sours JA. Narcolepsy and other disturbances in the sleep-waking rhythm: a study of 115 cases with review of the literature. *J. Nerv. Ment. Dis.* 1963;137:525-42.

[126] Reynolds CF 3rd, Christiansen CL, Taska LS, Coble PA, Kupfer DJ. Sleep in narcolepsy and depression. Does it all look alike? J Nerv Ment Dis. 1983;171(5):290-5.

[127] Kondziella D, Rlien-Soborg P. Diagnostic and therapeutic challenges in narcolepsy-related psychosis. *J. Clin. Psychiatry.* 2006;67(11):1817-9.

[128] Kishi Y, Konishi S, Koizumi S, Kudo Y, Kurosawa H, Kathol RJ. Schizophrenia and narcolepsy: a review with a case report. *Psychiatry Clin. Neurosci.* 2004;58(2):117-24.

[129] Walterfang M, Upjohn E, Velakoulis D. Is schizophrenia associated with narcolepsy? *Cogn. Behav. Neurol.* 2005;18(2):113-8.

[130] Vourdas A, Shneerson JM, Gregory CA, Smith IE, King MA, Morrish E, McKenna PJ. Narcolepsy and psychopathology: is there an association? *Sleep Med.* 2002;3(4):353-60.

[131] Fortuyn HA, Lappenschaar GA, Nienhuis FJ, Furer JW, Hodiamont PP, Rijnders CA, Lammers GJ, Renier WO, Buitelaar JK, Overeem S.Psychotic symptoms in narcolepsy: phenomenology and a comparison with schizophrenia. *Gen. Hosp. Psychiatry.* 2009;31(2):146-54.

[132] Arnulf I, Rico TJ, Mignot E. Diagnosis, disease course, and management of patients with Kleine-Levin syndrome. *Lancet Neurol.* 2012;11(10):918-28.

[133] Kleine W. Periodische Schlafsucht. Monatsschr Psychiatr Neurol 1925; 57:285–320.

[134] Levin M. Periodic somnolence and morbid hunger: a new syndrome. *Brain* 1936; 58:494–515.

[135] Billiard M. The Kleine Levin syndrome. In: Kryger MH, Roth T, Dement WC, eds. *Principles and Practice of Sleep Medicine.* Philadelphia: WB Saunders, 1989;377–8.

[136] Billiard M, Jaussent I, Dauvilliers Y, Besset A. Recurrent hypersomnia: a review of 339 cases. *Sleep Med. Rev.* 2011;15(4):247-57.

[137] Billiard M. Diagnosis of narcolepsy and idiopathic hypersomnia. An update based on the International classification of sleep disorders, 2nd edition. *Sleep Med. Rev.* 2007;11(5):377-88.

[138] Roth B, Nevsimalova S, Rechtschaffen A. Hypersomnia with "sleep drunkenness." *Arch. Gen. Psychiatry* 1972; 26:456–62.

[139] Billiard M, Dauvilliers Y. Idiopathic Hypersomnia. *Sleep Med. Rev.* 2001; 5(5):349–58.

[140] Rechtschaffen A, Dement WC. Narcolepsy and hypersomnia. In Kales A, ed. Sleep: *Physiology and Pathology. Philadelphia*: JB Lippincott Co., 1969:119–30.

[141] Vankova J, Stepanova I, Jech R, Elleder M, Ling L, Mignot E, Nishino S, Nevsimalova S. Sleep disturbances and hypocretin deficiency in Niemann-Pick disease type C. *Sleep.* 2003 15;26(4):427-30.

[142] Mignot E. Narcolepsy: pharmacology, pathophysiology, and genetics. In: Kryger MH, Roth T, Dement WC, eds. Principles and Practice of Sleep Medicine. 4th ed. Philadelphia, PA: *Elsevier Saunders*, 2005:761–79.

[143] Kanbayashi T, Kodama T, Kondo H, et al. CSF histamine and noradrenaline contents in narcolepsy and other sleep disorders. *Sleep* 2004; 27:A236.

[144] Dauvilliers Y. Differential diagnosis in hypersomnia. *Curr. Neurol. Neurosci. Rep.* 2006;6(2):156-62.

[145] Roehrs T, Zorick F, Sicklesteel J, et al. Excessive daytime sleepiness associated with insufficient sleep. *Sleep* 1983; 6:319–25.

[146] Van Dongen HP, Maislin G, Mullington JM, et al. The cumulative cost of additional wakefulness: dose–response effects of neurobehavioral functions and sleep physiology from chronic sleep restriction and total sleep deprivation. *Sleep* 2003; 26:117–26.

In: Sleep Medicine
Editors: A. Del Casale, R. Brugnoli and P. Girardi

ISBN: 978-1-62808-515-0
© 2013 Nova Science Publishers, Inc.

Chapter IV

Parasomnias

Daniele Serata, **Chiara Rapinesi**, **Antonio Del Casale**
and Roberto Tatarelli*

NESMOS (Neurosciences, Mental Health and Sensory Functions) Department,
School of Medicine and Psychology, Sapienza University,
Sant'Andrea Hospital, UOC Psychiatry

Abstract

Parasomnias are defined undesirable physical events or experiences that occur during entry into sleep, within sleep or during arousals from sleep. Parasomnias occur more frequently in children than in adults. All parasomnias can be diagnosed based on subjective reports from the patient, parent or caregiver, except for REM sleep behavior disorder where diagnosis requires polysomnographic investigation.

This chapter also addresses the main clinical features and most recent treatments of parasomnias.

Keywords: Parasomnias, Disorders of Arousal, REM sleep, REM Sleep Behavior Disorder

Introduction

The etymology of the term "parasomnia" comes from the Greek prefix $\pi\alpha\rho\alpha$, meaning "alongside from", combined with the Latin word *somnus*, meaning "sleep".

The International Classification of Sleep Disorders, 2nd edition (ICSD-2), defines parasomnias as undesirable physical events or experiences that occur during entry into sleep, within sleep, or during arousals from sleep [1]. They are classified into disorders of arousal

---

* Corresponding author:Dr. Daniele Serata"Sapienza" University, Rome.Email: seratadaniele@gmail.com.

from non-rapid eye movement (REM) sleep, parasomnias usually associated with REM sleep and other parasomnias (Table 1).

The approach to parasomnias requires attention to clinical history, age of onset, and duration and frequency of these "unusual episodes during sleep". Some predisposing factors like sleep deprivation, medications or drug abuse should be explored. Neurological and psychiatric examination should be carried out to exclude comorbidities or causal factors. Not all parasomnias require evaluation by polysomnography (PSG). PSG is an exam that should be taken into account when the disorder affects global functioning (excessive diurnal sleepiness or risk of injury and violent behavior) and to rule out medical, psychiatric and neurological comorbidities. Parasomnias occur more frequently in children than adults (with the exception of REM sleep behavior disorder, which is more common in men over 50).

All parasomnias can be diagnosed based on subjective reports from the patient, parent or caregiver, except for REM sleep behavior disorder where diagnosis requires polysomnographic investigation.

Many parasomnias produce manifestations on the central nervous system. Autonomic nervous system changes and skeletal muscle activity are the predominant features of this group of disorders.

Although there are notes on early descriptions of parasomnias in the ancient Greek literature [2], a recent paper by Golzari and colleagues [3] showed how Persians, in the 10th century, studied sleep paralysis and its relationship with epilepsy.

The lifetime prevalence of different parasomnias varied from about 4% to 67% [4].

Table 1. Classification of parasomnias (American Academy of Sleep Medicine, 2005)

Non-REM Parasomnias (Disorder of Arousal)	Parasomnias Usually Associated With REM Sleep (Stage R)	Other parasomnias
Confusional Arousal	REM sleep behavior disorder (including parasomnia overlap disorder and status dissociatus)	Sleep-Related Dissociative Disorder
Sleepwalking	Recurrent Isolated Sleep Paralysis	Sleep Enuresis
Sleep Terrors	Nightmare disorder	Sleep-Related Groaning
		Exploding Head Syndrome
		Sleep-Related Hallucinations
		Sleep-Related Eating Disorder

Non-REM Parasomnias

Non-REM parasomnia, known also as disorders of arousal, are grouped together because impaired arousal from sleep is a common feature of these disorders. The onset of these disorders in non-REM slow-wave sleep is typical (Stage III). The non-REM parasomnias include confusional arousals, sleepwalking and sleep terrors. There are some clinical overlaps in these parasomnias.

Non-REM parasomnias most commonly occur in children and have features in common with both sleepwalking and sleep terrors. Although not listed in the major ICSD-2 disorder, sexsomnia [5] and sleep-related violence are considered variants of non-REM parasomnias.

The differential diagnosis of these NREM parasomnias includes rapid eye movement sleep behavior disorder (RBD), nightmare disorder, nocturnal seizure activity, posttraumatic stress disorder (PTSD), and nocturnal panic attacks. Nightmare disorders (also called dream anxiety attacks) and RBD occur during REM sleep and are more common in the second part of the night. Body movements during RBD can result in patients leaving the bed, but rarely the bedroom. RBD usually does not begin until after age 40 and has a strong male predominance. The ICSD-2 [1] diagnostic criteria for non-REM parasomnias are summarized in Table 2.

Confusional Arousals

Confusional arousals consist of confusion during and following arousals from sleep, usually from deep sleep, in the first part of the night.

The individual is disoriented in time and space, is slow of speech and mentation, and responds poorly and slowly to stimuli. There is major memory impairment, and both retro- and anterograde amnesia. The duration of confusion may last from several minutes to several hours. Confusional arousals can be precipitated by forced awakenings, mainly in the first third of the night. The course of the childhood form is usually benign and confusional arousal improves with age [6]. The prevalence of confusional arousal in the 15 to 24-year-old population is 6%, and in those over the age of 65 it is 1% [7].

In adults, the condition is usually fairly stable, varying only with the main predisposing factors. Some predisposing factors include recovery from sleep deprivation, circadian rhythm sleep disorders (shift work, jet lag, etc.), use of medications (particularly central nervous system depressants, including hypnotics, sedatives, tranquilizers, alcohol, and antihistamines) or metabolic, hepatic, renal, toxic, and other encephalopathies. Confusional arousals are often seen in hypersomnia. Some organic causes of the disorder have also been described, such as lesions at the periventricular gray matter, midbrain reticular area and posterior hypothalamus. Polysomnographic recordings during confusional arousals have typically shown their onset in arousals from slow-wave sleep [1]. In general, confusional arousals are benign and require no treatment. Parents need to be reassured, and episodes should not be interrupted. Interruption may lead to increased agitation and possible injury [8].

Sleepwalking

Sleepwalking, also known as "somnambulism", consists of a series of complex behaviors that are initiated during slow-wave sleep and result in walking during sleep. Episodes can range from simple sitting up in bed to walking or running. When patients are awakened they are often disoriented and amnestic. Sleepwalking originates from slow-wave sleep and is therefore most often evident during the first third of the night. For these reasons, it can be distinguished from REM sleep behavior disorder that occurrs in REM sleep and from sleep-related epilepsy by the absence of clinical and electroencephalographic features of seizures.

The use of several medications, such as thioridazine, hydrochloride, lithium carbonate, perphenazine, zolpidem, and desipramine hydrochloride can exacerbate or induce sleepwalking.

Obstructive sleep apnea syndrome (OSAS) and other disorders that produce severe disruption of slow-wave sleep can be associated with sleepwalking episodes. Internal stimuli, such as a distended bladder, or external stimuli, such as noises, can also precipitate episodes. There is also a strong family association in some cases [9], and in particular the DQB1 gene is associated with sleepwalking [10]. The treatment of sleepwalking includes environmental precautions (e.g., closed doors and windows, sleeping on the f first level) and avoidance of predisposing factors. Benzodiazepines (clonazepam 0.5 to 2.0 mg) are used with considerable success [11].

Sleep Terrors

Sleep terrors (*pavor nocturnus*) occur in approximately 3% of children aged 4 to 12 years and may also commonly present around age 20 to 30 years [12]. These are dramatic sudden arousals from non-REM sleep with associated screaming, fear, and increased autonomic activity. In particular, the severe autonomic activity is characterized by tachycardia, tachypnea, flushing of the skin, diaphoresis, mydriasis, decreased skin resistance, and increased muscle tone. Patients may be disoriented and unresponsive to stimuli. Amnesia is generally present. In contrast, nightmares typically occur during REM sleep toward the end of the night and are not associated with autonomic activity or amnesia.

Regarding polysomnographic features, sleep terrors begin in sleep stage 3 or 4, usually in the first third of the major sleep episode. However, episodes can occur in slow-wave sleep at any time. Usually, no treatment is needed.

**Table 2. ICSD-2 diagnostic criteria for disorders of arousal
(American Academy of Sleep Medicine, 2005)**

Confusional Arousal	Sleepwalking	Sleep terrors
A. Recurrent mental confusion or confusional behavior during an arousal or awakening from nocturnal sleep or a daytime nap.	A. Ambulation during sleep.	A. A sudden episode of terror during sleep, usually initiated by a cry or loud scream that is accompanied by autonomic nervous system and behavioral manifestations of intense fear.
	B. Persistence of sleep, an altered state of consciousness, or impaired judgment during ambulation is demonstrated by at least one of the following: 1. Difficulty in arousing the person 2. Mental confusion when awakened from an episode 3. Routine behaviors that occur at inappropriate times 4. Inappropriate or nonsensical behaviors 5. Dangerous or potentially dangerous behaviors	B. At least 1 of the following associated features is present: 1. Difficulty in arousing the person 2. Mental confusion when awakened from an episode 3. Amnesia (complete or partial) for the episode 4. Dangerous or potentially dangerous behaviors
The disturbance is not better explained by another sleep disorder, medical or neurological disorder, mental disorder, medication use, or substance use disorder.		

Parasomnias Usually Associated with REM Sleep (Stage R)

Parasomnias usually associated with REM sleep (stage R) include REM Sleep Behavior Disorder (RBD), recurrent isolated sleep paralysis, and nightmare disorders. RBD has two variants: overlap parasomnia and *status dissociatus* (SD). "Stage R" is the new nomenclature proposed by the American Academy of Sleep Medicine to substitute the term Stage REM [13].

REM sleep Behavior Disorder (RBD, Including Parasomnia Overlap Disorder and Status Dissociatus)

Rapid eye movement sleep behavior disorder (RBD) is characterized by loss of normal skeletal muscle atonia during rapid eye movement (REM) sleep with prominent motor activity and dreaming.

There are three predominant clinical features of RBD: abnormal vocalizations, abnormal motor behavior, and altered dream mentation. The vocalizations of the RBD tend to be loud and suggest unpleasant dream mentation. Shouting, screaming, and swearing are different from the tone of voice during wakefulness. The abnormal motor behavior generally starts with some repetitive jerking or movements, followed seconds later by more dramatic and seemingly purposeful activity such as punching, flailing as if to protect oneself, running, jumping out of bed. Injuries have been reported. Altered dream mentation typically involves a chasing/attacking theme, with insects, animals or other humans being the aggressors and the patient as the defender. Behavior is often focused on dream content [14] and may be very bizarre, mimicking "oneiroid" states. Typically, patients with RBD are male between 40 and 70 years old. Those with RBD evolving before age 40 typically have narcolepsy (RBD and narcolepsy often coexist), although in some cases RBD that begins early in life has an association with some neurodegenerative diseases such as Parkinson's disease and dementia with Lewy bodies [15]. RBD is the only parasomnia requiring polysomnogram for diagnosis to confirm the lack of physiological REM atonia. Polysomnography (PSG) is also necessary to differentiate RBD patients from those with moderate to severe obstructive sleep apnea (OSA) and a history of recurrent dream enactment behavior [16]. There two main features of PSG in RBD: unstained muscle activity in REM sleep and excessive transient muscle activity in REM sleep.

There are two main variants of parasomnias: Parasomnia overlap disorder and Status Dissociatus. Parasomnia overlap disorder consists of a combination of RBD and NREM parasomnias (sleepwalking, confusional arousals, and sleep terrors) [17]. Status dissociatus is characterized by state dissociation without identifiable sleep stages, but with sleep and dream-related behaviors that resemble RBD [18]. It can lead to problems in differential diagnosis between disorder of arousal and RBD (Table 3)

Although the scientific literature lacks clinical trials on pharmacologic therapy of RBD, the most abundant published data are on the use of clonazepam. Melatonin use is increasing as a first-line treatment for RBD in patients with dementia and sleep apnea [19].

Since several antidepressant drugs including selective serotonin reuptake inhibitors, tricyclic antidepressants, venlafaxine, mirtazapine, and monoamine oxidase inhibitors, with the exception of bupropion, have all been associated with an increased risk of developing the acute forms of RBD. Consequently, it is better to avoid these drugs in patients with RBD, and bupropion should be the antidepressant of choice [8].

Table 3. Differential diagnosis between non-REM parasomnias-Disorder of arousal and REM Sleep Behavior Disorder

	Non-REM parasomnias-Disorder of arousal	REM Sleep Behavior Disorder
Sleep stage	Usually III	REM (stage R)
Sleep period	First third of sleep period	Final third of sleep period
Age group	Children	Adults (between 40-70 years old)
Family history	Yes	No
Confusion	Yes	No

Recurrent Isolated Sleep Paralysis

Recurrent Isolated Sleep Paralysis (RISP) consists of a period of inability to perform voluntary movements at sleep onset (hypnagogic form) or upon awakening, either during the night or the morning (hypnopompic form).

The transient inability to move or speak during in the absence of other clinical features of narcolepsy is observed. Eye movements are typically not affected. The experience is usually frightening, particularly if the patient senses difficulty in being able to breathe. Isolated events are a commonly reported phenomenon, with a reported lifetime prevalence of about 20-60%, depending on the study population [20]. RISP is a rarer form of sleep paralysis, varying in frequency and duration; in particular by the range and intensity of the perceived phenomena during the episodes. RISP generally affects females.

The treatment for RISP is avoidance of sleep deprivation and other identified precipitants. Serotonergic agents may reduce the frequency of episodes [21].

Nightmare Disorders

Nightmares are frightening dreams that usually awaken the sleeper from REM sleep. The nightmare is generally a long, complicated dream that becomes increasingly frightening towards the end. The long, dreamlike feature is essential in making clinical differentiation from sleep terrors. The awakening occurs out of REM sleep. On occasion there will not be an immediate awakening, but instead recall of a very frightening dream will occur at a later time. This latter situation is not common with nightmares. A large number of children (10-50% of the population) will suffer from nightmares between ages 3 and 6 years.

In the adult population nightmares may be idiopathic (without clinical signs of psychopathology) or associated with other disorders including Post-Traumatic Sleep Disorder (PTSD), substance abuse, stress and anxiety, and borderline personality, and other psychiatric illnesses such as schizophrenia-spectrum disorders. Eighty percent of PTSD patients report nightmares [22]. Prazosin is recommended for treatment of Posttraumatic Stress Disorder (PTSD)-associated nightmares. Non-pharmacological strategies such as Image Rehearsal Therapy (IRT) and Systematic Desensitization and Progressive Deep Muscle Relaxation training are suggested for treatment of idiopathic nightmares.

Other Parasomnias

Sleep-Related Dissociative Disorders

Sleep-Related Dissociative Disorder (SRDD) must fulfill Diagnostic and Statistical Manual of Mental Disorders, 4th ed. (DSM-IV) criteria for Dissociative Disorder (DD) and emerges in close association with the main sleep period. PSG demonstrates a dissociative episode or episodes that emerge during sustained EEG wakefulness, either in the transition from wakefulness to sleep or after an awakening from NREM or REM sleep. The DSM-IV states that "a dissociative disorder is characterized by a disruption in the usually integrated functions of consciousness, memory, identity, or perception of the environment" [23]. SRDD predominantly affects women. Its treatment involves therapy of the underlying DD.

Sleep Enuresis

Sleep enuresis is characterized by recurrent involuntary micturition that occurs during sleep. It is possible to differentiate primary sleep enuresis and secondary sleep enuresis. In primary enuresis, the patient has never been consistently established bladder control after age 5 years. In secondary enuresis, the patient was previously experienced consistent dryness, and there is a more strong association with medical causes or comorbidity. These can be represented by the inability to concentrate urine, increased urine production (due or not to caffeine or medications), neurological (seizures, neurogenic bladder), urinary tract disorders or OSA [24]. In fact, untreated OSA in children can worsen or cause enuresis [25] and the presence of sleep apnea should always be explored. After evaluation for sleep apnea and genitourinary pathology, especially in secondary sleep enuresis, treatments range from behavioral approaches (frequent daytime voiding, fluid restriction at night) to drug therapy (vasopressin, anticholinergic, tricyclic antidepressants).

Sleep-Related Groaning (Catathrenia)

Sleep-related groaning is a chronic disorder characterized by expiratory groaning, most often out of REM sleep (especially in the REM episodes in the second part of the night, but they can also occur in NREM sleep). It may be associated with bradypneic episodes (slow respiratory rate) with long exhalations. Habitual snoring is common, occurring in 44% of males and 28% of females between 30 and 60 years of age in the general population [26].

Differentiation from obstructive sleep apnea syndrome may require polysomnography. Not all cases require treatment, but there are contrasting results with Continuous Positive Airway Pressure (cPAP).

Exploding Head Syndrome

The exploding head syndrome (EHS) is characterized by a sudden loud imagined noise or sense of violent explosion in the head occurring as the patient is falling asleep on waking during the night. Onset in the fifth or sixth decade and the disorder is more frequent in women. The pathophysiology of the EHS is not known. The most important differential diagnosis is from the Sleep-Related Headache. Evidence for treatment comes only from case reports: nifedipine, [27] and clomipramine [28] resulted effective in single cases.

Sleep-Related Hallucinations

Sleep-related hallucinations (SRHs) include hypnagogic hallucinations (HGHs) at sleep onset, hypnopompic hallucinations (HPHs) on awakening from sleep, and complex nocturnal visual hallucinations (CNVHs) [1] (American Academy of Sleep Medicine, 2005). Generally SRHs consist of visual hallucinations, but these phenomena can involve all five senses (including kinetic experiences). Some predisposing factors are medications (beta-blockers, zolpidem) or drug of abuse (including past alcohol use), mood disorder or anxiety disorders. SRHs present an association with some neurological disorders like narcolepsy, idiopathic hypersomnia, Parkinson's disease, and dementia with Lewy bodies. There are few data on the treatment of SHRs. One approach is to protect the patients from predisposing factors or to treat the associated disorder.

Sleep-Related Eating Disorder

Sleep-related eating disorder (SRED) is characterized by recurrent episodes of involuntary eating and drinking occurring during the main sleep period. In this disorder, the awareness/alertness and the recall of the eating episodes may be variable. PSG may show multiple arousals from stage N3). SRED is more common in women (20-35 years old) and sometimes presents "binge eating" features in which patients prefer high-calorie food or unusual food (frozen or toxic).

Comorbidities with other sleep disorders (sleepwalking, restless leg syndrome, OSA) and eating disorders are also present. There is also a strong association with the current use of zolpidem [29]; the use of lithium or hypnotic benzodiazepines can also be associated with SRED.

Regarding treatment, if SRED is due to medications, these should be withdrawn. Sertraline [30], pramipexole [31], and topiramate [32] have been used in non-iatrogenic forms.

Unspecified parasomnia, Parasomnia due to Drug or Substance

When parasomnia is believed to be secondary to a psychiatric diagnosis, before this diagnosis can be made with certainty it is possible to use the term *Unspecified Parasomnia*. If there is a temporal association between the onset of a parasomnia and current medication or substance use it possible to use the term *Parasomnia Due to Drug or Substance.*

Parasomnia Due to Medical Condition

These can be caused by a neurological or medical condition. Some authors have used the term "secondary parasomnias" to emphasize the causal relationship with an underlying organic pathology. RBD is frequently associated with an underlying neurological condition ("symptomatic RBD") such as Parkinson's disease, Lewy body with dementia, and multiple system atrophy. Other medical conditions that lead to parasomnia are Delirium Tremens, Morvan Syndrome (an autoimmune limbic encephalopathy), fatal familial insomnia (an autosomal dominant disease clinically characterized by loss of sleep associated with autonomic and motor over activity), and sporadic Creutzfeldt-Jakob disease.

The term "*Agrypnia excitata*" describes a clinical syndrome characterized by the inability to sleep associated with a generalized motor and autonomic over-activation. It appears that this clinical entity may result from the three above-cited conditions associated with thalamo-limbic system dysfunction: Delirium tremens, Morvan syndrome and fatal familial insomnia [33].

Parasomnia-Like Disorders or Behaviors

The ICSD-2 classifies a number of nocturnal behaviors under other categories including *sleep-related movement disorders (bruxism and rhythmic movement disorder)* and others such as *sleep talking, hypnic jerks* and *propiospinal myoclonus.*

Sleep bruxism is a stereotyped movement disorder characterized by grinding or clenching of the teeth during sleep. The sounds made by friction of the teeth are usually perceived by a bed partner. Bruxism is more prevalent at the age of one year, soon after the eruption of the deciduous incisors. The prevalence of sleep bruxism in children is high. Approximately 40% of preschoolers and 50% of first graders were reported to experience bruxism once time per week. In adults, usually begins at 10 to 20 years of age. It is frequently associated with orofacial pain, headaches, and other more severe sleep disorders such as sleep-disordered breathing [34].

The aims of treatment are to reduce pain and prevent permanent damage to the teeth (using mouth guards or appliances). In more severe cases, benzodiazepines or Botulinum toxin (BTX) may be used.

Sleep-related rhythmic movement disorder is classified as a sleep-related movement disorder [1] (ICSD-2; American Academy of Sleep Medicine, 2005), which may involve large muscle groups in different parts of the body. The ICSD-2 characterizes this as repetitive, stereotyped, and rhythmic motor behaviors that occur predominantly during drowsiness or sleep that are typically seen in infants and children.

Resolution is normally spontaneous in children by 4 years of age and pharmacological treatment is usually not necessary.

Sleep Talking (Somniloquy) is usually reported by the bed partner or someone asleep near the affected individual. Although few sleep recordings have been performed, sleep talking can arise from NREM or REM sleep. Vocalizations have been described associated with sleepwalking, RBD, PTSD, SRED, on arousal from OSA, and with nocturnal seizures. An organic cause or psychopathology should be suspected if the disorder occurs in adulthood. Sleep talking is very common in the general population: is estimated that about the 50% of children of between 3 and 10 years old presented somniloquy at least once a year, but less than 10% presented it every day [35].

Sleep talking is a benign entity and does not require treatment; however, an exceptional organic cause or psychopathology should be suspected if the onset is in adulthood (after 25 years).

Another benign entity is the *Hypnic Jerks* (sleep starts), which are brief total body jerks that generally occur at sleep onset. They may be associated with a sense of falling. The jerks may affect the body asymmetrically. Caffeine or alcohol before bed and strenuous activities like exercise are predisposing factors. *Propiospinal Myoclonus* at sleep onset has similar characteristics. It consists of muscular jerks that occur in transition from wakefulness to light sleep. Jerks involve the abdominal and trunk muscles with spread to involve limbs and neck muscles. Jerks are typically slow, rhythmic, bilateral, and synchronous most represented in flexion.

Differential Diagnosis

There are some conditions that should be considered for differential diagnosis, one of which is nocturnal epilepsy.

The previous classification of parasomnias [36] included the disorders nocturnal paroxysmal dystonia (NPD). *Nocturnal Paroxysmal Dystonia* is characterized by repeated dystonia or dyskinetic episodes occurring during NREM sleep. There are two clinical varieties of Nocturnal Paroxysmal Dystonia classified by the length of duration of the episode (15 to 60 sec for the briefest known as Paroxysmal Arousals and the Episodic Nocturnal Wanderings, up to 60 min in duration). The duration of episodes and dystonic-dyskinetic features such as ballistic or choreoathetoid movement can distinguish sleep terrors from REM sleep behavior disorder [37]. These are now believed to be manifestations of nocturnal frontal lobe epilepsy.

In this disorder patients have seizures confined to the night and typical manifestations mimic parasomnias (for the complex motor manifestations or for the vocalizations). In these cases, PSG investigation is essential to exclude seizures.

Among psychiatric disorders, panic attacks can present as nocturnal spells. Panic attacks occur from wakefulness after arousal from sleep. The individual is alert and the severity builds with intense fear, tachycardia, dyspnea, chest pain, or flushing. Whereas nocturnal panic attacks usually occur in patients with known daytime attacks, a few patients may have panic attacks only at night.

PTSD patients may also complain of terrifying dreams and awaken with episodes similar to sleep terrors. They are usually not confused on awakening and may have vivid dream recall.

References

[1] American Academy of Sleep Medicine International classification of sleep disorders, 2nd ed.: Diagnostic and coding manual. Westchester, IL: *American Academy of Sleep Medicine*, 2005.

[2] Adler SR, ed. Sleep paralysis: nightmares, nocebos, and the mind–body connection. Piscataway, NJ: Rutgers University Press, 2011. pp. 37-58.

[3] Golzari SE, Khodadoust K, Alakbarli F, et al. Sleep paralysis in medieval Persia - the Hidayat of Akhawayni (?-983 AD). *Neuropsychiatr. Dis. Treat.* 2012;8:229-34.

[4] Bjorvatn B, Grønli J, Pallesen S. Prevalence of different parasomnias in the general population. *Sleep Med.* 2010;11:1031-4.

[5] Shapiro CM, Trajanovic NN, Fedoroff JP. Sexsomnia: A new parasomnia? *Can. J. Psychiatry.* 2003;48:311-7

[6] Ferber R. Sleep disorders in infants and children. In: Riley TL, ed. Clinical aspects of sleep and sleep disturbance. Boston: *Butterworth,* 1985. pp. 113-158.

[7] Ohayon MM, Guilleminault C, Priest RG. Night terrors, sleepwalking, and confusional arousals in the general population: Their frequency and relationship to other sleep and mental disorders. *J. Clin. Psychiatry.* 1999;60:268-76.

[8] Markov D, Jaffe F, Doghramji K. Update on Parasomnias: A Review for Psychiatric Practice. *Psychiatry* (Edgmont). 2006;3:69-76.

[9] Kales A, Soldatos CR, Bixler EO, et al. Hereditary factors in sleepwalking and night terrors. *Br. J. Psychiatry.* 1980;137:111-8.

[10] Mahowald MW, Cramer Bornemann MA. NREM sleep-arousal parasomnias. In: Kryger MH, Roth T, Dement WC, eds. *Principles and Practice of Sleep Medicine.* Philadelphia, PA: WB Saunders; 2005. pp. 889-96.

[11] Schenck CH, Milner DM, Hurwitz TD, et al: A polysomnographic and clinical report of sleep related injury in 100 adult patients. *Am. J. Psychiatry.* 1989;146:1166-72.

[12] Avidan A. Motor disorders of sleep and parasomnias. In: Avidan A, Zee PC, editors. *Handbook of sleep medicine.* Philadelphia: Lippincott Williams & Wilkins; 2006. pp. 98-136.

[13] Iber C, Ancoli-Israel S, Chesson S, et al. The American Academy of Sleep Medicine. *The AASM manual for the scoring of sleep and associated events: rules, terminology and technical specifications.* American Academy of Sleep Medicine, Chicago, IL, 2007.

[14] Boeve BF. REM sleep behavior disorder: Updated review of the core features, the REM sleep behavior disorder-neurodegenerative disease association, evolving concepts, controversies, and future directions. *Ann. N. Y. Acad. Sci.* 2010;1184:15-54.

[15] Schenck, C, Bundlie S, Mahowald M. REM behavior disorder (RBD): Delayed emergence of parkinsonism and/or dementia in 65% of older men initially diagnosed

with idiopathic RBD, and an analysis of the minimum & maximum tonic and/or phasic electromyographic abnormalities found during REM sleep. *Sleep.* 2003;26:316.

[16]   Iranzo A, Santamaria J. Severe obstructive sleep apnea/hypopnea mimicking REM sleep behavior disorder. *Sleep.* 2005;28:203-6.

[17]   Mahowald MW, Schenck CH: Status dissociatus : a perspective on states of being. *Sleep.* 1991;14:69-79.

[18]   Aurora RN, Zak RS, Maganti RK, et al. Best practice guide for the treatment of REM sleep behavior disorder (RBD). Standards of Practice Committee; American Academy of Sleep Medicine. *J. Clin. Sleep Med.* 2010;15:85-95.

[19]   Spanos NP, DuBreuil C, McNulta SA, et al. The frequency and correlates of sleep paralysis in a university sample. *J. Res. Pers.* 1995;29:285-305.

[20]   Koran LM, Raghavan S. Fluoxetine for isolated sleep paralysis. *Psychosomatics* 1993;34:184-7.

[21]   Kilpatrick D, Resnick H, Freedy J, et al. Posttraumatic stress disorder field trial: Evaluation of PTSD construct criteria A through E. In: Widiger T, Frances A, Pincus H, et al., eds. DSM-IV Sourcebook. Vol 4. Washington, D.C.: American Psychiatric Press; 1994.

[22]   American Psychiatric Association: *Diagnostic and Statistical Manual of Mental Disorders*, 4th ed. Washington, DC: American Psychiatric Association, 1994.

[23]   Robson WLM: Evaluation and management of enuresis. N Engl J Med. 2009;360:1429-36.

[24]   Brooks LJ, Topol HI: Enuresis in children with sleep apnea. *J. Pediatr.* 2003;142:515-18

[25]   Young T, Palta M, Dempsey J, et al. The occurrence of sleep-disordered breathing among middle-aged adults. *N. Engl. J. Med.* 1993;328:1230.

[26]   Jacome DE. Exploding head syndrome and idiopathic stabbing headache relieved by nifedipine. *Cephalagia.* 2001;21:617-8.

[27]   Sachs C, Svanborg E: The exploding head syndrome: polysomnographic recordings and therapeutic suggestions. *Sleep.* 1991;14:263-266.

[28]   Morgenthaler TI, Silber MH: Amnestic sleep-related eating disorder associated with zolpidem. *Sleep Med.* 2002;3:323-327.

[29]   O'Reardon JP, Allison KC, Martino NS, et al: A randomized, placebo-controlled trial of sertraline in the treatment of night eating syndrome. *Am. J. Psychiatry.* 2006;163:893–898.

[30]   Provini F, Albani R, Vetrugno R, et al: A pilot double-blind placebo-controlled trial of low-dose pramipexole in sleep related eating disorder. *Eur. J. Neurol.* 2005;12:432-6.

[31]   Winkelmann JW: Efficacy and tolerability of open-label topiramate in the treatment of sleep-related eating disorder: a retrospective case series. *J. Clin. Psychiatry.* 2006;67:1729-34.

[32]   Lugaresi E, Provini F, Cortelli P. Agrypnia excitata. Sleep Med. 2011;2:3-10

[33]   Carra MC, Bruni O, Huynh N. Topical review: sleep bruxism, headaches, and sleep-disordered breathing in children and adolescents. *J. Orofac. Pain.* 2012;26:267-76.

[34]   Reimão RN, Lefévre AB. Prevalence of sleep-talking in childhood. *Brain Dev.* 1980;2:353-7.

[35] American Academy of Sleep Medicine International classification of sleep disorders, revised: *Diagnostic and coding manual.* Westchester, IL: American Academy of Sleep Medicine, 2001.

[36] Lugaresi E, Cirignotta F, Montagna P. Nocturnal paroxysmal dystonia. *J. Neurol. Neurosurg. Psychiatry.* 1986;49:375-380.

In: Sleep Medicine
Editors: A. Del Casale, R. Brugnoli and P. Girardi

ISBN: 978-1-62808-515-0
© 2013 Nova Science Publishers, Inc.

Chapter V

Sleep-Related Breathing and Movement Disorders

Luigi Ferini-Strambi, Sara Marelli and Andrea Galbiati*
Department of Clinical Neurosciences, Sleep Disorders Center,
Università Vita-Salute San Raffaele, Milan, Italy

Abstract

Sleep-related breathing disorders (SRBDs) are a significant health problem associated with important morbidity. The large spectrum of respiratory disturbances include conditions resulting in complete or partial upper airway obstruction, those that alter breathing patterns and those that lead to hypoventilation or hypoxemia. Obstructive sleep apnea (OSA), which represents cessation of airflow, develops because of factors such as anatomic obstruction of the upper airway related to obesity, excess tissue bulk in the pharynx, and changes in muscle tone and nerve activity during sleep. Central sleep apnea represents cessation of airflow along with absence or significant reduction in respiratory effort during sleep and is more commonly found in the setting of congestive heart failure, neurologic disorders, or cardiopulmonary disease.

A complete sleep history should be obtained on all patients suspected of having a SRBD. Objective evaluation is mandatory for SRBD diagnosis. Because of the high prevalence of SRBD, the high cost, and technical requirements of in-laboratory polysomnography, portable monitoring approaches have been widely investigated and used in the last several years.

Several studies have demonstrated that vascular changes related to OSA can lead to chronic cardiovascular consequences such as hypertension. Moreover, one of the other major consequences of OSA is an impact on neurocognitive functioning. Recent studies have used functional and structural neuroimaging to delineate the brain areas affected in patients with OSA with neurocognitive dysfunction. These changes can be reversed at least partially with the use of CPAP, which highlights the importance of early recognition and treatment of OSA.

---

* Email: ferinistrambi.luigi@hsr.it.

Sleep-related movement disorders (SRMD) constitute a class of movements that are simple, usually stereotyped, and associated with undesirable effects such as impaired sleep quantity or quality, and/or impairment in daytime functioning. Restless leg syndrome (RLS), periodic limb movements (PLMS), sleep-related leg cramps, and sleep-related bruxism are included in this relatively new category of sleep disorders. SRMD vary considerably in their overall as well as gender- and age-dependent prevalence, and some of the disorders in this category do not have prevalence estimates. Nocturnal sleep disturbances or complaints of daytime sleepiness or fatigue are mandatory for a diagnosis of a sleep-related movement disorder. The history may be usually telling; however, polysomnography (or video-polysomnography in some cases) may be necessary to make a firm diagnosis of sleep-related movement disorders. Extensive or detailed analyses of the impact of SRMD on economics and society are largely lacking, although there are studies that explore the consequences of RLS.

Sleep-Related Breathing Disorders

Diagnostic Definition

Sleep-related breathing disorders (SRBDs) are a significant public health problem associated with important morbidity. The large spectrum of respiratory disturbances include conditions resulting in complete or partial upper airway obstruction, those that alter breathing patterns and those that lead to hypoventilation or hypoxemia. In the early 19th century, the clinical observation of a pattern of breathing called Cheyne–Stokes was described [1,2]. Subsequently, clinical descriptions of patients with obesity and excessive sleepiness were noted, and in 1956 Burwell and colleagues applied the term "Pickwickian syndrome" to describe individuals with obesity, hypersomnolence, and chronic hypoventilation [3]. Gastaut and co-workers in 1966 discovered that cessation of respiration during sleep in the patients with the Pickwickian syndrome was due to intermittent upper airway obstruction [4]. This work is credited as the initial recognition of obstructive sleep apnea (OSA) as a distinct clinical syndrome. Subsequently, the connection between nocturnal obstructive respiratory events and daytime sleepiness became generally accepted with some authors describing the OSA syndrome as a disorder with daytime sleepiness and obstructive apneas on polysomnography (PSG) [5]. More recently, Guilleminault and colleagues described a group of patients who had daytime sleepiness, but no apneas or hypopneas on PSG [6] : esophageal manometry in these patients demonstrated episodes of increasingly negative intrathoracic pressure without reductions in tidal volume. These findings were evidence of periodic increased upper airways resistance. This led to the appellation of "upper airways resistance syndrome" (UARS) to describe these patients and the use of "respiratory effort–related arousals (RERAs)" as the corresponding nomenclature for these episodes of increased upper airways resistance.

In the International Classification of Sleep Disorders-2 (ICSD-2) published in 2005 [7], the broad category of SRBDs encompasses the following five groups: (i) central sleep apnea syndromes (CSA), (ii) OSA syndromes, (iii) sleep-related hypoventilation/ hypoxemic syndromes, (iv) sleep-related hypoventilation/hypoxemia due to medical conditions, and (v) other sleep-related breathing disorders.

Central Sleep Apnea Syndromes are divided into six subcategories: the idiopathic form, or primary CSA, and five other with defined underlying causes (CSA secondary to Cheyne–Stokes breathing pattern or periodic breathing, CSA due to high-altitude periodic breathing, CSA due to a medical condition exclusive of Cheyne–Stokes respiration, CSA due to a drug or substance, and primary sleep apnea of infancy).

Obstructive Sleep Apnea Syndromes are divided into adult and pediatric forms.

Sleep-Related Hypoventilation/Hypoxemic Syndromes include two subcategories, the idiopathic sleep-related nonobstructive alveolar hypoventilation syndrome and the congenital central alveolar hypoventilation syndrome. Alternate names for the idiopathic disorder are central alveolar hypoventilation or primary alveolar hypoventilation.

Sleep-Related Hypoventilation/Hypoxemia due to Medical Conditions include three subcategories of medical conditions that lead to sleep-related hypoventilation or hypoxemia: pulmonary parenchymal or vascular pathology, lower airways obstruction, and neuromuscular and chest wall disorders. The obesity-hypoventilation syndrome (OHS) is included in this category.

Other Sleep-Related Breathing Disorder is a category used for forms of SRBD that cannot be classified elsewhere or do not clearly fit into one of the above categories, but they are felt to be disorders of respiratory sleep disturbance.

OSA syndrome is characterized by frequent repetitive episodes of complete (apnea) or partial (hypopnea) upper airway obstruction during sleep, but not always leading to reduction in oxygen saturation. In adults, these episodes last a minimum of 10 seconds, during which there is effort to breathe and can occur at any stage of sleep. Generally, OSA is felt to be present when there are five or more episodes per hour of sleep (Medicine AAoS, 2005) [8]. Most affected individuals have a mixture of both apneic and hypopneic events during their sleep. Frequently, bed partners report loud, disruptive snoring, breathing pauses, or episodes of choking or gasping in the night. Excessive daytime sleepiness and chronic fatigue are very commonly present symptoms, although a high prevalence (39%-58%) of insomnia symptoms have been reported in patients with OSA [9]. Individuals often complain of feeling unrested with a headache upon awakening in the morning [10].

OSA is often present concurrently with a number of other medical conditions including hypertension, atherosclerotic cardiovascular disease, stroke, diabetes mellitus, depression, and gastroesophageal reflux [11-13].

OSA is increasingly recognized in children [14]. However, because of the child's increased respiratory rate, the minimum event duration is the length of two breath cycles. There is as yet no consensus on the minimum event frequency, but a number of studies consider that one or more apnea or hypopnea events per hour of sleep is diagnostic of OSA in a child. Moreover, hypopneas are the predominant event type rather than the mixture of frank apnea and hypopneas observed in adults. Like adults, children with OSA may present with loud snoring, however frequently they paradoxically exhibit hyperactive behaviour and no excessive daytime sleepiness. Poor school performance also is frequently observed [15].

In UARS, many of the symptoms overlap with those in OSA. However, there are some important differences. Chronic insomnia tends to be more common in patients with UARS[16]. Many patients complain of sleep onset as well as sleep maintenance insomnia. This is thought to be a result of conditioning, as a consequence of frequent sleep disruption. Fatigue is a more likely complaint than sleepiness. Some authors emphasized that patients with UARS tend to have more complaints of functional somatic problems such as headaches, sleep-onset insomnia, and irritable bowel syndrome [17]. Unfortunately, often the patients are misdiagnosed with chronic fatigue syndrome or fibromyalgia, attention deficit or psychiatric disorder [18]. Autonomic dysfunction is seen more often in patients with UARS than in those with OSA. Patients complain of cold hands and feet, and a quarter of them will complain of lightheadedness. Hypotension may be associated with UARS and can account for the lightheadedness [19].

Cheyne–Stokes breathing during sleep occurs if there are at least three consecutive cycles of a cyclical crescendo and decrescendo change in breathing amplitude, and there are five or more central sleep apneas or hypopneas per hour of sleep or the cyclic crescendo and decrescendo change in breathing amplitude has a duration of at least 10 consecutive minutes [8]. CSA with Cheyne–Stokes breathing, that is markedly more prevalent in men older than 60 years, generally occurs in the setting of impairment in left ventricular function or cerebrovascular disease [20-22]. CSA with Cheyne–Stokes breathing occurs more commonly in those with severe left ventricular dysfunction, however it can be observed in those with milder heart disease as well [23]. It has been recently reported that whereas obstructive apnoea is considered injurious to the cardiovascular system, the effects of CSA with Cheyne–Stokes breathing are less clear and may be a compensatory response to severe heart failure [24].

In addition to symptoms of the underlying disorder, individuals with Cheyne–Stokes breathing may complain of nonrestorative sleep, morning headaches, paroxysmal nocturnal dyspnea, and insomnia more frequently than daytime sleepiness.

OHS is defined as a combination of obesity (body mass index $\geq$ 30 kg/m^2), daytime hypercapnia (Pa$_{CO2}$ $\leq$ 45 mm Hg) and sleep-disordered breathing after ruling out other disorders that may cause alveolar hypoventilation. The clinical presentation may be similar to that of OSA syndrome as patients may present with excessive daytime sleepiness, fatigue, or morning headaches. Patients with OHS also have daytime hypercapnia and hypoxemia, which leads to the development of pulmonary hypertension and cor pulmonale [25].

Incidence and Prevalence

Obstructive Sleep Apnea Syndromes

There is little available data documenting the incidence of OSA in adults. The Cleveland Family Study evaluated 286 eligible patients to determine the five-year incidence of SRBD and the influence of risk factors [26]. The five-year incidence was 10% for OSA defined as >15 apneas or hypopneas per hour (apnea-hypopnea index, AHI) and 16% for OSA with an AHI > 5. In this study, the incidence of OSA was influenced independently by age, sex, BMI, waist-hip ratio, and serum cholesterol concentration: incidence of OSA was greater in men and in those who were obese, but these effects diminished and eventually became inconsequential with increasing age.

The incidence of OSA in children is unknown. However, some authors recently described the prevalence, persistence, and characteristics associated with sleep disordered breathing (SDB) symptoms in a population-based cohort of 12,447 children followed from 6 months to 6.75 years [27]. In this study, the prevalence of apnea ("Always") was 1%-2% at all ages assessed. In contrast, snoring "Always" ranged from 3.6% to 7.7%, and snoring "Habitually" ranged from 9.6% to 21.2%, with a notable increase from 1.5- 2.5 years. At 6 years old, 25% were habitual mouth-breathers. The "Always" and "Habitual" incidence of each symptom between time points was 1%-5% and 5%-10%, respectively.

A fundamental contribution to understanding the prevalence of OSA among middle-aged adults was published in 1993 by Young and colleagues [28]. In this study, the estimated prevalence of OSA, defined as an AHI on polysomnography of five or higher, was 9% for women and 24% for men. In addition, this study estimated that 2% of women and 4% of men met the minimal diagnostic criteria for the OSA syndrome (an AHI of 5 or higher and daytime hypersomnolence). Some years later, there have been two additional large cohort studies in predominantly white men and women from Pennsylvania and Spain that utilized in laboratory polysomnography and similar methodology and design [29-31]. On the basis of the average of prevalence estimates from these three studies, approximately 1 of every 5 adults has at least mild OSA and 1 of every 15 has at least moderate OSA [32]. Other investigations in non-white populations also have shown a similarly high prevalence of OSA. Ip and colleagues studied 784 Hong Kong men and estimated the prevalence of OSA syndrome (defined as an AHI > 5) to be 4.1% [33]. Another study of middle-aged Korean men and women noted that the prevalence of polysomnographic OSA (AHI > 5) was 27% in men and 16% in women; for the OSA syndrome (AHI > 5 with excessive daytime sleepiness), its prevalence was 4.5% in men and 3.2% in women [34].

Also in more recent studies the estimated prevalence of OSA was comparable to previous estimates from general populations in the USA, Asia and Europe [35].

In contrast to earlier epidemiological studies that reported that OSA was eight to 10 times more common in men than women referred to sleep clinics, general population studies show that men are only two to three times more likely to have OSA than women. The diagnosis of OSA may be missed in women because they complain of different symptoms than men. Habitual snoring has less predictive value for OSA in women than men. Women with OSA often present to sleep specialists complaining of insomnia, nightmares or depression [36].

Central Sleep Apnea Associated with Cheyne–Stokes Breathing Pattern

CSA secondary to Cheyne–Stokes breathing pattern is the most common form of CSA that is clinically observed. The prevalence in the general population is low, but it is increased in patients with congestive heart failure (CHF) and stroke [37]. This SRBD has a strikingly higher prevalence in patients with heart failure as compared with those with normal left ventricular function: the prevalence varied from 21 to 66% in patients with CHF. Moreover, it is not limited to severe heart failure but may also occur at moderate stages of CHF with a left-ventricular ejection fraction (LVEF) between 35 and 45% with milder functional impairment [38].

Cheyne–Stokes breathing pattern is generally seen in patients who are male and over age 60 years of age.

Obesity-Hypoventilation Syndrome (OHS)

The prevalence of OHS in the general population is unknown because it has not been studied. According to Chau and colleagues [39] the prevalence of OHS among the general adult population in the United States is estimated to be 0.15–0.3%, because approximately 1.5% of the general United States population has severe obesity and OSA, and 10–20% of the severely obese patients with OSA have OHS. The prevalence of OHS is 11% in patients with known OSA and 8% in bariatric surgical patients [39].

Pathophysiology

Obstructive Sleep Apnea

In OSA, there are several factors which, when coupled with the physiologic changes in normal sleep, predispose them to airway obstruction. OSA patients are more likely to have an anatomically smaller airway during sleep. This may be coupled with increased pharyngeal fat pads further narrowing the airway, which renders it vulnerable to increased intraluminal pressure [40]. Moreover, this patient population may have increased activation of pharyngeal dilator muscles during wakefulness, and therefore, there is a relatively larger reduction in muscle activation during sleep [41]. Lastly, there is a significant reduction in the degree and speed of the pharyngeal reflex activation in response to brief impulses of negative intraluminal pressure, further rendering OSA patients enable to counteract upper airway collapse. Maximal negative intraluminal pressure occurs during midinspiration. However, on endoscopic examinations of OSA patients, the minimal cross-sectional area of the airway occurs at end expiration. Consequently, if there is a delay in the reflex activation of the dilator muscles, there is increased likelihood of airway obstruction. It has been proposed that chronic snoring and continuous trauma to the pharyngeal muscles may lead to permanent lesions and neuropathy causing the decrease, and potentially lack of, reflex response and activation of the muscles [42]. Biopsies from OSA patients demonstrated atrophy and an abnormal distribution of fiber types in the upper airway muscles [43, 44].

There are several risk factors associated with increased upper airway obstruction. In addition to age, male gender has been consistently associated with a two- to threefold increased risks of sleep apnea Hormonal differences are theorized to be the reason for the gender difference. Menopause, pregnancy and polycystic ovarian syndrome increase the risk for OSA in women. Neck fat and BMI influence apnea-hypopnea index (AHI) severity in women; abdominal fat and neck-to-waist ratio do so in men [36]. The degree of BMI and neck circumference and waist-tohip ratio has been correlated to the prevalence and the severity of OSA [45]. In a longitudinal study, it was found that a 10% increase in weight was associated with a six fold increase in the risk for developing OSA [46]. A 3% change in AHI is expected for each 1% increase in BMI, and similar change in the opposite direction is noted with decrease in BMI. However, not all patients with OSA are obese. Craniofacial and upper airway anatomy may play a significant role, especially in the Asian population and in the pediatric population. [36] Enlarged adenoids and tonsils during childhood will often lead to mouth breathing, which can cause abnormal growth of the lower face and jaw resulting in "adenoidal faces," predisposing the child to development of OSA [47].

Although adenotonsillar hypertrophy has never fully accounted for OSA in the pediatric population, the relative contributions of adiposity and airway lymphoid tissue in the emerging epidemic of obese pediatric OSA patients are unclear. Recently, Arens and colleagues [48] performed magnetic resonance imaging of the upper airway and abdomen in obese children with OSA and without OSA. They found greater adenoid and tonsil tissue volumes in those with OSA, leading to a 28% reduction in the oropharyngeal volume. They also identified retropharyngeal lymph node hypertrophy as an important contributor to airway restriction. Individual lymphoid tissue sizes were highly correlated with OSA severity, whereas BMI was not, suggesting that lymphoid tissue hypertrophy is due to local or systemic inflammation in children with OSA and not obesity itself. With regard to excess adiposity, two important findings emerged that could further promote airway collapse in those with OSA: greater parapharyngeal fat pad size and greater visceral abdominal fat. Although OSA and visceral fat have a highly confounded relationship, the negative effects of parapharyngeal fat pads on the upper airway caliber were similar to obese adults with OSA.

Central Apnea

Central Apnea Related to Ventilatory Control Instability

Sleep onset central apneas are not a rare condition that can be observed, especially in subjects with frequent sleep-wake transition, as insomniac patients. If the PCO_2 drops below a certain level, the "apnea threshold", breathing is likely to become dysrhythmic. The PCO_2 level that was adequate to stimulate ventilation during wakefulness, may be inadequate to do this during sleep, and an apnea occurs. The subsequent resumption of ventilation may arouse the subject, and the process may repeat itself when the individual falls back to sleep. Once a stable sleep is reached, breathing should become regular under metabolic control system. Occasional central apneas in the sleep-wake transition must be considered normal events.

Patients with idiopathic central sleep apnea tend to have a high hypercapnic response and low arterial PCO_2 levels during wakefulness [49]. The particular steep hypercapnic response in these patients led to a high loop gain with respiratory instability, yielding a waxing and waning of ventilation. As a result of the lower awake PCO_2, these patients are breathing closer to their PCO_2 apnea threshold during sleep [50]. Even if the high waking hypercapnic response is the most consistent finding, other mechanisms may be involved in idiopathic central sleep apnea. In these patients, the respiratory pauses are terminated with an abrupt, large breath, not with a gradual increment in ventilation. This finding suggests a failure of the expiratory-to-inspiratory switch, which may be influenced by not only the chemoreceptors but other mechanisms, as lung volume and chest wall mechanoreceptors.

As previously reported, CHF is associated with Cheyne-Stokes respiration. The breathing pattern is characterized by crescendo-decrescendo respiratory pattern with a central apnea/hypopnea at the nadir. The prolonged circulation time and the increased ventilatory responsiveness to rising Pco2 causes a breathing control system instability [51]. The abrupt onset and offset change in ventilation that is observed in idiopathic central apnea is not seen in Cheyne-Stokes respiration. This last abnormality has been also reported in patients with neurologic disease: [52] however, the actual breathing pattern in these patients has been less well characterized than in CHF patients.

Central Apneas Related to Upper Airway Changes

Nasal obstruction of different etiologies can affect breathing pattern during sleep, by causing both central and obstructive apneas [53]. It has been suggested that airflow may be detected by receptors in the nose and that these receptor mechanisms can influence respiration [54]. Moreover, the increased negative airway pressures generated by breathing through a partially occluded nasal passage collapse the pharynx and cause apneas. However, most such events are likely to be obstructive in nature. On the other hand, it has been reported that in patients with predominantly central sleep apnea, the events occurred more frequently when in supine posture, a position likely to produce pharyngeal collapse, and high levels of nasal CPAP eliminated the central apneas [55].

Central Apneas Related to Neurologic Disorders

The neurologic disorders that affect the control system of ventilation may cause central sleep apnea [56]. Respiratory rhythm is generated in the brainstem. Damage to the brainstem, particularly the medullary area, may affect ventilation during sleep. Tumors, vascular processes (infarction or hemorrhage), or encephalitis can damage directly the medullary areas, leading to breathing dysrhytmias during sleep, with central events. Moreover, these processes or other conditions, such as multiple sclerosis or cervical cordotomy, may only interrupt the neural pathways from the medullary respiratory neurons to the motoneurons of the ventilatory muscles: this interruption, without damage to the brainstem itself, affects the metabolic control of breathing, yielding central apneas. Moreover, in chronic neuromuscular diseases, such as myasthenia gravis or muscular dystrophy, hypoventilation during sleep is the more prominent finding, but central apneas may be also observed [57].

Diagnostic Tools

History and Physical Examination

An extensive sleep history should be obtained on all patients suspected of having a sleep-related breathing disorder (SRBD). The sleep history should include questions regarding the patient's sleep habits and symptoms of other common sleep disorders, especially insomnia, restless leg syndrome and narcolepsy, that can frequently coexist with a SRBD. A full medical history should be obtained as a diagnosis of congestive heart failure or neurologic disease may indicate the presence of Cheyne–Stokes respiration as the underlying cause of the SRBD. Moreover, a complete list of medications should be ascertained as many medications may affect sleep and/or respiration. The list includes sedatives, hypnotics, narcotics, and stimulants. A family history of SRBD should be sought as OSA appears to display a familial aggregation [58]. Finally, a complete history of alcohol and/or tobacco use, which worsens OSA, should also be obtained [59]. Symptoms suggestive of a SRBD are generally divided into two groups: nocturnal and daytime. Snoring is the most common nocturnal complaint and is generally described as loud, irregular, habitual, and disturbing to a bed or room partner (who sometimes moves out of the bedroom to avoid the noise). A bed or room partner will also often notice pauses in the snoring or breathing (witnessed apneas) that may end with a snorting sound. Other nocturnal symptoms include gasping, gagging, or choking sensations, restless sleep, and frequent unexplained awakenings. Nicturia is another symptom frequently reported in OSA patients [60]. The most common daytime symptom is excessive sleepiness. The sleepiness in OSA patients is most evident when the patient is in a relaxing inactive situation. With extreme sleepiness, the patient may fall asleep while actively conversing, eating, walking, or driving. Some studies showed that the degree of sleepiness, whether measured using the Epworth Sleepiness Scale or the multiple sleep latency test (MSLT) does not correlate with the degree of OSA [9]. Moreover, a no trivial percentage (39-54 %) of OSA patients may refer insomnia symptoms, and no diurnal hypersomnia [9]. Patients also frequently complain of fatigue, tiredness, and lack of energy. Interestingly, in one investigation, when asked to choose their most significant symptom, more patients chose lack of energy (40%) compared to sleepiness (22%) [61]. Other daytime symptoms include morning headache, morning dry or sore throat, and impaired memory and concentration.

In patients with central apnea, daytime sleepiness has been described, [62] however several studies reported that these subjects less commonly complain of daytime hypersomnolence than do patients with obstructive sleep apnea [49]. The primary complaint of many patients with central apnea tends to be insomnia, restless sleep, or frequent awakenings during the night. Such awakenings may be accompanied by gasping for air.

The physical examination of the patient with a suspected SRBD generally starts with measures of body habitus. The body mass index and neck circumference both are predictive of the presence and severity of OSA and are the most commonly used measures of body habitus. However, it should be noted that some other measures of body habitus, including measures such as waist-hip ratio and skin-fold thicknesses, are also predictive of OSA. [28] It has been recently observed that waist-hip ratio is more predictive of severity of OSA in men than in women [63].

The physical examination of the patient with a suspected SRBD is concentrated on the upper airway examination. A common finding in children and thin adults with suspected OSA is tonsillar enlargement. Other upper airway findings that have been associated with OSA include an overjet (horizontal relationship of upper and lower central incisors), retrognathia, tongue and/or uvula enlargement, a low-lying palate, a high-arched palate, and a high Mallampati score [64,65].

Two physical examination findings have been found to be independent predictors of the presence of OSA: the Mallampati score (Figure 1) and lateral narrowing. The Mallampati score is a simple airway-classification scheme developed to identify patients at risk for difficult intubation. It has been reported that each 1-point increase in the Mallampati score was associated with a two-fold increase in the odds of having OSA and a 5-point increase in the apnea-hypopnea index (AHI) [66]. Lateral narrowing is the finding of airway narrowing by the lateral pharyngeal walls. In a study of 420 subjects with suspected OSA, some authors found that narrowing of the airway by the lateral pharyngeal walls and tonsillar enlargement are independent predictors for the presence of OSA after controlling the body mass index and neck circumference, but only in men [64]. The reason for the gender difference in the occurrence of lateral narrowing is unclear.

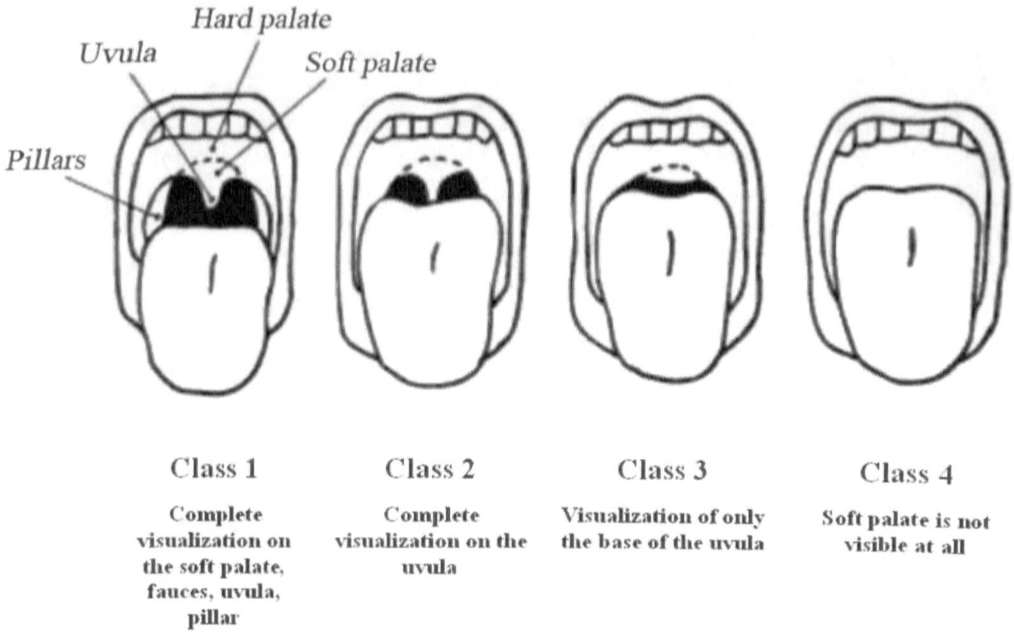

Figure 1. Mallampati Score.

Subjective Assessment Tools

The Berlin Questionnaire (BQ) was first developed in 1996 at the Conference on Sleep in Primary Care in Berlin, Germany. This questionnaire was validated as an authentic tool for identifying patients who are at high risk for OSA in some countries, [67, 68] and this questionnaire is composed of three categories: snoring, wake-time sleepiness or tiredness, and the presence of obesity or hypertension [68]. The BQ has been frequently used in the screening for OSA and is well-known as a convenient and inexpensive tool [69]. In a recent study, using a general population sample (n=793) with no history of OSA, case and control status for moderate-severe OSA was determined by home-based nasal flow and oximetry-derived apnoea-hypopnoea index using a cut-off value of $\geq$15 events/h to define cases. The age-standardised prevalence estimate of moderate-severe OSA was 9.1 % (12.4 % in men, 5.7 % in women). Sensitivity of the BQ in this population was 54 %, and specificity, 70 %. A combination of questions regarding snoring frequency and hypertension provided maximal post-test probability of OSA and greatest post-screen sample size [70].

The STOP-Bang model has been validated as an easy and effective screening method to exclude pre-surgical patients with undiagnosed severe sleep apnea from going to the operating room. Consisting of 8 yes or no questions based upon snoring, tiredness/sleepiness, observed apneas, hypertension, BMI > 35 kg/m2, age > 50 years, neck circumference > 40 cm, and male gender, a score of any 3 affirmative responses was used to dichotomize the population. The sensitivities measured 83.6%, 92.9%, and 100%, respectively, for patients with at least mild (AHI > 5/h), moderate (AHI > 15/h), and severe (AHI > 30/h) sleep apnea. The predictive values negative measured 60.8%, 90.2%, and 100%, respectively. Thus, one could confidently exclude the possibility of at least moderate or severe OSA with a score of 0-2 affirmative responses; however, the test was less reliable in excluding mild sleep apnea [71]. Questionnaire surveys of sleepiness are useful in epidemiological research in OSA, but they can also serve as screening instruments in clinical practice. Epworth Sleepiness Scale and the Stanford Sleepiness Scale have been discussed in the Chapter 2 of the present book.

Objective Assessment Tools

Overnight polysomnography is the most widely used test for the diagnosis of SRBDs.

During polysomnography, multiple physiologic parameters are continuously monitored and recorded. Respiratory parameters generally include flow channel (both oronasal thermal sensors and nasal pressure transducers), thoracic and abdominal effort channels (ideally inductance plethysmography), snoring channel, and continuous pulse oximetry [72]. For sleep studies in children, it is also recommended that end-tidal carbon dioxide monitoring should also be performed as many children present with obstructive hypoventilation rather than obstructive apneas and hypopneas [73].

Airflow through the upper airway can be measured by some different methods [74]. Most of the available methods are adequate for detecting apneas (the absence of flow) but have varying ability to detect hypopneas (reduction in flow). The pneumotachometer, which measures airflow by measuring the pressure drop across a linear resistance, is considered the gold standard for measuring and quantifying airflow through the upper airway. Tidal volume can be computed by integration of the flow signal. However, the use of the pneumotachometer requires collection of all exhaled air via a closed breathing circuit; thus, it is primarily used in the research setting.

Respiratory effort has traditionally been monitored by measuring rib cage and abdominal movement using piezo sensors or strain gauges. These devices provide qualitative information on changes in rib cage and abdominal movement and cannot be used to reliably distinguish between central and obstructive events, particularly hypopneas [74]. In contrast, measurement of pleural pressure using an esophageal pressure monitor (esophageal manometry), is considered the gold standard for measuring respiratory effort. The use of esophageal pressure monitoring has two major clinical applications. First, it can be used to verify central apnea and hypopnea episodes with a high degree of certainty [75]. Second, esophageal pressure monitoring is necessary to detect RERAs and the upper airway resistance syndrome [74]. The updated guidelines on polysomnography recommend either esophageal manometry or inductance plethysmography for the detection of respiratory effort [72]. As the identification of a hypopnea generally requires a desaturation of 3% to 4%, the accuracy of the oximeter is important. Because of the high prevalence of SRBD, the high cost, and technical requirements of in laboratory polysomnography and the limited availability of sleep centers in some but not all countries, alternative approaches, such as portable monitoring, to the diagnosis of SRBD have been widely investigated in the last several years. The most common of these approaches is the use of portable monitoring. The American Academy of Sleep Medicine defined four types of monitors: type 1 is defined as in-laboratory standard polysomnography; type 2, comprehensive portable polysomnography (similar number of channels as type 1 monitors including EEG; there is limited evidence for these devices and they will not be discussed further); type 3, generally four channels, including flow, effort, ECG, and oximetry; type 4, limited monitoring with generally 1–2 channels, and often oximetry alone.

Based upon the available evidence, guidelines have been recently updated regarding the use of portable monitors in the diagnosis of OSA [76]. For patients with a high pretest probability of moderate to severe OSA, Type 3 monitors may be used as an alternative to polysomnography in the unattended setting. Physicians should recognize the following limitations: the studies need to be scored and reviewed manually, the patient should not have any significant comorbidity (particularly significant pulmonary disease or congestive heart failure), and that a negative study should be followed by a full Type 1 sleep study.

The termination of apnea or hypopnea is often associated with transient arousal from sleep. Repetitive arousals lead to sleep fragmentation and daytime sleepiness. Visual inspection of the cortical EEG is time-consuming and fraught with subjective variability. Therefore, development of objective, even if indirect, markers of arousal would be greatly beneficial. Changes in heart rate or blood pressure may serve as reliable surrogates of arousal, even if cortical changes are minimal or absent [77]. One technique for detecting acute changes in blood pressure is pulse transit time (PTT), an indirect method of measuring beat-to-beat blood pressure change [77-79]. Pulse-transit time reflects the interval from the ECG R-wave until the pulse pressure wave reaches the finger. The normal interval is about 250 milliseconds, and is determined primarily by the stiffness/tension in the arterial walls and hence blood pressure. Accordingly, an increase in blood pressure leads to increased arterial wall stiffness, a faster pulse wave, and a shorter PTT. The essential components required to measure beat-to-beat are three thoracic electrodes and a modified oximeter finger probe. Several studies have shown that PTT is a sensitive marker of the arousal process in normal subjects. PTT has not yet been incorporated in commercial polysomnographic recordings; however, it is of potential benefit and can be applied in an objective, reproducible, and automated fashion.

Transient arousals from sleep are associated with increased bursts of sympathetic nerve activity in adults that lead to increased heart rate, blood pressure, and peripheral vasoconstriction. Peripheral arterial tonometry (PAT) is a new technique that uses a plethysmographic technique to measure the peripheral vasoconstriction. PAT uses a fingermounted pneumo-optical sensor that measures the digital arterial pulse wave volume. Attenuation of the PAT signal indicates digital vasoconstriction and can be used as a marker for arousals associated with respiratory events [80, 81]. The PAT signal has been combined with pulse oximetry and wrist actigraphy in a wrist-worn portable monitor that is being studied as a home-based methodology for the diagnosis of OSA. In laboratory-based investigations comparing the PAT device with standard polysomnography performed simultaneously, there is excellent correlation between the PAT index and the AHI with high sensitivities and specificities [82, 83]. The PAT device has also been studied in the home and was found to have a high positive likelihood ratio for diagnosing moderate OSA [84].

Consequences of OSA

The significant consequences of OSA include comorbid medical conditions such as hypertension, and cognitive impairment.

Hypertension

The prevalence of hypertension is higher than expected in patients with OSA. The association has been known since 1970s; however, only some years later several studies showed OSA to be an independent risk factor for hypertension [85, 86]. The Wisconsin Sleep Cohort Study examined the development of hypertension as a function of OSA and found the unadjusted odds ratio for developing hypertension was 4.5 in patients with AHI greater than 15. When adjusted for age, sex, smoking, body habitus, and alcohol consumption, the odds ratio was 2.9. About of patients with one half OSA are affected by hypertension [87] and a linear relationship was identified between the severity of OSA and the prevalence of hypertension [88]. OSA and hypertension share several risk factors such as age, male gender, obesity, alcohol intake and smoking [89]. Negative effects of OSA on blood pressure appear to be more relevant in middle-aged compared with older subjects and are predominantly associated with increased systolic blood pressure [90]. Interestingly, OSA is the most common condition associated with drug-resistant hypertension with an estimated prevalence of 64% among subjects with resistant hypertension [91]. Not only systemic hypertension, but also high blood pressure in pulmonary circulation can complicate the course of the disease. In the most recent pulmonary hypertension guidelines, sleep-disordered breathing is included among the causes of secondary pulmonary hypertension [92].

The mechanisms linking sleep apnea and hypertension have been extensively reviewed [93]. There is increased sympathetic activity, which has been demonstrated in OSA patients using sympathetic micro-neurography of the nerves supplying muscles, and also using plasma and urinary catecholamine assays. Several potential mechanisms contributing to OSA-related hypertension have been described: endothelial dysfunction leading to inhibition of nitric oxide production, decreased vasodilatation, and increased vasoconstriction; systemic inflammation, which favours endothelial dysfunction; oxidative stress, which results in the production of reactive oxygen species and causes vasoconstriction as a result of nitric oxide synthase blockade, increased generation of endothelin-1, and activation of angiotensin II; activation of the renin–angiotensin–aldosterone system, which increases plasma aldosterone levels; and metabolic anomalies leading to hyperinsulinism and resistance to the metabolic effects of leptin, the adipocyte-derived hormone. Activation of the endothelin system results in vasoconstriction and depressed baroreflexes. Concerning the possible genetic contribution to the association between OSA and hypertension there is currently only a limited amount of available data. Animal models [94] and more recently a model developed in normal volunteers, [95, 96] showed the role of hypoxia in promoting an increase in blood pressure appears prominent. In the human model, it has been demonstrated that intermittent hypoxia during the night did not produce an immediate increase in blood pressure, presumably due to vasodilatation occurring in response to intermittent hypoxia counteracting the effects of sympathetic activation [96]. However, there was a sustained increase in sympathetic activity that seems to be responsible for the daytime increase in blood pressure observed in these subjects after only one night of intermittent hypoxia, which is more pronounced after 13 nights, and still tending to persist after 5 days of intermittent hypoxia exposure withdrawal [96]. Blood pressure lowering response to continuous positive airway pressure (CPAP) treatment appears to be dependent on sleep apnoea severity [97-99]. Recently, it has been clearly found that a reduction in blood pressure, as well as a reduced incidence of hypertension, cannot be achieved unless a minimum of 4–6 h of CPAP usage is achieved [100].

Cognitive Impairment

The extent of cognitive dysfunction in OSA is not fully understood, [101-103] however the literature data showed that OSA patients exhibit significant impairment on several neuropsychological tests [104-107]. Authors who have previously reviewed the evidence on OSA and cognitive functions have categorized cognition into four discrete domains: intellectual function, memory, attention, and executive function [104, 105]. Concerning the influence of OSA on intellectual function, deficits in measures of global intellectual function have been reported by individual studies [108-110]. However, a meta-analysis of twenty-five studies conducted by [111] showed no significant impairment in intellectual function in OSA patients compared with control subjects and normative data [111]. Alchanatis and co-workers (2005) [112] reported that OSA patients with intellectual function scores in the 90th percentile maintained normative attentional capacity: the authors suggested that high intellectual function may protect against the deterioration of some other cognitive abilities in OSA [112]. More extensively, researchers have investigated whether OSA has an impact within the different domains of memory. Several individual studies have suggested that OSA patients experience impairments in both short-term and long-term memory [110, 113-115]. More recent papers suggest that OSA may impair only some aspects of memory: patients perform significantly worse on tests of verbal memory, but not visual memory, when compared with controls [116,117]. Taken together, these studies underscore the importance of extensive testing of specific memory subdomains to fully understand memory deficits in OSA. The ability to maintain alertness over time is important in order to perform adequately during wakefulness. OSA has been identified as a contributing factor to increased daytime sleepiness in the population and a risk factor for falling asleep at the wheel [118]. Driving simulation instruments are designed to mimic real-world driving conditions and thus measure the reaction time and sustained attention of subjects [119]. OSA patients have clearly exhibited worse performance in these simulations compared with controls [118, 120-122]. Differences between individual with OSA and controls have been shown on more traditional neuropsychological tests of attention [123-125]. Executive functions collectively manage higher order cognitive processes, and are responsible for volition, planning, purposeful action and monitoring effective performance [126,127]. Some studies have shown that executive function may be significantly impacted by OSA [128,124]. One systematic review posited that executive function may be the cognitive domain most impaired in OSA [129]. Specifically, patients show impairment on tests that require set shifting, mental flexibility, and planning [130]. Other authors have reported disturbances in some, but not all, measures of executive function in individuals affected by OSA [114].

Several different mechanisms linking OSA to cognitive dysfunction have been proposed, and multiple processes may contribute to this impairment [131,104]. Excessive daytime somnolence (EDS), particularly in the domains of attention and executive function, is one proposed cause of cognitive dysfunction in OSA [132]. Lis and colleagues (2008) [128] showed that slower reaction time was correlated with increased subjective sleepiness in a sample of OSA patients [128]. A second proposed mechanism for cognitive dysfunction in

OSAS is intermittent hypoxemia. Several studies of patients with OSA typically have suggested that greater hypoxemia is associated with poorer memory performance. Recently, Yaffe and colleagues (2011) [133] aimed to determine the prospective relationship between OSA and cognitive impairment as well as the potential underlying mechanisms in a sample of 298 women without dementia. Overnight in-home polysomnography provided data on hypoxia, sleep-fragmentation, and sleep duration at the study baseline, while cognitive assessment (normal, mild cognitive impairment, or dementia) was performed approximately 5 years later via neuropsychological tests. In a multivariate logistic regression adjusting for age, body mass index, education level, presence of diabetes, and baseline cognitive scores, sleep-disordered breathing was associated with development of cognitive impairment (odds ratio, 1.85; 95% confidence interval, 1.11-3.08). Measures of intermittent hypoxia (oxygen desaturation index and high percentage (>7%) of sleep time in apnea or hypopnea) were associated with mild cognitive impairment or dementia, suggesting that hypoxia is a likely mechanism through which OSA increases risk for cognitive impairment. Yaffe and co-workers (2011) [133] also found that sleep fragmentation (arousal index and wake after sleep onset) or sleep duration (total sleep time) were not associated with risk of mild cognitive impairment or dementia. However, their study focused on older women, and it is known that older adults appear somewhat less sensitive than young adults to sleep fragmentation or sleep reduction [134].

The current literature examining neuroimaging-derived neural correlates in patients with OSA has made some important preliminary contributions. Techniques including MRI and magnetic resonance spectroscopy can provide unique information about brain structures, function, and metabolic composition that are affected by the disorder. While conventional structural neuroimaging studies in OSA patients have reported inconclusive findings, imaging studies using voxel-based morphometry (VBM) reported alterations in several gray matter regions, including areas that regulate memory, executive function, and affect (e.g. frontal cortex, anterior cingulate, and hippocampus). One study compared gray matter in 21 males with OSA with 21 controls, and found significant reductions in gray matter in several brain region (i.e. anterior cingulate, hippocampus, frontal, parietal, and temporal lobes) that correlated with OSA severity [135]. In another study, gray matter loss was demonstrated in the hippocampus, a key area for cognitive processing [136]. Yaouhi and co-workers (2009) [137] reported gray matter loss in frontal and temporo–parieto–occipital cortices and hippocampal and cerebellar regions despite minor memory and motor impairments. Canessa and co-workers (2011) [138] found that reduced gray matter volume in the left hippocampus, left posterior parietal cortex, and right superior frontal gyrus of severe OSA patients was associated with cognitive dysfunctions. As regard to the detection of subtle structural white matter alterations in OSA patients, Macey and co-workers (2008) [139] used Diffusion Tensor Imaging (DTI) to examine Fractional Anisotropy (FA), a measure of white matter integrity, among 41 OSA patients. Patients showed several areas of abnormal FA when compared to controls, suggesting a bilateral and nearly global white matter involvement in OSA. Recently, Kumar and co-workers (2012) [140] assessed global mean and regional brain MD values in newly-diagnosed, treatment-naïve OSA over age- and gender-matched control subjects using DTI procedures. The authors hypothesized that global mean MD values will be reduced in OSA patients compared with control subjects, and localized declines in MD values will appear in multiple brain areas, indicative of acute injury at those sites. Mean global brain MD values were significantly reduced in OSA compared with controls. Multiple brain sites in

OSA, including medullary, cerebellar, basal ganglia, prefrontal and frontal, limbic, insular, cingulum bundle, external capsule, corpus callosum, temporal, occipital, and corona radiata regions showed reduced regional MD values compared with controls. The results suggest that global brain MD values are significantly reduced in OSA, with certain regional sites especially affected, presumably a consequence of axonal, glial, and other cell changes in those areas. According to the authors, these findings likely represent acute pathological processes in newly-diagnosed OSA subjects. It is known that CPAP normalizes both sleep disruption and oxygen desaturation in OSA patients. The effects of CPAP on cognitive function have been an area of interest for many apnea researchers. In the 1980s, some researchers provided first evidence of short-term effect of CPAP on improvement in a variety of cognitive deficits. In a review of CPAP treatment studies in peer reviewed journals from 1985 to 2002, Aloia and co-workers examined whether pre-treatment cognitive impairments were permanent or if they remitted with CPAP treatment [106]. Overall, a positive association between treatment adherence and improved cognitive performance has been reported in these studies More recently, significant improvement in cognitive performance following CPAP treatment was reported in studies.

Table 1. Results of some studies on cognition and OSA before and after CPAP treatment

Author	Sample/Age	Methods	Results
Engleman et al., 1999 [141]	34 Pts (13 W) average age 44± 8	A randomized, placebo controlled crossover design, in which all patients spent 4 weeks on CPAP and 4 weeks on an oral placebo therapy with no washout period, with randomization of treatment order.	Cognitive improvements with CPAP (on digit symbol substitution and PASAT, with a trend in Trail Making A) were small in size and obtained from test drawing on attention skills.
Muñoz et al., 2000 [142]	80 Pts (mean age 49±1, Sex M/F 78/2) vs 80 HC (mean age 46±1, Sex M/F 78/2) AHI/RDI=60±2	In Pts and HC, measures were obtained at the beginning of the study and 12±1 months later.	Results showed that before treatment, Pts had a longer reaction time and poorer vigilance. The use of CPAP improved significantly. Reaction time changes were minor.
Bardwell et al., 2001 [143]	20 CPAP treated Pts, mean age 47±1.9 16 Placebo Group, 48±2.2 AHI/RDI= Placebo Group 43.6±6.4 CPAP 56.8±5.4	OSA Pts were randomized for 1 week treatment to CPAP or placebo and were tested before and after treatment with a neuropsychological battery	Only one (Digit Vigilance Time) of the 22 scores showed significant changes specific to CPAP treatment.
Aloia et al., 2003 [144]	12 Pts 6 COMPLIANT (>6 h usage per night) mean age 64.8±6.4 NON COMPLIANT (< 6 h usage per night) 64.8±2.6 AHI/RDI= COMPLIANT 51.2±19.8 NON COMPLIANT 45.9±21.7	Participants were administered a full NP battery before and 3 months after treatment with CPAP	Compliant use of CPAP at 3 months was associated with greater improvement in attention, psychomotor speed, executive functioning and non-verbal delayed recall.
Ferini-Strambi et al., 2003 [115]	23 OSA Pts, mean age 56.52±6.13 AHI/RDI=54.95±13.37	Neuropsychological evaluation was performed in the OSA Pts before the	After 15-days CPAP treatment attentive, visuospatial learning, and

Author	Sample/Age	Methods	Results
		beginning of CPAP treatment, and after 15 days and 4 months of CPAP.	motor performances returned to normal levels. A 4-months CPAP treatment did not result in any further improvement in cognitive tests.
Barnes at al., 2004 [145]	114 OSA pts (mean age 47.0±0.9) AHI/RDI 21.3±1.3	The responses to 3 months of treatment with nasal CPAP, a mandibular advancement splint and placebo tablet were compared. At the beginning of the trial and at the end of each 3-month treatment period, all subjects underwent overnight polysomnography, comprehensive neurobehavioral testing.	A broad range of neuropsychological function was assessed, CPAP increased vigilance, and both CPAP and mandibular advanced splint were superior to placebo in improving executive cognitive function. No other treatment effects on neurocognitive function were observed.
Zimmerman et al., 2006 [146]	58 Pts (mean age 48.1±10.1) AHI/RDI=46.1±27.9	Participants were administered neuropsychological testing prior to the initiation of PAP treatment and at 3 month follow-up visit. (sample divided in POOR USERS (n=14) averaged <2 h of PAP; MODERATE USERS (n=25) 2 to 6h; OPTIMAL (n=19) users > 6h per night).	Impaired verbal memory performance in Pts with OSA may be reversible with optimal levels of PAP treatment. OSA Pts exhibiting verbal memory impairments may experience a clinically meaningful benefit in their memory abilities when they use PAP for at least 6h per night.
Lim et al., 2007 [147]	17 CPAP treated Pts, mean age 46.7±2.4, 15 Oxygen treated Pts 47.1±2.3 14 Placebo 48.9±3.2 AHI/RDI= Placebo 65.8±8.2 CPAP 63.5±7.8 Oxygen 58.6±8.3	Subject received one of the 3 treatments (therapeutic C-PAP, supplemental oxygen, and placebo-CPAP) in a random fashion and were tested with a neuropsychological test battery before and after treatment.	2 weeks of CPAP treatment might be helpful in terms of speed of information processing, vigilance, or sustained attention and alertness.
Antic et al., 2011 [148]	174 OSA patients 50.1 ± 12.0	Participants were assessed pre-treatment and again after 3 months of CPAP therapy.	Greater percentage of patients achieve normal functioning with longer
		At the beginning and at the conclusion of the trial, participants completed a day of testing that included measures of objective and subjective daytime sleepiness, neurocognitive function, and quality of life.	nightly CPAP duration of use, but a substantial proportion of patients will not normalize neurobehavioral responses despite seemingly adequate CPAP use.

M=male; W= women, Pts= patients, OSA= obstructive sleep apnea, HC= healthy controls,

Table 2. Results of some studies on neuroimaging and OSA before and after CPAP treatment

Author	Sample/Age	Methods	Results
O'Donoghue et al., 2005 [149]	27 OSA Pts, mean age 45.7±10.1, 24 HC mean age 43.3±9.4 AHI/RDI= 71.7±17.0	27 M, untreated Pts with severe sleep apnea without comorbidities, and 24 age-matched HC had T1-weighted brain imaging in a high resolution magnetic resonance scanner. 23 Pts with sleep apnea had repeat imaging after 6 months of CPAP.	No gray matter volume deficits or focal structural changes in severe OSA. Whole brain volume decreases without focal changes after 6 months of CPAP.
Tonon at al., 2007 [150]	14 OSA Pts vs 10 matched HC AHI/RDI=58	CPAP Pts underwent a single voxel 1H-MRS in the parietal-occipital cortex before and after 6 months of CPAP	OSAS Pts have cortical metabolic changes that persisted after CPAP treatment
Castronovo et al., 2009 [151]	17 OSA Pts never treated, M, mean age 43.93±7.78, 15 HC, M, age- and education matched, 42.15±6.64 AHI/RDI= 50.14±24.84	OSA Pts and HC underwent fMRI scanning. They were compared on performance and brain activation during a 2-back working-memory task. Pts were also re-evaluated after 3-months treatment with PAP.	OSA Pts showed an over recruitment of brain regions compared to HC, in the presence of the same level of performance on a working-memory task. Decreases of activation in prefrontal and hippocampal structures were observed after treatment in comparison to baseline.
Aloia et al., 2009 [152]	9 OSA Pts (4 W), mean age 51.1±9.3 AHI/RDI= 42.4±28.2	Pts performed a 2-back verbal working memory paradigm during repeated fMRI. Counterbalanced fMRI sessions were under conditions of PAP treatment or non-treatment.	Treatment effects on 2-back-related brain activity were significant, with greater deactivation in the right posterior insula and overactivation in the right inferior parietal lobe.
Sweet et al., 2010 [153]	10 OSA pts (4W), mean age 51.1±9.3 AHI/RDI 42.4±28.2	Ten OSA patients performed a 2-Back working memory task during functional magnetic resonance imaging in two separate conditions, following regular CPAP use, and after two nights of CPAP withdrawal.	Withdrawal of CPAP treatment alters the brain response in regions normally deactivated during a verbal working memory challenge in OSA patients.
Canessa et al., 2011 [138]	17 OSA Pts, mean age 44±7.63, 15 HC mean age 42.15±6.64 AHI/RDI = 55.83±19.08	All Pts underwent a MRI at baseline and after 3 months to assess therapy efficacy.	Focal reduction of gray-matter volume in the left hippocampus (enthorinal cortex), left posterior parietal cortex, and right superior frontal gyrus. After treatment, gray matter volume increases in hippocampal and frontal structures.

Author	Sample/Age	Methods	Results
O'Donoghue et al., 2012 [154]	30 severe OSA Pts, mean age 45.2±9.6, 23 HC, mean age 41.3±9.3 AHI/RDI=71.5±16.2	Single voxel bilateral hippocampal and brainstem, and multivoxel frontal metabolite concentrations were measured using MRS (magnetic resonance spectroscopy), and repeated after 6 months CPAP.	OSA Pts have brain metabolite changes detected by MRS, suggestive of decreased frontal lobe neuronal viability and integrity, and decreased hippocampal membrane turnover. These regions have previously been shown to have no gross structural lesion using VBM. Little change was seen with CPAP treatment after 6 months.

M=male; W= women, Pts= patients, OSA= obstructive sleep apnea, HC= healthy controls.

Growing evidence suggest the OSA-related changes in brain morphology may improve with CPAP treatment. A recent study [139] evaluated the cognitive deficits and the corresponding brain morphology changes in OSA, and the modifications after 3-month CPAP treatment, using combined neuropsychologic testing and voxel-based morphometry. In pretreatment OSA they found that the cognitive impairments in most cognitive areas were associated with focal reductions of gray-matter volume in the left hippocampus (entorhinal cortex), left posterior parietal cortex, and right superior frontal gyrus. After treatment, the significant improvements involving memory, attention, and executive-functioning paralleled gray-matter volume increases in hippocampal and frontal structures.

Sleep-Related Movement Disorders

Diagnostic Definition

Sleep related movement disorders (SRMDs) are conditions that are primarily characterized by relatively simple, usually stereotyped, movements that can disturb sleep or by other sleep related monophasic movement disorders such as nocturnal cramps.

Nocturnal sleep disturbances or complaints of daytime sleepiness or fatigue are mandatory for a diagnosis of a SRMD. The history is usually telling, however polysomnography may be necessary to make a firm diagnosis of SRMDs. Since body movements that disturb sleep are also seen in other sleep disorder categories, e.g., in NREM and REM parasomnias, in some cases it is necessary to perform a video-polysomnography for the differential diagnosis.

Restless Legs Syndrome

Restless legs syndrome (RLS) is a sensorimotor disorder characterized by an unpleasant and uncomfortable feeling in the legs that leads to an urge to move. The diagnosis of RLS is largely based on the patient's report of clinical symptoms [155]. Individuals often have difficulty describing the unpleasant sensations experienced with RLS. Some of the terms used include "creepy crawling", "jittery", "soda bubbling in the veins", "worms moving", and "itching bones". A common thread appears to be the sensation of movement deep within the leg rather than superficially or on the surface of the leg. In some patients, RLS symptoms may also involve the arms. With increasing severity, symptoms may spread to the trunk and face. However, by definition, RLS must involve the legs. The need to move the legs and the unpleasant sensations are exclusively present or worsen during periods of rest or inactivity such as lying or sitting. Physical stimulation (e.g., rubbing the legs, walking) or intense, concentrated mental activity appear to reduce the symptoms. Factors that lead to reduced arousal (e.g., restricted or confined activity, drowsiness) tend to exacerbate or precipitate the symptoms. Another important clinical feature is the circadian variation of symptoms, which are worse in the evening and at night. In addition to the four essential criteria for an RLS diagnosis (Table 3), there are supportive clinical features that can help resolve diagnostic uncertainty and avoid misdiagnosis [156].

These include a positive family history of RLS and a positive therapeutic response to dopaminergic compounds. Both of these features may strongly help in the differential diagnosis. More than 50% of patients with primary RLS report familial pattern, and early onset of RLS symptoms (before the age of 45 years) indicates an increased risk of RLS occurrence in the family. Indeed, family history and age at onset appear to differentiate 2 phenotypes of RLS. Early-onset RLS, in which symptoms occur before 45 years of age, has an autosomal dominant mode of inheritance. Patients with earlier- rather than later-onset RLS generally have much slower progression of symptoms with age, have milder symptoms, and tend to have less relation between body iron stores and severity of disease.

Table 3. The four minimal criteria for the diagnosis of RLS

1.	a desire to move legs associated with a sensory discomfort;
2.	a motor restlessness that consists of moving;
3.	leg discomfort occurring predominantly at rest with at least temporary relief of discomfort occurring with movement;
4.	leg discomfort that is worse in the evening and at night. RLS can lead to severe sleep disruption, with daytime fatigue and other functional consequences

In subjects with a latter onset of RLS symptoms (>45 years of age), the symptoms progress more rapidly with advancing age. For this reason, the most severely affected individuals tend to be middle aged or elderly [157].

RLS may be divided into primary and secondary forms. Primary, or idiopathic, RLS refers to patients without associated conditions that may explain the symptoms. Secondary causes of RLS include pregnancy, and iron deficiency. RLS occurs more commonly in subjects that present these conditions; however, only approximately one third to one half of patients with these conditions develops RLS. Symptoms also resolve with resolution of the condition. For example, RLS occurs in approximately 20% of pregnant women, but symptoms usually resolve within 1-4 weeks after delivery. Successful kidney transplantation and treatment of iron deficiency anemia have also resulted in resolution of RLS symptoms [158].

RLS appears to be a chronic condition, however little is known about the pattern of expression of mild or intermittent RLS because most patients with this subtype typically do not seek treatment. It is also unknown whether this group experiences periods of remission.

The clinical course varies according to the age of onset. For those with more severe disease who seek medical attention, the severity and frequency of exacerbations usually increase over time. For those with late-onset RLS, there generally is a more rapid development of symptoms. In patients with early-onset RLS, symptoms develop more insidiously over many years and may not become persistent until the patient is 40 to 60 years of age. Although secondary RLS appears to remit with correction of the secondary condition, long-term studies are lacking [159]. In most of the cases, RLS patients are not aware of periodic limb movements (PLM), but occasionally they can refer of sudden involuntary movements or shakes of the limbs, usually involving the legs and occurring during the night especially in the transition from relaxed awake to sleep. When PLM occur during sleep, the patient complaining of frequent awakenings of bed-partner observations may help to in the clinical suspect of PLM. Subjects with PLM may report some generic associated symptoms such as non refreshing sleep, insomnia, excessive daytime sleepiness or weakness. However the medical history it is usually insufficient in sensitivity or specificity to supplant instrumental investigations in the diagnosis of PLM.

Sleep Related Leg Cramps

Leg cramps during sleep has been accepted as an individual nosological disorder characterized by a painful sensation in the leg or foot associated with sudden and strong muscle contraction, which occurs during sleep and is relived by forceful stretching of the affected muscles [160,7]. A detailed medical history is fundamental in the diagnosis of nocturnal leg cramps. In these cases the patients usually complain of abrupt involuntary and sustained contractions of one or a group of muscles associated with painful sensations and relived by stretching the affected region [160]. Leg cramps arise during night period either in wake or sleep and remit spontaneously after seconds or few minutes. Possible persistent leg discomfort after the cramp may delays the following return to sleep. Massages or heat applications may be other possible strategies used by the patients to improve the symptoms. Leg cramps occur more often in elderly people and in patients with neuromuscular, metabolic, endocrine and peripheral vascular disorders; and in young subjects after prolonged and intense exercise.

Bruxism

Sleep bruxism (SB) is defined as a stereotyped movement disorder occurring during sleep and characterized by tooth grinding (TG) and/or clenching [161]. The last International Classification of Sleep Disorders [7] categorizes SB as a sleep-related movement disorder. SB should be distinguished from the daytime-awake bruxism that is mainly related to "stress/anxiety" reactivity and expressed as a jaw muscle clenching habit/tic., TG is described as secondary or iatrogenic, when medical disorders, medication or drug use are present [162, 163]. Well-known consequences of SB are tooth destruction, temporomandibular joint and muscle pain or jaw lock, temporal headaches and cheek-biting [161, 162]. The odds ratio (OR) of reporting temporomandibular disorders or chronic myofascial pain of masticatory muscles, when clenching and/or grinding are concomitant, have been estimated at between 4.2 and 8.4 [164]. Up to 65% of SB patients of all ages report headaches [165]. The noise made by the TG can greatly disturb the sleep of bedroom partners. The following risk factors may exacerbate SB-TG: (1) smoking, caffeine and heavy alcohol drinking; (2) type A personality—anxiety; (3) sleep disorders such as snoring (OR:1.4), sleep apnea (OR:1.8) or PLMs (concomitant in 10%) [161, 162].

Prevalence

Restless Legs Syndrome

Ekbom initially estimated a 5% prevalence of RLS in the general population [166]. The largest epidemiological study of RLS involved more than 23,000 persons from five countries [167]. Similar to smaller reports, 9.6% of all people met criteria for RLS. In general, northern European countries demonstrated higher prevalence compared to Mediterranean countries. The vast majority of these subjects were not previously diagnosed, despite frequently reporting symptoms to their physicians.

Recently, some authors reviewed the nearly 50 community-based studies have been published in the last decade around the world [168]. The development of strict diagnostic criteria in 1995 and their revision in 2003 helped to stimulate research interest on this syndrome. In community-based surveys, RLS has been studied as: 1) a symptom only, 2) a set of symptoms meeting minimal diagnostic criteria of the international restless legs syndrome study group (IRLSSG), 3) meeting minimal criteria accompanied with a specific frequency and/or severity, and 4) a differential diagnosis. In the first case, prevalence estimates in the general adult population ranged from 9.4% to 15%. In the second case, prevalence ranged from 3.9% to 14.3%. When frequency/severity is added, prevalence ranged from 2.2% to 7.9% and when differential diagnosis is applied prevalence estimates are between 1.9% and 4.6%. In all instances, RLS prevalence is higher in women than in men. It also increases with age in European and North American countries but not in Asian countries. Symptoms of anxiety and depression have been consistently associated with RLS. In a recent study in depressed patients [169] RLS was reported by 31.48% of sample. There was no gender difference in prevalence of RLS (X^2 =0.46; P=0.33). There was no difference in the age , total duration of depressive illness and number of depressive episodes between RLS and non-RLS groups (F=0.44; P=0.77; Wilk's Lambda=0.96). The Hamilton depression score was higher in the non-RLS group. Concerning the epidemiology of secondary forms of RLS, there are new interesting data.

A survey investigated whether restless legs syndrome during pregnancy represented a risk factor for later development of RLS [170]. After a mean interval of 6.5 years, 207 parous women were contacted again to compare the incidence of RLS among subjects who never experienced the symptoms with those who reported RLS during the previously investigated pregnancy. The incidence of restless legs syndrome was 56% person/year in women who experienced the transient pregnancy restless legs syndrome form, and 12.6% person/year in subjects who did not, with a significant 4-fold increased risk of developing chronic restless legs syndrome in women who presented restless legs in the previous pregnancy. Thus, the transient pregnancy RLS form is a significant risk factor for the development of a future chronic RLS, and for a new transient symptomatology in a future pregnancy.

Another recent study evaluated the prevalence and clinical significance of RLS in iron-deficient anemic (IDA) population [171]. In this study all new patients referred for anemia to a community-based haematology practice over a 1-year period (March 2011-2012) were included if they had IDA and no RLS treatment. Patients completed a validated questionnaire identifying RLS, blood tests, and a sleep-vitality questionnaire (SVQ). Patients with RLS were compared to patients with no RLS for differences on SVQ, blood tests, baseline characteristics, and sleep quality. Three hundred forty-three patients were evaluated and 251 included in the study. The prevalence of clinically significant RLS was 23.9%, nine times higher than the general population. IDA-RLS sufferers reported poorer quality of sleep, decreased sleep time, increased tiredness, and decreased energy during the day compared to patients with IDA without RLS. Blood tests did not relate to RLS diagnosis but RLS was less likely for African-American than Caucasian patients. Clinically significant RLS occurs commonly with IDA producing much greater disruption of sleep and shorter sleep times than does IDA alone. Another recent study evaluated the prevalence of RLS in the chronic kidney disease (CKD) population and determine the relationship between severity of renal dysfunction and risk of RLS [172]. The prevalence of positive RLS in the CKD subjects was significantly higher than that in the controls (3.5% vs. 1.5%, $p = 0.029$). The proportion of renal failure (RF) in CKD subjects with RLS was significantly higher than in those without RLS, and multiple logistic regression analysis revealed that the presence of RLS symptoms was associated only with the existence of RF. In addition, the presence of both RLS and CKD was significantly associated with the presence of depression and sleep disturbance.

The incidence of PLM in the general population increases with age and is reported to occur in as many as 57% of elderly people [173-175]. Bixler reported that 29% of people over the age of 50 had PLM, whereas only 5% of those aged between 30 and 50 and almost none under 30 were affected [176]. PLMs in normal children are uncommon.

Sleep Related Leg Cramps

Leg cramps are a common condition with reported prevalence rates of 7.3% in children [177], 15% in young adults [178], 20% to 30% in middle-aged adults [179], and up to 60% in the elderly [180, 181]. Incidence rates in the elderly are considerably lower and range between 14% (4 weeks incidence [182]) and 30% (two months incidence [183]). In one study, frequent awakenings due to leg cramps were reported by 8.7% of men and 12.1% of women in the Sleep Heart Health Study comprising 6440 men and women aged 40 years or older [184]. There seems to be a slightly higher prevalence in women as evidenced by significant differences only emerging in very large-scale studies [179, 184].

Bruxism

Sleep bruxism is a frequent habit. In normal subjects, primary sleep bruxism is reported by 8% of the adult population. Its prevalence decreases with age from 14% in childhood to 3% in the elderly [185, 186] and no gender difference is observed. However, the exact prevalence of the disorder is difficult to estimate because, in most cases, there are no clinical symptoms.

Pathogenesis

Restless Legs Syndrome

Neuroimaging studies, autopsy investigations and experimental studies using animal models have been conducted to investigate the potential causes of RLS, resulting in the generation of multiple pathophysiological hypotheses. Dopamine dysfunction within basal ganglia pathways and iron deficiency have consistently been found to be involved. Pharmacological trials have provided evidence that the dopamine system may play a central role in the pathophysiology of RLS. L-dopa and dopaminergic agonists were highly effective in alleviating RLS symptoms and dopamine antagonists induced or worsened RLS [187], indicating that reduced central dopaminergic neurotransmission may underlie RLS. However, the abnormalities of the central dopaminergic neurotransmission in RLS might be more complex than only a simple decrease. Recent studies on postmortem brain and cerebrospinal fluid (CSF) have found that dopamine synthesis was increased in patients with severe RLS. Increased tyrosine hydroxylase activity was found both in autopsies of patients with RLS [188] and in the rodent iron-deprivation model of RLS [189]. D2 receptors in the putamen were significantly decreased in postmortem brains of patients with severe to very severe RLS [190]. Abnormally increased levels of CSF 3-O-methyldopa (3-OMD) and homovanillic acid were observed only in patients with severe RLS, suggesting that dopamine synthesis may be increased in more severe, but perhaps not mild, RLS [191]. Thus, the dopamine pathology underlying RLS can be different according to the phases or subtypes of RLS, and, therefore, different results pertaining to the dopaminergic dysfunction in patients with RLS might be obtained depending on the severity of the RLS of the tested subjects. A recent study evaluated whether reduced striatal dopaminergic neurotransmission was associated with moderate to moderately severe RLS [192]. Dopamine transporter density of patients with RLS was increased in the caudate (P = 0.037), posterior putamen (P = 0.041), and entire striatum (P = 0.046) compared with that of normal controls. DAT density was higher in the anterior putamen of patients with RLS than controls, although statistically not significant (P = 0.079). There was no difference in the D2 receptor density between patients with RLS and normal controls in the whole striatum or any of subregions. The authors concluded that dysregulation rather than simple upregulation or downregulation of central dopaminergic neurotransmission may underlie the pathogenesis of RLS, and decreased dopaminergic neurotransmission may cause moderate to moderately severe RLS.

There is evidence to suggest that defect in the brain iron metabolism may contribute to the pathogenesis of the disease. A lower cerebrospinal fluid (CSF) ferritin was reported in RLS cases [193]. Pathologic data in RLS autopsied brains show not only reduced ferritin staining, iron staining, and increased transferrin, but also reduced staining for transferrin receptors. Thy-1 expression, which is activated by iron, is also reduced [194] MRI studies have demonstrated low iron concentration in the substantia nigra and decrease in ferritin concentrations in the cerebrospinal fluid of patients of RLS. [195,196] Another study revealed a decrease in transferrin receptor expression in the microvasculature of blood brain interface [197]. These findings along with the significant response observed after initiation of iron therapy—intravenous or oral—and erythropoietin, further supports the iron-RLS relation [198, 199]. An inverse relationship has been suggested between symptom severity and serum ferritin levels finding, which is observed in children as well [200]. Interestingly, iron is a cofactor for tyrosine hydroxylase, which is a rate-limiting step in the conversion of levodopa to dopamine. Therefore decrease in iron may affect the availability of dopamine. It has been identified that there is a circadian variation in the activity of tyrosine hydroxylase that may account for the worsening of symptoms in the night [201]. A genetic contribution to primary RLS has been well documented, is substantial, and has been consistently recognized from population and family studies. Ekbom, who first described RLS in 1945, described familial aggregation in one third of RLS patients in 1960 [166]. To date, nine major susceptibility loci for RLS have been identified by linkage analysis [202-209]. Only one locus has been reported under an autosomal recessive (AR) model. Originally reported in a French Canadian family, AR RLS linked to chromosome 12q has since been reported in several other French Canadian families as well as in the Icelandic population [210, 211]. Evidence of linkage in all other instances assumed an autosomal dominant inheritance model and is limited to single or a small number of kindreds. Genome-wide association studies have identified variants suspected to be involved in RLS. Single nucleotide polymorphisms (SNPs) in the BTBD9 gene on chromosome 6p21 have been found to be associated with RLS [212, 213]. Additionally, variants in the intronic and intergenic regions of the MEIS1, MAP2K5/LBXCOR1, PTPRD, and NOS1 genes have been identified in association studies [212, 214-215]. These molecular findings suggest substantial genetic heterogeneity in RLS. Another recent investigation of an Irish family with autosomal dominant RLS reported a novel RLS locus on chromosome 19p13.3, providing further evidence of genetic heterogeneity of RLS [216].

Periodic Limb Movements (PLM)

The exact pathophysiology of PLM is not known. From their initial description, similarities with the Babinski sign lead to speculation that they result from cortical disinhibition. Subsequent research has generally supported this. First, back-averaging techniques triggered from the movements do not elicit any cortical potentials, suggesting that they are not generated from the cortex [217]. Second, functional MRI demonstrates increased pontine and red nucleus activity during PLM in RLS patients [218]. The cortex was not abnormal. The spinal cord is implicated by the phenomenology of the movements, the fact that spinal cord injury often causes PLM, and evidence of spinal cord disinhibition and spatial spread [219, 220]. PLM are also associated with other rhythmic, often autonomic activities. They are often accompanied by K-complexes, and by increases in pulse and blood pressure [217]. The K complexes usually precede the PLMS and may persist even if PLMS are reduced with L-dopa [221]. PLM may also correlate with the cyclic alternating pattern seen in electroencephalogram [222].

Dopamine systems are strongly suggested by the response to dopaminergic treatments [223].

Inhibition of dopaminergic tracts that descend to the spinal cord may be involved. These are reciprocally inhibited by descending serotonergic systems, which may explain why serotonergic reuptake inhibitors precipitate PLM [224, 225]. Indeed, it has been reported in 274 consecutive patients taking antidepressants that venlafaxine and selective serotonin reuptake inhibitors had significantly higher mean PLMIs than control and bupropion groups [225]. Interestingly, a very recent study evaluated the influence of amitriptyline on PLMS during sleep in healthy subjects [226]. Amitriptyline can induce or even increase the number of PLM during sleep in healthy subjects. When treating sleep disturbances with amitriptyline, PLM should be considered as a possible cause of insufficient improvement.

Bruxism

Several hypotheses have been proposed for the sleep bruxism (SB), but no single mechanism or theory may fully explain the pathophysiology of this motor activity.

Stress and anxiety have been suggested as possible cause of SB [227, 228], but rigorous evidence is lacking to support the notion that SB is an anxiety-related disorder [229]. The possible involvement of the dopaminergic system remains to be confirmed. It is known that dopamine has a role in the execution of movement and in maintaining vigilance during wakefulness. During sleep the dopaminergic system is probably minimally active at the exception of brief period of arousal related movements such as periodic limb movements [230]. Some authors hypothesized that in SB there is an asymmetry in the dopamine uptake level of D2 receptors in the basal ganglia. This asymmetry could favour the appearance of SB in stressful conditions that stimulate the production and secretion of dopamine in the substantia nigra of the midbrain (mesocorticolimbic and nigrostriatal pathways). However, in most randomized experimental trials with dopaminergic medications (e.g., l-dopa, bromocriptine), the onset of SB episodes is only marginally reduced [230, 231].

Another catecholamine-related medication reported to reduce SB and teeth grinding is propanolol, a beta-blocker [232]. However, a controlled study in young patients with SB showed that propanolol did not reduce teeth grinding nor did it influence the frequency or duration of jaw muscle contraction [233].

Researches with the recording of masseter electromyographic activity to assess rhythmic masticatory motor activity (RMMA) in the jaw-closer muscles found that about 60% of normal sleepers showed RMMA during sleep [162]. In SB, RMMA probably represents an extreme manifestation of an ongoing or natural activity during sleep. An hypothesis on genesis of nocturnal RMMA is that, conversely to wake state, cortico-bulbar influences are not dominant during sleep. The top-down circuits seem to be partially de-activated during sleep to preserve the so-called sleep continuity [234]. Some evidences support this hypothesis in the physiopathology of SB: (1) a specific increase in the cortical activity, over the motor cortex, precedes most limb movements. This brief and large deflection of brain wave activity is termed pre-motor potential. It has been reported that RMMA are not preceded by such pre-motor cortical potential during sleep [229]. Thus, SB is not generated by a clear pattern of cortical activation; (2) SB episodes are not associated with the so-called cortical K-complexes that are electroencephalographic (EEG) marker of sudden changes in brain activity [235]; (3) In the macaca fascicularis, the intracortical microstimulation (ICMS) threshold did not evoke RMMA (or a rhythmic jaw movements = RJM) responses from the cortical masticatory area (CMA) during light non-REM sleep in comparison to the quiet awake state [236]. However, as soon as the animal wakes up, there is a rapid return of RJM at ICMS threshold levels comparable to pre-sleep. These data suggest that the geneses of RJM or RMMA during sleep are probably not directly under the influence of the cortical network as seen during wake condition.

Another hypothesis is that the onset of RMMA and SB episodes during sleep are under the influences of transient activity of the brainstem arousal. It is possible that the sudden onset of RMMA during sleep is occurring in brief time windows at which the brain is switching from sleep to an aroused state. These periods are termed micro-arousal which is defined as 3–15 s abrupt shifts in EEG activity accompanied by a rise in heart rate and muscle tone. Micro-arousals (MA) tends to recur 8–15 times per hour of sleep in young healthy subjects [237].

To initiate non-REM sleep, a massive inhibition of GABA on brain arousal ascending system is needed to reverse the influences of arousal related orexin/hypocretin, from the hypothalamus, and on acetylcholine, noradrenalin, histamine and serotonin brain networks238. Moreover, from the sleep onset, a reduction in muscle tone to a clear hypotonia in the REM sleep stages is observed. It is further suggested that the reduction of muscle tone during REM sleep is under the influences of noradrenergic neurons of the peduculopontine tegmentum neurons and of GABA and glycine inhibition on both brainstem and spinal cord motoneurons [238, 239].

SB tends to occur in relation to recurrent MA within the so-called cyclic alternating pattern or CAP240. MA are characterized by a repetitive rise in heart and brain activity within sleep and they represent a natural process for maintaining body homeostasis [241]. Some authors explored the role of MA, as a physiological state that may increase the probability of initiating an episode of SB, with the use of a sensory vibrator during sleep [242]. Experimentally induced RMMA related MA were followed by TG in over 70% of trials in SB patients only and not in control subjects. The same research group also demonstrated that the onset of SB is related to a sequence of physiological activations in relation to the MA243. A rise in sympathetic cardiac activity around 4 min before RMMA; b) A rise in the frequency of EEG activity 4 s before RMMA; c) A tachycardia starting one heart beat before RMMA.

Subjective Assessment Tools

Restless Legs Syndrome

Three validated scales are usually used to quantify RLS symptom severity. One was developed by the IRLSSG [244]. It is a 10-question scale; the questionnaire typically is completed by a person trained in administering the scale, who records the patient's responses during an interview. The scale is divided into 5 questions that ask about symptom frequency and intensity, and 5 questions that address the impact of symptoms on daily life and sleeping. Each item is rated on a 5-point scale; higher scores represent greater RLS severity. Therefore, the sum score ranges from 0 (no RLS symptoms present) to 40 (maximum severity in all symptoms).

The second scale was developed by the Johns Hopkins RLS Research Group [155]. It focuses on the circadian characteristics, or the time of onset of symptoms. It is easier to use and has only 4 ratings (from 0 = none to 3 = severe). A 0 score means the patient has no symptoms. A score of 3 means the symptoms begin in early afternoon or may be present all day.

The third scale is the RLS-6 that consists of 6 subscale [245]. The subscales assess severity of symptoms at the following times of the day/evening: falling asleep, during the night, during the rest at day, and during the day when engaged in daytime activities. In addition, the subscales assess satisfaction with sleep and severity of daytime tiredness/sleepiness. Scores for each subscales ranges from 0 (completely satisfied) to 10 (completely dissatisfied).

The RLS-QoL is used to evaluate changes in quality of life due to RLS symptoms [246]. This disease-specific instrument consists of 12 items. In general, the items address the effects of RLS symptoms on sleep, activities of daily living, mood, social interactions, and coping behaviors. Scores for each item range from 0 (not at all) to 5 (extremely).

A recent study tried to validate the use of a single standard question for the rapid screening of RLS [247]. The question is the following: "When you try to relax in the evening or sleep at night, do you ever have unpleasant restless feelings in your legs that can be relieved by walking or movement?" The authors found that, in comparison to the four standard criteria, the single question had 100% sensitivity and 96.8% specificity for the diagnosis of RLS. This study represents the effort to simplify both the clinical and the epidemiological approaches to the diagnosis of RLS.

Objective Assessment

Restless Legs Syndrome and Periodic Limb Movements

Given that the four essential criteria for the diagnosis of RLS are ascertainable by an accurate clinical approach, objective investigations are not really mandatory to verify the presence of RLS [248, 249]. However, instrumental evaluations may be useful in several situations such as in doubtful RLS cases, differential diagnosis, distinction between primary and secondary RLS forms, sleep impact estimation, diagnosis and quantification of PLM, and valuation of treatment efficacy on sleep and PLM.

The gold standard in documenting the above mentioned RLS features is considered the full night polysomnographic study (PSG), which should always include the monitoring of both tibialis anterior (TA) muscles for the PLM detection. The actigraphy, the suggestion and the forced immobilization tests, have been proposed as possible cost-effective substitute of PSG.

Other neurophysiological techniques, such as electromyography and motor/somato-sensitive evoked potentials represent second line instrumental tools helpful in identifying neurological symptomatic RLS forms [250].

Methods for recording and scoring PLM were first established by Coleman and colleague [251], accepted by the American Association of Sleep Disorders in 1993 [252], and recently revised [72].

The final polysomnographic report usually include the absolute number of PLM, and the PLM index (number of PLM per hour of sleep), both of the parameters may be considered separately for wakefulness and sleep time and eventually for each sleep stages. PLM arousal index stands for the number of PLM associated with an arousal per hour of sleep. A PLM index greater than 5 for the entire night is usually considered pathologic, despite data supporting this feature are very limited. When a PLMS index of 5 or greater associates with otherwise unexplained sleep-wake complaint the diagnosis of the periodic limb movement disorder (PLMD) can be defined.

The suggested immobilization test (SIT) and the forced immobilization test (FIT) were validated in 1998 as two polysomnographic tests able to identify and score PLM during wakefulness (PLMW) [253]. During the SIT the patients are asked to sit at a 45-degree angle in bed with their legs outstretched, and were instructed not to move. During the FIT, the patient sits at a 45-degree angle in bed with the legs immobilized in a stretcher. The number of PLMW index (number of PLMW per hour) represents the main outcome measure. If a patient, due to the RLS symptoms, is unable to maintain the rest position till the end of the test, the movement index has to be calculated as the number of the PLMW multiplied for 60 minutes and divided for the duration in minutes of the test until that moment. According to

Montplaisir and colleague [253] a SIT movement index greater than 40 is considered abnormal, while it should be greater than 25 for the FIT. Using these pathological thresholds, the clinical RLS diagnosis is correctly predicted in 81% of subjects [254]. SIT has been used more than FIT, probably because it does not need any special equipment to hold the legs. The low cost and the possibility to repeat the tests more time during the day are the two major advantages associated with SIT and FIT.

General evidences for eventual RLS or PLM's related insomnia may come from the ordinary actigraphic monitoring by placing the device at the not dominant wrist of the patient [255]. This analysis usually shows an increase of the mean motor activity during the first part of the night usually proportionally with severity of the symptoms. By attaching the accelerometer to one, or better, to both the ankles (to both the big toes for particular versions), also PLM can be reliably diagnosed [256]. This method has few advantages, such as the low cost, the portability, and the possibility to record for long period, but does not collect any other information regarding sleep.

Sleep Related Leg Cramps

Sleep related leg cramps may coexist with other sleep disorders, especially in elderly and may be confused with RLS/PLM [160, 257, 258]. Only in case of hard differential diagnosis with other sleep related movement disorder a full-night PSG including EMG of both TA and eventually the affected movements, together with the video-recording, is indicated. The typical cramp lasts usually from 1 to several minutes and appears as a tonic stereotyped EMG activity.

Bruxism

In most of the cases clinicians can diagnose sleep bruxism by an accurate medical history supported by a visual inspection of orofacial structures [7, 257-259]. The typical teeth grinding or tapping is usually noted by the patient's partner or family members. Orofacial discomfort, such as pain, fatigue, muscular tension, and teeth hypersensitivity to cold food or beverages are often reported by the patient [260, 261]. Instrumental techniques are recommended only in specific cases: confirmation of diagnosis in uncertain patients; severe bruxism; differential diagnosis, especially with other sleep disorders; scoring of bruxism episodes for a better severity quantification or for research purpose; documentation of teeth and oro-mandibular damage.

The first level of instrumental diagnosis is represented by the ambulatory assessment of bruxism by the detection of sound, EMG activity of masticatory muscles or pressure exerted by jaw movements. Self-made audio-video recordings may be useful in confirm bruxism and verify its frequency of occurrence. Ambulatory polygraphic monitoring is available with different levels of complexity. Ambulatory polygraphy may provide a good quality of signal and, depending on the number of recorded parameters, a high reliable diagnosis. Moreover ambulatory techniques allow a low-cost monitoring of even more than one night in the habitual environment of the patient. The lower specificity of ambulatory compared to laboratory polysomnography in differentiate bruxism to other orofacial physiological (talking, yawning, coughing, swallowing) or pathological (oro-mandibular myoclonus, nocturnal groaning, epileptic bursts) activities, mainly depend of the absence of the audio-video recording during ambulatory studies [262].

The typical polysomnographic pattern of bruxism (figure 2) is characterized by rhythmic bursts of masticatory muscle activity, usually at 1 Hz of frequency, with a duration ranging between 0.25 to 2 s, accompanied by muscular artifacts on EEG channels. When the single burst of masseter exceed 2 s in duration, generally is classified as tonic bruxism, while shorter contractions as phasic.

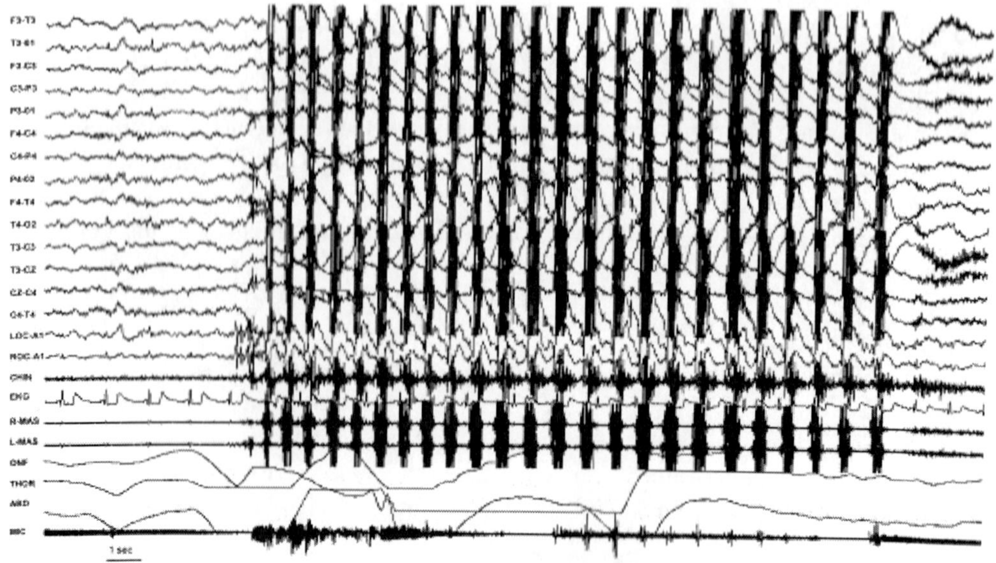

Abbreviations: LOC, ROC =left and right electro-oculogram; A1, A2 = left and right earlobes; EKG = electrocardiogram; R-MAS, L-MAS = right and left masseter muscles; ONF = oro-nasal flow; THOR = thoracic movements; ABD = abdominal movements; MIC = microphone.

Figure 2. Polysomnographic example of bruxism during NREM stage 2.

Consequences

Mild RLS may have relatively few consequences; however, severe RLS can result in a marked reduction in quality of life. Sleep deprivation greatly contributes to this as does the learned helplessness and frustration derived from the sensations themselves. Abetz and colleague demonstrated a selected group of RLS subjects who sought treatment at a tertiary referral center and had quality of life score (Medical Outcomes Study Short Form-36 [SF-36]) as bad or worse to those in-patients with congestive heart failure, diabetes mellitus, and osteoarthritis [263].

Berger and colleague [264] used a cross-sectional survey and a face-to-face interview. This was a population-based health study cohort that involved a little over 4000 subjects, with 433 people having been identified as having RLS. SF-12 mental health and SF-12 physical health scores were used as well as individual patients' ratings of their overall health. The study by Allen [265] was a general population survey and involved a little over 15,000 subjects from the United States and several European countries. The SF-36 was used for quality of life in the United States and involved 158 RLS patients who completed that questionnaire. Kushida [266] did a random-digital dial telephone interview with stratification across the US population using trained interviewers from which 158 individuals were identified as having RLS. He used the SF-36 and the physical and mental summary scores. For this population, the author's criteria for RLS included the four essential diagnostic criteria plus symptom severity of two or more times per week and a reporting of moderate or severely distressing.

Several studies overall have been fairly consistent in demonstrating increased prevalence or risk of depressive and anxiety symptoms in RLS patients. Some inconsistencies across the data have been on the basis of gender with some studies reporting the increased risk of depression only in men with RLS. These were primarily surveys in elderly populations (>64 years) in which men and not women with RLS had increased risk for depression [267-268].

There is some concern in interpreting these data that that there may be an overlap in the symptomatology of depression and RLS. Of the nine criteria considered in making a diagnosis of major depression (five out of the nine need to be present to make the diagnosis), at least four and possibly five of those criteria could be reported by most RLS patients with at least some sleep disturbance. Those would include psychomotor agitation, diminished concentration, fatigue/loss of energy, insomnia and diminished interests. These symptoms have been better defined and characterized on the SF-36, and, as noted above, patients with even mild RLS symptoms have markedly lower scores. Most research on the association between RLS and depression has involved cross-sectional data. A recent study [269] evaluated this issue prospectively among Nurses' Health Study participants. A total of 56,399 women (mean age = 68 years) who were free of depression symptoms at baseline (2002) were followed until 2008.

Physician-diagnosed RLS was self-reported. During 300,155 person-years of follow-up, the authors identified 1,268 incident cases of clinical depression (regular use of antidepressant medication and physician-diagnosed depression). Women with RLS at baseline were more likely to develop clinical depression (multivariate-adjusted relative risk (RR) = 1.5, 95% confidence interval (CI): 1.1, 2.1; P = 0.02) than those without RLS.

There have been several studies that have looked at the risk of cardiovascular disease in RLS populations. Ulfberg [270] used a randomized sampling of 4000 men in a Swedish population using self-reporting questionnaires on sleep habits, somatic issues, health and neuropsychiatric complaints. There were 2801 respondents of which 181 were considered to have RLS. The RLS group compared to those without RLS had a significant odds ratio (OR) of 2.5 for "heart problems" and a non-significant OR of 1.5 for hypertension.

Ohayon and Roth [271], using telephone interview techniques across five European countries, administered a broad-based sleep survey (Sleep-EVAL). The population was any non-institutionalized residents age 15 years or older. The final sample included nearly 19,000 subjects, of whom 732 were defined as having RLS symptoms. There was a significantly greater percentage of hypertension, heart disease and diabetes in the RLS population. Winkelman [272] utilized the Wisconsin Sleep Cohort, which is a community-based, questionnaire-driven population in which sleep studies were performed. A total of 2821 subjects were surveyed and 898 subjects had in-laboratory evaluations. There were 137 subjects who had daily RLS symptoms, 163 RLS who had between 1 and 6 episodes per week, 903 persons identified with leg complaints without RLS and 1618 subjects with no RLS symptoms and no leg complaints. The RLS group with daily symptoms, but not those with less frequent symptoms, in comparison with the "no-RLS group," had a significant increased risk (OR = 2.58) of cardiovascular disease (CVD), which was defined broadly in this study. The risk of hypertension was not significant for either of the RLS groups.

In the Sleep Heart Health Study (a cross-sectional, community-based prospective cohort), Winkelman [273] identified over 3000 subjects without RLS and 179 subjects with RLS. They found a higher risk of both coronary artery disease (OR = 2.05) and cardiovascular disease (OR = 2.07) in the RLS population, after controlling for age, sex, race, BMI, diabetes, systolic blood pressure, anti-hypertension medication use, total cholesterol, LDL cholesterol ratio and smoking history. Patients with RLS symptoms occurring more than half the month and those with moderate to severe RLS had the highest risk for coronary artery disease (CHD) or cerebrovascular disease. This study also did not find a RLS-attributed risk for hypertension.

A recent study prospectively examined whether RLS was associated with an increased risk of CHD in women who participated in the Nurses' Health Study, taking into account the duration of RLS symptoms [274].

A total of 70 977 women (mean age, 67 years) who were free of CHD and stroke at baseline (2002) were followed up until 2008. Physician-diagnosed RLS was collected via questionnaire. CHD was defined as nonfatal myocardial infarction or fatal CHD. Women with RLS at baseline had a marginally higher risk of developing CHD (multivariable-adjusted hazard ratio, 1.46; 95% confidence interval, 0.97–2.18) compared with women without RLS. The risk was dependent on duration of symptoms: 0.98 (95% confidence interval, 0.44–2.19) for women with RLS for <3 years and 1.72 (95% confidence interval, 1.09–2.73) for women with RLS for ≥3 years (P trend=0.03). The multivariable-adjusted hazard ratios of women with RLS for ≥3 years were 1.80 (95% confidence interval, 1.07–3.01) for nonfatal myocardial infarction and 1.49 (95% confidence interval, 0.55–4.04) for fatal CHD relative to women without RLS.

That RLS/PLMS may be associated with an increase in CVD is not surprising. It is well known that insomnia and OSA also contribute to an increased risk for hypertension and CVD, albeit likely through different mechanisms. Disorders such as RLS/PLMS, insomnia, and OSA do share commonalities such as reduced sleep and increased arousals during the night, all of which have been shown to increase blood pressure through sympathetic activation and reduce nocturnal blood pressure dipping.

Concerning the consequences for the other SRMDs there are no systematic and extensive data. It is well known that sleep bruxism can cause tooth destruction, temporomandibular dysfunction (e.g., jaw pain or movement limitation), headaches, and the disruption of the bed partner's sleep because of the grinding sounds.

References

[1]   Cheyne J. A case of apoplexy in which the fleshy part of the heart was converted into fat. *Dublin. Hosp. Rep.* 1818; 2: 216–223.

[2]   Stokes W. The Diseases of the Heart and Aorta. Dublin: Hodges and Smith, 1854.

[3]   Burwell CS, Robin ED, Whaley RD, et al. Extreme obesity associated with alveolar hypoventilation: a Pickwickian syndrome. *Am. J. Med.* 1956; 21: 811–818.

[4] Gastaut H, Tassinari CA, Duron B. Polygraphic study of the episodic diurnal and nocturnal (hypnic and respiratory) manifestations of the Pickwick syndrome. *Brain Res.* 1966; 1: 167–186.

[5] Guilleminault C, Tilkian A, Dement WC. The sleep apnea syndromes. *Annu. Rev. Med.* 1976; 27: 465–484.

[6] Guilleminault C, Stoohs R, Clerk A, et al. A cause of excessive daytime sleepiness. The upper airwayresistance syndrome. *Chest* 1993; 104: 781–787.

[7] American Academy of Sleep Medicine. International Classification of Sleep Disorders, 2nd ed. *Diagnostic and Coding Manual.* Westchester, IL: American Academy of Sleep Medicine, 2005.

[8] Medicine AAoS, . The Interntional Classicfication of Sleep Disorders: *Diagnostic and Coding Manual.* Westchester, IL: American Academy of Sleep Medicine, 2005.

[9] Luyster FS, Buysse DJ, Strollo PJ Jr. Comorbid insomnia and obstructive sleep apnea: challenges for clinical practice and research. *J. Clin. Sleep Med.* 2010; 6(2): 196-204.

[10] Rains JC, Poceta JS. Sleep-related headaches. *Neurol. Clin.* 2012; 30(4): 1285-98.

[11] Flemons WW. Clinical practice. Obstructive sleep apnea. *N. Engl. J. Med* 2002; 347: 498–504.

[12] Priou P, Le Vaillant M, Meslier N, et al; IRSR Sleep Cohort Group. Independent association between obstructive sleep apnea severity and glycated hemoglobin in adults without diabetes. *Diabetes Care.* 2012; 35(9): 1902-6.

[13] Wheaton AG, Perry GS, Chapman DP, et al. Sleep disordered breathing and depression among U.S. adults: National Health and Nutrition Examination Survey, 2005-2008. *Sleep.* 2012 1; 35(4): 461-7.

[14] Marcus CL, Brooks LJ, Draper KA, et al; American Academy of Pediatrics. Diagnosis and management of childhood obstructive sleep apnea syndrome. *Pediatrics.* 2012; 130(3): e714-55

[15] Brockmann PE, Urschitz MS, Schlaud M, et al. Primary snoring in school children: prevalence and neurocognitive impairments. *Sleep Breath.* 2012; 16(1): 23-9.

[16] Pépin JL, Guillot M, Tamisier R, et al. The upper airway resistance syndrome. *Respiration.* 2012; 83(6): 559-66.

[17] Gold A, Dipalo F, Gold M, et al. The symptoms and signs of upper airway resistance syndrome: a link to the functional somatic syndromes. *Chest* 2003; 123: 87–95.

[18] Lewin D, Pinto M. Sleep disorders andADHD: shared and common phenotypes. *Sleep* 2004; 27: 188–189.

[19] Guilleminault C, Faul J, Stoohs R. Sleep-disordered breathing and hypotension. *Am. J. Respir. Crit. Care Med* 2001; 164: 1242–1247.

[20] Bradley TD, Floras JS. Sleep apnea and heart failure: Part II: central sleep apnea. *Circulation* 2003; 107: 1822–1826.

[21] Mohsenin V. Sleep-related breathing disorders and risk of stroke. *Stroke* 2001; 32: 1271–1278.

[22] Javaheri S. Central sleep apnea in congestive heart failure: prevalence, mechanisms, impact, and therapeutic options. *Semin. Respir. Crit Care Med* 2005; 26: 44–55.

[23] Javaheri S, Parker TJ, Liming JD, et al. Sleep apnea in 81 ambulatory male patients with stable heart failure. Types and their prevalences, consequences, and presentations. *Circulation* 1998; 97: 2154–2159.

[24] Naughton MT. Cheyne-Stokes respiration: friend or foe?. *Thorax.* 2012;67(4):357-60.

[25] Mokhlesi B. Obesity hypoventilation syndrome: a state-of-the-art review. *Respir. Care* 2010; 55: 1347–1362.

[26] Tishler PV, Larkin EK, Schluchter MD, et al. Incidence of sleep-disordered breathing in an urban adult population: the relative importance of risk factors in the development of sleep-disordered breathing. *JAMA* 2003; 289: 2230–2237.

[27] Bonuck KA, Chervin RD, Cole TJ, et al. Prevalence and persistence of sleep disordered breathing symptoms in young children: a 6-year population-based cohort study. *Sleep.* 2011 Jul 1; 34(7): 875-84.

[28] Young T, Palta M, Dempsey J, et al. The occurrence of sleep-disordered breathing among middle-aged adults. *N. Engl. J. Med.* 1993; 328: 1230–1235.

[29] Duran J, Esnaola S, Rubio R, et al. Obstructive sleep apnea-hypopnea and related clinical features in a population-based sample of subjects aged 30 to 70 yr. *Am. J. Respir. Crit. Care Med* 2001; 163: 685–689.

[30] Bixler EO, Vgontzas AN, Lin HM, et al. Prevalence of sleep-disordered breathing in women: effects of gender. *Am. J. Respir. Crit. Care Med* 2001; 163: 608–613.

[31] Bixler EO, Vgontzas AN, Ten Have T, et al. Effects of age on sleep apnea in men: I. Prevalence and severity. *Am. J. Respir. Crit. Care Med* 1998; 157: 144–148.

[32] Young T, Shahar E, Nieto FJ, et al. Predictors of sleep-disordered breathing in community-dwelling adults: the Sleep Heart Health Study. *Arch. Intern. Med.* 2002; 162: 893–900.

[33] Ip MS, Lam B, Lauder IJ, et al. A community study of sleep-disordered breathing in middle-aged Chinese men in Hong Kong. *Chest* 2001; 119: 62–69.

[34] Kim J, In K, You S, et al. Prevalence of sleep-disordered breathing in middle-aged Korean men and women. *Am. J. Respir. Crit. Care Med* 2004; 170: 1108–1113.

[35] Lurie A. Obstructive sleep apnea in adults: epidemiology, clinical presentation, and treatment options. *Adv. Cardiol.* 2011; 46: 1-42.

[36] Ralls FM, Grigg-Damberger M. Roles of gender, age, race/ethnicity, and residential socioeconomics in obstructive sleep apnea syndromes. *Curr. Opin. Pulm Med.* 2012 Nov; 18(6): 568-73.

[37] Pepin JL, Chouri-Pontarollo N, Tamisier R, et al. Cheyne-Stokes respiration with central sleep apnoea In chronic heart failure: proposals for a diagnostic and therapeutic strategy. *Sleep Med. Rev.* 2006; 10: 33–47.

[38] Brack T, Randerath W, Bloch KE. Cheyne-Stokes respiration in patients with heart failure: prevalence, causes, consequences and treatments. *Respiration.* 2012; 83(2): 165-76.

[39] Chau EH, Lam D, Wong J, et al. Obesity hypoventilation syndrome: a review of epidemiology, pathophysiology, and perioperative considerations. *Anesthesiology.* 2012 Jul; 117(1): 188-205.

[40] Horner R, Mohiaddin R, Lowell D, et al. Sites and sizes of fat deposits around the pharynx in obese patients with obstructive sleep apnea and weight matched controls. *Eur. Respir. J.* 1989; 2: 613–622.

[41] Mezzanotte W, Tangel D, White D. Waking geioglossal electromyogram in sleep apnea patients versus normal controls (a neuromuscular compensatory mechanism). *J. Clin. Invest.* 1992; 89: 1572–1579.

[42] Kimoff R, Sforza E, Champagne V, et al. Upper airway sensation in snoring and obstructive sleep apnea. *Am. J. Respir. Cri.t Care Med* 2001; 164: 250–255.

[43]   Smirne S, Iannaccone S, Ferini-Strambi L, et al. Muscle fiber type and habitual snoring. *Lancet* 1991; 337: 597–599.

[44]   Frieberg D, Answed T, Borg K. Histological indications of a progressive snorer disease in upper airway muscle. *Am. Respir. Crit Care Med* 1998; 157: 586–593.

[45]   Newman A, Nieto F, Guidry U, et al. Relation of sleep-disordered breathing to cardiovascular disease risk factors: the Sleep Heart Health Study. *Am. J. Epidemiol.* 2001; 154(1): 50–59.

[46]   Peppard P, Young T, Palta M, et al. Longitudinal study of moderate weight change and sleepdisordered breathing. *JAMA* 2000; 284: 3015–3021.

[47]   Riley R, Powell N, Li K, et al. Surgery and obstructive sleep apnea: long-term clinical outcomes. *Otolaryngol. Head Neck Surg.* 2000; 122: 415–421.

[48]   Arens R, Sin S, Nandalike K, et al. Upper airway structure and body fat composition in obese children with obstructive sleep apnea syndrome. *Am. J. Respir. Crit. Care Med.* 2011; 183: 782–787.

[49]   White D. Central sleep apnea. In: Kryger MH, Roth T, Dement WC (Eds), Principles and Practice of Sleep Medicine, IV Edition, *Elsevier Saunders*, Philadelphia, PA, 2005: 969-982.

[50]   Xie A, Rutherford R, Rankin F, et al. Hypocapnia and increased ventilatory responsiveness in patients with idiopathic central sleep apnea. *Am. J. Respir. Crit. Care Med.* 1995 Dec; 152(6 Pt 1): 1950-5.

[51]   Javaheri S. A mechanism of central sleep apnea in patients with heart failure. *N. Engl. J. Med.* 1999 Sep 23; 341(13): 949-54.

[52]   Nachtmann A, Siebler M, Rose G, et al. Cheyne-Stokes respiration in ischemic stroke. *Neurology.* 1995 Apr; 45(4): 820-1.

[53]   Suratt PM, Turner BL, Wilhoit SC. Effect of intranasal obstruction on breathing during sleep. *Chest.* 1986 Sep; 90(3): 324-9.

[54]   Ramos J, On the integration of respiratory movements: III. The fifth nerve afferents. *Acta Physiol. Lat. Am.* 1960; 10: 104-113.

[55]   Hoffstein V, Slutsky AS. Central sleep apnea revesed by continous positive airway pressure. *Am. Rev. Respir. Dis.* 1987; 135: 1210-12.

[56]   Ferini-Strambi, Luigi. "Sleep disorders in multiple sclerosis". *Handbook of clinical neurology* 2011; (0072-9752), 99: 1139.

[57]   Kennedy JD, Martin AJ. Chronic respiratory failure and neuromuscular disease. *Pediatric Clin. North Am.* 2009; 56: 261-73.

[58]   Redline S, Tishler P, Tosteson T, et al. The familial aggregation of obstructive sleep apnea. *Am. J. Respir. Crit. Care Med* 1995; 151: 682–687.

[59]   Kim KS, Kim JH, Park SY, et al. Smoking induces oropharyngeal narrowing and increases the severity of obstructive sleep apnea syndrome. *J. Clin. Sleep Med.* 2012 Aug 15; 8(4): 367-74.

[60]   Kang SH, Yoon IY, Lee SD, et al. The impact of sleep apnoea syndrome on nocturia according to age in men. *BJU Int.* 2012 Dec; 110(11 Pt C): E851-6.

[61]   Chervin RD. Sleepiness, fatigue, tiredness, and lack of energy in obstructive sleep apnea. *Chest* 2000; 118(2): 372–379.

[62]   Bradley TD, McNicholas WT, Rutherford R, et al. Clinical and physiological heterogeneity of the central sleep apnea syndrome. *Am. Rev. Respir. Dis.* 1986; 134: 217-21.

[63]   Subramanian S, Jayaraman G, Majid H, et al. Influence of gender and anthropometric measures on severity of obstructive sleep apnea. Sleep Breath. 2012 Dec;16(4): 1091-5.

[64]   Schellenberg JB, Maislin G, Schwab RJ. Physical findings and the risk for obstructive sleep apnea. *Am. J. Respir. Crit Care Med* 2000; 162: 740–748.

[65]   Tsai WH, Remmers JE, Brant R, et al. A decision rule for diagnostic testing in obstructive sleep apnea. *Am. J. Respir. Crit. Care Med* 2003; 167(10): 1427–1432.

[66]   Nuckton TJ, Glidden DV, Browner WS, et al. Physical examination: Mallampati score as an independent predictor of obstructive sleep apnea. *Sleep* 2006; 29: 903–908.

[67]   Sharma SK, Vasudev C, Sinha S, et al. Validation of the modified Berlin questionnaire to identify patients at risk for the obstructive sleep apnoea syndrome. *Indian J. Med. Res.* 2006; 124: 281–290.

[68]   Netzer NC, Stoohs RA, Netzer CM, et al. Using the Berlin questionnaire to identify patients at risk for the sleep apnea syndrome. *Ann. Intern. Med.* 1999; 131: 485–491.

[69]   Ahmadi N, Chung SA, Gibbs A, et al. The Berlin questionnaire for sleep apnea in a sleep clinic population: relationship to polysomnographic measurement of respiratory disturbance. *Sleep Breath* 2008; 12: 39–45.

[70]   Simpson L, Hillman DR, Cooper MN, et al. High prevalence of undiagnosed obstructive sleep apnoea in the general population and methods for screening for representative controls. *Sleep Breath.* 2012 Nov 16. [Epub ahead of print].

[71]   Farney RJ, Walker BS, Farney RM, et al. The STOP-Bang Equivalent Model and Prediction of Severity of Obstructive Sleep Apnea: Relation to Polysomnographic Measurements of the Apnea/Hypopnea Index. *J. Clin. Sleep Med.* 2011; 7(5): 459–465.

[72]   Iber C, Ancoli-Israel S, Chesson AL Jr., et al. *The AASM Manual for the Scoring of Sleep and Associated Events.* Westchester, IL: American Academy of Sleep Medicine, 2007.

[73]   Katz ES, Marcus CL. Diagnosis of obstructive sleep apnea syndrome in infants and children. In: Sheldon SH, Ferber R, Kryger MH, eds. Principles and Practice of Pediatric Sleep Medicine. Philadelphia, PA: *Elsevier Saunders*, 2005:197–210.

[74]   American Academy of Sleep Medicine Task Force. Sleep-related breathing disorders in adults: recommendations for syndrome definition and measurement techniques in clinical research. The Report of an American Academy of Sleep Medicine Task Force. *Sleep* 1999; 22(5): 667–689.

[75]   Boudewyns A, Willemen M, Wagemans M, et al. Assessment of respiratory effort by means of strain gauges and esophageal pressure swings: a comparative study. *Sleep* 1997; 20(2): 168–170.

[76]   Collop NA, Anderson WA, Boehlecke B, et al. Clinical guidelines for the use of unattended portable monitors in the diagnosis of obstructive sleep apnea in adult patients. *J. Clin. Sleep Med* 2007; 3: 737–747.

[77]   Pitson DJ, Stradling JR. Autonomic markers of arousal during sleep in patients undergoing investigation for obstructive sleep apnoea, their relationship to EEG arousals, respiratory events and subjective sleepiness. *J. Sleep Res.* 1998; 7(1): 53–59.

[78]   Pitson DJ, Sandell A, van den HR, et al. Use of pulse transit time as a measure of inspiratory effort in patients with obstructive sleep apnoea. *Eur. Respir. J.* 1995; 8(10): 1669–1674.

[79]   Pepin JL, Delavie N, Pin I, et al. Pulse transit time improves detection of sleep respiratory events and microarousals in children. *Chest* 2005; 127(3): 722–730.

[80] Grote L, Zou D, Kraiczi H, et al. Finger plethysmography—a method for monitoring finger blood flow during sleep disordered breathing. *Respir. Physiol. Neurobiol.* 2003; 136(2–3): 141–152.

[81] O'Donnell CP, Allan L, Atkinson P, et al. The effect of upper airway obstruction and arousal on peripheral arterial tonometry in obstructive sleep apnea. *Am. J. Respir. Crit Care* Med 2002; 166(7): 965–971.

[82] Ayas NT, Pittman S, MacDonald M, et al. Assessment of a wrist-worn device in the detection of obstructive sleep apnea. *Sleep Med* 2003; 4(5): 435–442.

[83] Bar A, Pillar G, Dvir I, et al. Evaluation of a portable device based on peripheral arterial tone for unattended home sleep studies. *Chest* 2003; 123(3): 695–703.

[84] Pittman SD, Ayas NT, MacDonald MM, et al. Using a wrist-worn device based on peripheral arterial tonometry to diagnose obstructive sleep apnea: in-laboratory and ambulatory validation. *Sleep* 2004; 27(5): 923–933.

[85] Peppard PE, Young T, Palta M, et al. Prospective study of the association between sleep-disordered breathing and hypertension. *N. Engl. J. Med* 2000; 342: 1378–1384.

[86] Lavie P, Herer P, Hoffstein V. Obstructive sleep apnea syndrome as a risk factor for hypertension: population study. *BMJ* 2000; 320: 479–482.

[87] Silverberg DS, Oksenberg A, Iaina A. Sleep-related breathing disorders as a major cause of essential hypertension: fact or fiction?. *Curr. Opin. Nephrol. Hypertens* 1998; 7: 353–357.

[88] Nieto FJ, Young TB, Lind BK, et al. Association of sleep-disordered breathing, sleep apnea, and hypertension in a large community-based study: Sleep Heart Health Study. *JAMA* 2000; 283: 1829–1836.

[89] Silverberg DS, Oksenberg A. Essential hypertension and abnormal upper airway resistance during sleep. *Sleep* 1997; 20: 794–806.

[90] Haas DC, Foster GL, Nieto FJ, et al.. Age-dependent associations between sleep disordered breathing and hypertension: importance of discriminating between systolic/diastolic hypertension and isolated systolic hypertension in the Sleep Heart Health Study. *Circulation* 2005; 111: 614–621.

[91] Pedrosa RP, Drager LF, Gonzaga CC, et al.. Obstructive sleep apnea: the most common secondary cause of hypertension associated with resistant hypertension. *Hypertension* 2011; 58: 811–817.

[92] Galiè N, Hoeper MM, Humbert M, et al.. Guidelines for the diagnosis and treatment of pulmonary hypertension: the Task Force for the Diagnosis and Treatment of Pulmonary Hypertension of the European Society of Cardiology (ESC) and the European Respiratory Society (ERS), endorsed by the International Society of Heart and Lung Transplantation (ISHLT). ESC Committee for Practice Guidelines (CPG). *Eur. Heart J.* 2009; 30: 2493–2537.

[93] Lévy P, McNicholas WT. Sleep apnoea and hypertension: time for recommendations. *Eur. Respir. J.* 2013 Mar; 41(3): 505-6.

[94] Tamisier R, Pepin JL, Remy J, et al. Fourteen nights of intermittent hypoxia elevate daytime blood pressure and sympathetic activity in healthy humans. *Eur. Respir. J.* 2011; 37: 119–128.

[95] Pepperell JC, Ramdassingh-Dow S, Crosthwaite N, et al. Ambulatory blood pressure after therapeutic and subtherapeutic nasal continuous positive airway pressure for obstructive sleep apnoea: a randomised parallel trial. *Lancet* 2002; 359: 204–210.

[96]   Becker HF, Jerrentrup A, Ploch T, et al. Effect of nasal continuous positive airway pressure treatment on blood pressure in patients with obstructive sleep apnea. *Circulation* 2003; 107: 68–73.

[97]   Haentjens P, Van Meerhaeghe A, Moscariello A, et al. The impact of continuous positive airway pressure on blood pressure in patients with obstructive sleep apnea syndrome: evidence from a meta-analysis of placebo-controlled randomized trials. *Arch. Intern. Med* 2007; 167: 757–764.

[98]   Barbe F, Mayoralas LR, Duran J, et al. Treatment with continuous positive airway pressure is not effective in patients with sleep apnea but no daytime sleepiness: a randomized, controlled trial. *Ann. Intern. Med.* 2001; 134: 1015–1023.

[99]   Robinson GV, Smith DM, Langford BA, et al. Continuous positive airway pressure does not reduce blood pressure in nonsleepy hypertensive OSA patients. *Eur. Respir. J.* 2006; 27: 1229–1235.

[100] Logan AG, Perlikowski SM, Mente A, et al. High prevalence of unrecognized sleep apnoea in drug-resistant hypertension. *J. Hypertens* 2001; 19: 2271–2277.

[101] Quan SF, Wright R, Baldwin CM, et al. Obstructive sleep apnea-hypopnea and neurocognitive functioning in the Sleep Heart Health Study. *Sleep Medicine* 2006; 7: 498–507.

[102] Sforza E, Roche F, Thomas-Anterion C, et al. Cognitive function and sleep related breathing disorders in a healthy elderly population: The SYNAPSE study. *Sleep* 2010; 33: 515–521.

[103] Quan SF, Chan CS, Dement WC, et al. The association between obstructive sleep apnea and neurocognitive performance-the apnea positive pressure long-term efficacy study (APPLES). *Sleep* 2011; 34: 303–314.

[104] Décary A, Rouleau I, Montplaisir J. Cognitive deficits associated with sleep apnea syndrome: A proposed neuropsychological test battery. *Sleep* 2000; 23: 369–381.

[105] Sateia, MJ. Neuropsychological impairment and quality of life in obstructive sleep apnea. *Clinics in Chest Medicine* 2003; 24: 249–259.

[106] Aloia MS, Arnedt JT, Davis JD, et al. Neuropsychological sequelae of obstructive sleep apnea- hypopnea syndrome: A critical review. *Journal of the International Neuropsychological Society* 2004; 10: 772-785.

[107] El-Ad B, Lavie P. Effect of sleep apnea on cognition and mood. International Review of Psychiatry 2005; 17: 277–282.

[108] Findley LJ, Barth JT, Powers DC, et al. Cognitive impairment in patients with obstructive sleep apnea and associated hypoxemia. *Chest* 1986; 90: 686–690.

[109] Greenberg GD, Watson RK, Deptula D. Neuropsychological dysfunction in sleep apnea. *Sleep* 1987; 10: 254–262.

[110] Bédard M, Montplaisir J, Richer F, et al. Obstructive sleep apnea syndrome: Pathogenesis of neuropsychological deficits. *Journal of Clinical and Experimental Neuropsychology* 1991 ; 13: 950–964.

[111] Beebe DW, Groesz L, Wells C, et al. The neuropsychological effects of obstructive sleep apnea: A meta-analysis of norm-referenced and case-controlled data. *Sleep* 2003; 26: 298–307.

[112] Alchanatis M, Zias N, Deligiorgis N, et al. Sleep apnea-related cognitive deficits and intelligence: An implication of cognitive reserve theory. *Journal of Sleep Research* 2005; 14: 69–75.

[113] Naëgelé B, Thouvard V, Pépin JL. Deficits of cognitive executive functions in patients with sleep apnea syndrome. *Sleep* 1995; 18: 43–52.

[114] Salorio CF, White DA, Piccirillo J, et al. Learning, memory, and executive control in individuals with obstructive sleep apnea syndrome. *Journal of Clinical and Experimental Neuropsychology* 2002; 24: 93–100.

[115] Ferini-Strambi L, Baietto C, Di Gioia MR, et al. Cognitive dysfunction in patients with obstructive sleep apnea (OSA): Partial reversibility after continuous positive airway pressure (CPAP). *Brain Research Bulletin* 2003; 61: 87–92.

[116] Kloepfer C, Riemann D, Nofzinger EA, et al. Memory before and after sleep in patients with moderate obstructive sleep apnea. *Journal of Clinical Sleep Medicine* 2009; 5: 540–548.

[117] Twigg GL, Papaioannou I, Jackson M, et al. Obstructive sleep apnea syndrome is associated with deficits in verbal but not visual memory. *American Journal of Respiratory and Critical Care Medicine* 2010; 182: 98–103.

[118] Masa JF, Rubio M, Findley LJ. Habitually sleepy drivers have a high frequency of automobile crashes associated with respiratory disorders during sleep. *American Journal of Respiratory and Critical Care Medicine* 2000; 162: 1407–1412.

[119] Pichel F, Zamarróna C, Magánb F, et al. Sustained attention measurements in obstructive sleep apnea and risk of traffic accidents. *Respiratory Medicine* 2006; 100: 1020–1027.

[120] George CF, Boudreau AC, Smiley A. Simulated driving performance in patients with obstructive sleep apnea. *American Journal of Respiratory and Critical Care Medicine* 1996; 154: 175–181.

[121] Juniper M, Hack MA, George CF, et al. Steering simulation performance in patients with obstructive sleep apnoea and matched control subjects. *European Respiratory Journal* 2000; 15: 590–595.

[122] Tippin J, Sparks J, Rizzo M. Visual vigilance in drivers with obstructive sleep apnea. *Journal of Psychosomatic Research* 2009; 67: 143–151.

[123] Mazza S, Pépin JL, Naëgelé B, et al. Most obstructive sleep apnoea patients exhibit vigilance and attention deficits on an extended battery of tests. *European Respiratory Journal* 2005; 25: 75–80.

[124] Bawden FC, Oliveira CA, Caramelli P. Impact of obstructive sleep apnea on cognitive performance. *Arquivos de Neuro-Psiquiatria* 2011; 69: 585–589.

[125] Shpirer I, Elizur A, Shorer R, et al. Hypoxemia correlates with attentional dysfunction in patients with obstructive sleep apnea. *Sleep Breath* 2012; 16: 821-827.

[126] Strauss E, Sherman EMS, Spreen O. A Compendium of Neuropsychological Tests: Administration, Norms, and Commentary. 3rd edn, 2006 Oxford University press, Oxford.

[127] Lezak MD, Howieson DB, Loring DW. *Neuropsychological Assessment.* 4th edn, 2004 Oxford University Press, New York.

[128] Lis S, Krieger S, Hennig D, et al. Executive functions and cognitive subprocesses in patients with obstructive sleep apnoea. *Journal of Sleep Research* 2008; 17: 271–280.

[129] Saunamäki T, Jehkonen M. A review of executive functions in obstructive sleep apnea syndrome. *Acta Neurol. Scand.* 2007; 115: 1-11.

[130] Saunamäki T, Himanen SL, Polo O, et al. Executive dysfunction in patients with obstructive sleep apnea syndrome. *Eur. Neurol.* 2009; 62: 237-42.

[131] Valencia-Flores M, Bliwise DL, Guilleminault C, et al. Cognitive function in patients with sleep apnea after acute nocturnal nasal continuous positive airway pressure (CPAP) treatment: Sleepiness and hypoxemia effects. *Journal of Clinical and Experimental Neuropsychology* 1996; 18: 197–210.

[132] Naismith S, Winter V, Gotsopoulos H, et al. Neurobehavioral functioning in obstructive sleep apnea: Differential effects of sleep quality, hypoxemia and subjective sleepiness. *Journal of Clinical and Experimental Neuropsychology* 2004; 26: 43–54.

[133] Yaffe K, Laffan AM, Harrison SL, et al. Sleep-disordered breathing, hypoxia, and risk of mild cognitive impairment and dementia in older women. *Journal of the American Medical Association* 2011; 306: 613–619.

[134] Canessa N, Ferini-Strambi L. Sleep-disordered breathing and cognitive decline in older adults. *Journal of the American Medical Association* 2011; 306: 654-655.

[135] Macey PM, Henderson LA, Macey KE, et al. Brain morphology associated with obstructive sleep apnea. *American Journal of Respiratory and Critical Care Medicine* 2002; 166: 1382-1387.

[136] Morrel MJ, McRobbie DW, Quest RA, et al. Changes in brain morphology associated with sleep apnea. *Sleep Medicine* 2003; 4: 451-454.

[137] Yaouhi K, Bertran F, Clochon P, et al. A combined neuropsychological and brain imaging study of obstructive sleep apnea. *Journal of Sleep Research* 2009; 18: 36-48.

[138] Canessa N, Castronovo V, Cappa SF, et al. Obstructive sleep apnea: brain structural changes and neurocognitive function before and after treatment. *American Journal of Respiratory and Critical Care Medicine* 2011; 183: 1419-1426.

[139] Macey PM, Kumar R, Woo MA, et al. Brain structural changes in obstructive sleep apnea. *Sleep* 2008; 31: 967-977.

[140] Kumar R, Chavez AS, Macey PM, et al. Altered global and regional brain mean diffusivity in patients with obstructive sleep apnea. *Journal of Neuroscience Research* 2012; 90: 2043-2052.

[141] Engleman HM, Kingshott RN, Wraith PK, et al. Randomized placebo-controlled crossover trial of continuous positive airway pressure for mild sleep Apnea/Hypopnea syndrome. *American Journal of Respiratory and Critical Care Medicine* 1999; 159: 461–467.

[142] Muñoz A, Mayoralas LR, Barbé F, et al. Long-term effects of CPAP on daytime functioning in patients with sleep apnoea syndrome. *European Respiratory Journal* 2000; 15: 676–681.

[143] Bardwell WA, Ancoli-Israel S, Berry CC, et al. Neuropsychological effects of one-week continuous positive airway pressure treatment in patients with obstructive sleep apnea: A placebo-controlled study. *Psychosomatic Medicine* 2001; 63: 579–584.

[144] Aloia MS, Ilniczky N, Di Dio P, et al. Neuropsychological changes and treatment compliance in older adults with sleep apnea. *Journal of Psychosomatic Research* 2003; 54: 71–76.

[145] Barnes M, McEvoy RD, Banks S, et al. Efficacy of Positive Airway Pressure and Oral Appliance in Mild to Moderate Obstructive Sleep Apnea. *Am. J. Respir. Crit. Care Med.* 2004; 170; 656–664.

[146] Zimmerman ME, Arnedt JT, Stanchina M, et al. Normalization of memory performance and positive airway pressure adherence in memory-impaired patients with obstructive sleep apnea. *Chest* 2006; 130: 1772–1778.

[147] Lim W, Bardwell WA, Loredo JS, et al. Neuropsychological effects of 2-week continuous positive airway pressure treatment and supplemental oxygen in patients with obstructive sleep apnea: A randomized placebo-controlled study. *Journal of Clinical Sleep Medicine* 2007; 3: 380–386.

[148] Antic NA, Catcheside P, Buchan C, et al. The Effect of CPAP in Normalizing Daytime Sleepiness, Quality of Life, and Neurocognitive Function in Patients with Moderate to Severe OSA. *Sleep* 2011; 34(1): 111-119.

[149] O'Donoghue FJ, Briellmann RS, Rochford PD, et al. Cerebral structural changes in severe obstructive sleep apnea. *American Journal of Respiratory and Critical Care Medicine* 2005; 171: 1185-1190.

[150] Tonon C, Vetrugno R, Lodi R, et al. Proton magnetic resonance spectroscopy study of brain metabolism in obstructive sleep apnoea syndrome before and after continuous positive airway pressure treatment. *Sleep* 2007; 30: 305–311.

[151] Castronovo V, Canessa N, Ferini Strambi L, et al. Brain activation changes before and after PAP treatment in obstructive sleep apnea. Sleep 2009; 32: 1161-72.

[152] Aloia MS, Sweet LH, Jerskey BA, et al. Treatment effects on brain activity during a working memory task in obstructive sleep apnea. *Journal of Sleep Research* 2009; 18: 404-410.

[153] Sweet LH, Jerskey BA, Aloia MS. Default Network Response to a Working Memory Challenge after Withdrawal of Continuous Positive Airway Pressure Treatment for Obstructive Sleep Apnea. *Brain Imaging and Behavior* 2010; 4: 155–163.

[154] O'Donoghue FJ, Wellard RM, Rochford PD, et al. Magnetic resonance spectroscopy and neurocognitive dysfunction in obstructive sleep apnea before and after CPAP treatment. *Sleep* 2012; 35: 41-48.

[155] Allen RP, Earley CJ. Restless legs syndrome: a review of clinical and pathophysiologic features. *J. Clin. Neurophysiol.* 2001; 18: 128–147.

[156] Ferini-Strambi L. RLS-like symptoms: differential diagnosis by history and clinical assessment. Sleep Med 2007; 8(suppl 2): S3–S6.

[157] Milligan SA, Chesson AL. Restless legs syndrome in the older adult: diagnosis and management.*Drugs Aging* 2002; 19(10): 741–751.

[158] Kushida CA. Clinical presentation, diagnosis, and quality of life issues in restless legs syndrome. *Am. J. Med* 2007; 120(1 suppl 1): S4–S12.

[159] Allen RP, Picchietti D, Hening WA, et al. Restless legs syndrome: diagnostic criteria, special considerations, and epidemiology. A report from the restless legs syndrome diagnosis and epidemiology workshop at the National Institutes of Health. *Sleep Med.* 2003; 4(2): 101–119.

[160] Riley JD, Antony SJ. Leg cramps: differential diagnosis and management. *Am. Fam. Physcian* 1995; 52: 1794–1798.

[161] Bader G and G. Lavigne GJ. Sleep bruxism; an overview of an oromandibular sleep movement disorder. Review article. *Sleep Med. Rev.* 2000, 4: 27–43.

[162] Lavigne GJ, Manzini C, Huynh N. Sleep bruxism. In: M.H. Kryger, T. Roth and W.C. Dement, Editors, Principles & Practice of Sleep Medicine, *Elsevier Saunders*, Philadelphia (2011), pp. 1128–1139.

[163] Ferini-Strambi L, Pozzi P, Manconi M, et al. Bruxism and nocturnal groaning. *Arch. Ital. Biol.* 2011 Dec 1; 149(4): 467-77.

[164] Velly AM , Gornitsky M, Philippe P. Contributing factors to chronic myofascial pain: a case-control study. *Pain* 2003; 104: 491–499.

[165] Camparis CM, Siqueira JT. Sleep bruxism: clinical aspects and characteristics in patients with and without chronic orofacial pain. *Oral. Surg. Oral. Med. Oral. Pathol. Oral. Radiol. Endod* 2006; 101: 188–193.

[166] Ekbom KA. Restless legs syndrome. *Neurology* 1960; 10: 868–873.

[167] Hening W, Walters AS, Allen RP, Montplaisir J, Myers A, Ferini-Strambi L.Impact, diagnosis and treatment of restless legs syndrome (RLS) in a primary care population: the REST (RLS epidemiology, symptoms, and treatment) primary care study. *Sleep Med.* 2004 May; 5(3): 237-46.

[168] Ohayon MM, O'Hara R, Vitiello MV. Epidemiology of restless legs syndrome: a synthesis of the literature. *Sleep Med. Rev.* 2012 Aug; 16(4): 283-95.

[169] Gupta R, Lahan V, Goel D. Prevalence of restless leg syndrome in subjects with depressive disorder. *Indian J. Psychiatry.* 2013 Jan; 55(1): 70-3.

[170] Cesnik E, Casetta I, Turri M, et al. Transient RLS during pregnancy is a risk factor for the chronic idiopathic form. *Neurology* 2010 Dec 7; 75(23): 2117-20.

[171] Allen RP, Auerbach S, Bahrain H, et al. The prevalence and impact of restless legs syndrome on patients with iron deficiency anemia. *Am. J. Hematol.* 2013 Apr; 88(4): 261-4.

[172] Aritake-Okada S, Nakao T, Komada Y, et al. Prevalence and clinical characteristics of restless legs syndrome in chronic kidney disease patients. *Sleep Med.* 2011 Dec; 12(10): 1031-3.

[173] Ancoli-Israel S, Kripke DF, Klauber MR, et al. Periodic limb movements in sleep in community dwelling elderly. *Sleep* 1991; 14(6): 496–500.

[174] Mosko SS, Dickel MJ, Paul T, et al. Sleep apnea and sleep-related periodic leg movements in community resident seniors. J Am Geriatr Soc 1988; 3 6(6): 502–508.

[175] Roehrs T, Zorick F, Sicklesteel J, et al. Age-related sleep-wake disorders at a sleep disorder center. *J. Am. Geriatr. Soc.* 1983; 31(6): 364–370.

[176] Bixler EO, Kales A, Vela-Bueno A. Nocturnal myoclonus and nocturnal myoclonic activity in a normal population. *Res. Commun. Chem Pathol. Pharmacol.* 1982; 36: 129–140.

[177] Leung AK, Wong BE, Chan PY, et al. Nocturnal leg cramps in children: incidence and clinical characteristics. *J. Natl. Med. Assoc.* 1999; 91: 329–332.

[178] Norris FH, Gasteiger EL, Chatfield PO. An elctromyographic study of induced and spontaneous muscle cramps. *Electroencephalogr. Clin. Neurophysiol.* 1957; 9: 139–147.

[179] Gulich M, Heil P, Zeitler HP. Epidemiology and determinants of nocturnal calf cramps. *Eur. J. Gen. Pract.* 1998; 4: 109–113.

[180] Hall AJ. Cramp and salt balance in ordinary life. *Lancet* 1947; 3: 231–233.

[181] Oboler SK, Prochazka AV, Meyer TJ. Leg symptoms in outpatient veterans. *West J. Med.* 1991; 155: 256–259.

[182] Gentili A, Weiner DK, Kuchibhatla M, et al. Factors that disturb sleep in nursing home residents. *Aging Clin. Exp. Res.* 1997; 9: 207–213.

[183] Naylor JR, Young JB. A general population survey of rest cramps. *Age Ageing* 1994; 23: 418–420.

[184] Baldwin CM, Kapur VK, Holberg CJ, et al. Associations between gender and measures of daytime somnolence in the Sleep Heart Health Study. *Sleep* 2004; 27:305–311.

[185] Lavigne GJ, Montplaisir JY. Restless legs syndrome and sleep bruxism: prevalence and association among Canadians. *Sleep* 1994; 17: 739–743.

[186] Ohayon MM, Li KK, Guilleminault C. Risk factors for sleep bruxism in the general population. *Chest* 2001; 119: 53–61.

[187] Wetter TC, Brunner J, Bronisch T. Restless legs syndrome probably induced by risperidone treatment. *Pharmacopsychiatry* 2002; 35: 109–111.

[188] Connor JR, Wang XS, Allen RP, et al. Altered dopaminergic profile in the putamen and substantia nigra in restless leg syndrome. *Brain* 2009; 132: 2403–2412.

[189] Nelson C, Erikson K, Pinero DJ, et al. In vivo dopamine metabolism is altered in iron-deficient anemic rats. *J. Nutr.* 1997; 127: 2282–2288.

[190] Connor JR, Wang XS, Allen RP, et al. Altered dopaminergic profile in the putamen and substantia nigra in restless leg syndrome. *Brain* 2009; 132: 2403–2412.

[191] Allen RP, Connor JR, Hyland K, et al. Abnormally increased CSF 3-Ortho-methyldopa (3-OMD) in untreated restless legs syndrome (RLS) patients indicates more severe disease and possibly abnormally increased dopamine synthesis. *Sleep Med.* 2009; 10: 123–128.

[192] Kim KW, Jhoo JH, Lee SB, et al. Increased striatal dopamine transporter density in moderately severe old restless legs syndrome patients. *Eur. J. Neurol.* 2012 Sep; 19(9): 1213-8.

[193] Earley CJ, Allen RP, Beard JL, et al. Insight into the pathophysiology of restless legs syndrome. *J. Neurosci. Res.* 2000; 62: 623–628.

[194] Wang X, Wiesinger J, Beard J, et al. Thy1 expression in the brain is affected by iron and is decreased in Restless Legs Syndrome. *J. Neurol. Sci.* 2004; 220(1–2): 59–66.

[195] Earley CJ, Connor JR, Beard JL, et al. Abnormalities in CSF concentrations of ferritin and transferrin in restless legs syndrome. *Neurology* 2000; 54: 1698–700.

[196] Allen RP, Barker PB, Wehrl F, et al. MRI measurement of brain iron in patients with restless legs syndrome. Neurology 2001; 56: 263–5.

[197] Krieger J, Schroeder C. Iron, brain and restless legs syndrome. *Sleep Med. Rev.* 2001; 5: 277–86.

[198] Earley CJ, Heckler D, Allen RP. The treatment of restless legs syndrome with intravenous iron dextran. *Sleep Med* 2004; 5: 231–5.

[199] Kemlink D, Sonka K, Pretl M, et al. Suggestive evidence of erythropoietin level abnormality in patients with sporadic and familial cases of the restless legs syndrome. *Neuro endocrinology letters* 2007; 28: 643–6.

[200] Allen RP. Race, iron status and restless legs syndrome. Sleep Med 2002; 3: 467–8.

[201] Allen RP, Earley CJ. The role of iron in restless legs syndrome. *Mov. Disord.* 2007; 22: S440–8.

[202] Desautels A, Turecki G, Montplaisir J, et al. Identification of a major susceptibility locus for restless legs syndrome on chromosome 12q. *Am. J. Hum. Genet.* 2001; 69: 1266–1270.

[203] Bonati MT, Ferini-Strambi L, Aridon P, et al. Autosomal dominant restless legs syndrome maps on chromosome 14q. *Brain* 2003; 126: 1485–1492.

[204] Chen S, Ondo WG, Rao S, et al. Genomewide linkage scan identifies a novel susceptibility locus for restless legs syndrome on chromosome 9p. *Am. J. Hum. Genet.* 2004; 74: 876–885.

[205] Levchenko A, Provost S, Montplaisir JY, et al. A novel autosomal dominant restless legs syndrome locus maps to chromosome 20p13. *Neurology* 2006; 67: 900–901.

[206] Pichler I, Marroni F, Beu Volpato C, et al. Linkage analysis identifies a novel locus for restless legs syndrome on chromosome 2q in a south Tyrolean population isolate. *Am. J. Hum. Genet.* 2006; 79: 716–723.

[207] Winkelmann J, Lichtner P, Kemlink D, et al. New loci for restless legs syndrome map to chromosome 4q and 17p. *Mov. Disord.* 2006; 21: 304.

[208] Kemlink D, Plazzi G, Vetrugno R, et al. Suggestive evidence for linkage for restless legs syndrome on chromosome 19p13. *Neurogenetics* 2008; 9: 75–82.

[209] Levchenko A, Montplaisir J-Y, Asselin G, et al. Autosomal-dominant locus for restless legs syndrome in French-Canadians on chromosome 16p12.1. *Mov. Disord.* 2009; 24: 40–50.

[210] Desautels A, Turecki G, Montplaisir J, et al. Restless legs syndrome: confirmation of linkage to chromosome 12q, genetic heterogeneity, and evidence of complexity. *Arch. Neurol.* 2005; 62: 591–596.

[211] Winkelmann J, Lichtner P, Putz B, et al. Evidence for further genetic locus heterogeneity and confirmation of RLS-1 in restless legs syndrome. *Mov. Disord.* 2006; 21: 28–33.

[212] Winkelmann J, Schormair B, Lichtner P, et al. Genome-wide association study of restless legs syndrome identifies common variants in three genomic regions. *Nat. Genet.* 2007; 39 : 1000–1006.

[213] Stefansson H, Rye DB, Hicks A, et al. A genetic risk factor for periodic limb movements in sleep. *N. Engl J. Med* 2007; 357: 639–647.

[214] Schormair B, Kemlink D, Roeske D, et al. PTPRD (protein tyrosine phosphatase receptor type delta) is associated with restless legs syndrome. *Nat. Genet.* 2008; 40: 946–948.

[215] Winkelmann J, Lichtner P, Schormair B, et al. Variants in the neuronal nitric oxide synthase (nNOS, NOS1) gene are associated with restless legs syndrome. *Mov. Disord.* 2008; 23: 350–358.

[216] Skehan EB, Abdulrahim MM , Parfrey NA, et al. A novel locus for restless legs syndrome maps to chromosome 19p in an Irish pedigree. *Neurogenetics.* 2012 May; 13(2): 125-32.

[217] Lugaresi E, Coccagna G, Mantovani M, et al. Some periodic phenomena arising during drowsiness and sleep in man. Electroencephalogr *Clin. Neurophysiol.* 1972; 32(6): 701–705.

[218] Wetter TC, Eisensehr I, Trenkwalder C. Functional neuroimaging studies in restless legs syndrome. *Sleep Med* 2004; 5(4): 401–406.

[219] De Mello MT, Lauro FA, Silva AC, et al. Incidence of periodic leg movements and of the restless legs syndrome during sleep following acute physical activity in spinal cord injury subjects. *Spinal Cord* 1996; 34(5): 294–296.

[220] Bara-Jimenez W, Aksu M, Graham B, et al. Periodic limb movements in sleep: state-dependent excitability of the spinal flexor reflex. *Neurology* 2000; 54(8): 1609–1616.

[221] Montplaisir J, Boucher S, Gosselin A, et al. Persistence of repetitive EEG arousals (K-alpha complexes) in RLS patients treated with L-DOPA. *Sleep* 1996; 19(3): 196–199.

[222] Terzano MG, Mancia D, Salati MR, et al. The cyclic alternating pattern as a physiologic component of normal NREM sleep. *Sleep* 1985; 8(2): 137–145.

[223] Manconi M, Ferri R, Zucconi M, et al. Dissociation of periodic leg movements from arousals in restless legs syndrome. *Ann. Neurol.* 2012 Jun;71(6): 834-44.

[224] Clemens S, Rye D, Hochman S. Restless legs syndrome: revisiting the dopamine hypothesis from the spinal cord perspective. *Neurology* 2006; 67(1): 125–130.

[225] Yang C, White DP, Winkelman JW. Antidepressants and periodic leg movements of sleep. *Biol. Psychiatry* 2005; 58(6): 510–514.

[226] Goerke M, Rodenbeck A, Cohrs S, et al. The Influence of the Tricyclic Antidepressant Amitriptyline on Periodic Limb Movements during Sleep. *Pharmacopsychiatry*. 2013 Jan 4. [Epub ahead of print].

[227] Pierce CJ, Chrisman K, Bennett ME, et al. Stress, anticipatory stress, and psychologic measures related to sleep bruxism. *J. Orofacial. Pain* 1995; 9: 51–56.

[228] Major M, Rompre PH, Guitard F et al. A controlled daytime challenge of motor performance and vigilance in sleep bruxers. *J. Dent Res.* 1999; 78: 1754–1762.

[229] Lavigne GJ, Huynh N, Kato T et al. Genesis of sleep bruxism: motor and autonomic-cardiac interactions. *Arch. Oral. Biol.* 2007; 52: 381-84.

[230] Lavigne GJ, Soucy JP, Lobbezoo F, et al. Double-blind, crossover, placebo-controlled trial of bromocriptine in patients with sleep bruxism. *Clin. Neuropharmacol.* 2001; 24: 145–149.

[231] Lobbezoo F, Lavigne GJ , Tanguay R, et al. The effect of catecholamine precursor l-dopa on sleep bruxism: a controlled clinical trial. *Mov. Disord.* 1997; 12: 73–78.

[232] Sjoholm T, Lowe AA, Miyamoto K, et al. Sleep bruxism in patients with sleep-disordered breathing. *Arch. Oral. Biol.* 2000; 45: 889–896.

[233] Huynh N, Lavigne GJ, Lanfranchi P, et al. The effects of two sympatholytic medications_ propanolol and clonidine- on sleep bruxism: experimental randomized controlled studies. *Sleep* 2006; 29: 307-316.

[234] Massimini M, Ferrarelli F, Huber R, et al. Breakdown of cortical effective connectivity during sleep. *Science* 2005; 309: 2228–2232.

[235] Lavigne GJ, Rompre PH, Guitard F, et al. Lower number of K-complexes and K-alphas in sleep bruxism: a controlled quantitative study. *Clin. Neurophysiol.* 2002; 113: 686–693.

[236] Adachi K, Rompre S, Yao D, et al. Loss of corticobulbar motor excitability during sleep in primates: preliminary findings, Society for Neuroscience 35th meeting Washington, DC (2005), p. 399.

[237] Parrino L, Smerieri A, Rossi M, et al. Relationship of slow and rapid EEG components of CAP to ASDA arousals in normal sleep. *Sleep* 2001; 24: 881–885.

[238] Saper CB, Scammell TE, Lu J. Hypothalamic regulation of sleep and circadian rhythms. *Nature* 2005; 437: 1257–1263.

[239] Pal D, Mallick BN. Role of noradrenergic and GABA-ergic inputs in pedunculopontine tegmentum for regulation of rapid eye movement sleep in rats. *Neuropharmacology* 2006; 51: 1–11.

[240] Macaluso GM, Guerra P, Di Giovanni G, et al. Sleep bruxism is a disorder related to periodic arousals during sleep. *J. Dent. Res.* 1998; 77(4): 565-73 .

[241] Terzano MG, Parrino L. Origin and significance of the cyclic alternating pattern (CAP): review article. *Sleep Med.* 2000; 4: 101–123.

[242] Kato T, Montplaisir JY, Guitard F, et al. Evidence that experimentally induced sleep bruxism is a consequence of transient arousal. *J. Dent Res.* 2003; 82: 284–288.

[243] Huynh N, Kato T, Rompré PH, et al. Sleep bruxism is associated to micro-arousals and an increase in cardiac sympathetic activity. *J. Sleep Res.* 2006; 15: 339–346.

[244] Walters AS, LeBrocq C, Dhar A, et al. Validation of the International Restless Legs Syndrome Study Group rating scale for restless legs syndrome. *Sleep Med* 2003; 4(2): 121-132.

[245] Kohnen R, Oertel WH, Stiasny-Kolster K. Severity rating of RLS: review of 10 years experienced with the RLS-6 scale in clinical trials. *Sleep* 2003; 26 (Abstract).

[246] Kohnen R, Benes H, Heinrich B, et al. Development of the disease-specific restless legs syndrome quality of life (RLS-QoL) questionnaire. *Mov. Disord.* 2002; 232(5): 743. (Abstract).

[247] Ferri R, Lanuzza B, Cosentino FI, et al. A single question for the rapid screening of restless legs syndrome in the neurological clinical practice. *Eur. J. Neurol.* 2007; 14(9): 1016-1021.

[248] Allen RP, Picchietti D, Hening WA, et al. Restless legs syndrome: diagnostic criteria, special considerations, and epidemiology. A report from the restless legs syndrome diagnosis and epidemiology workshop at the National Institutes of Health. *Sleep Med.* 2003; 4(2): 101–119.

[249] Walters AS. Toward a better definition of the restless legs syndrome. The International Restless Legs Syndrome Study Group. *Mov. Disord.* 1995; 10(5): 634-642.

[250] Radtke R. Sleep disorders in neurology. *J. Clin. Neurophysiol.* 2001; 18(2): 77.

[251] Coleman RM. Periodic movements in sleep (nocturnal myoclonus) and restless legs syndrome. In: Guilleminault C, editor. *Sleeping and waking disorders: indications and techniques.* Menlo Park, Calif.: Addison-Wesley, 1982: 265-295.

[252] Recording and scoring leg movements. The Atlas Task Force. *Sleep* 1993; 16(8): 748-759.

[253] Montplaisir J, Boucher S, Nicolas A, et al. Immobilization tests and periodic leg movements in sleep for the diagnosis of restless leg syndrome. *Mov. Disord.* 1998; 13(2): 324-329.

[254] Michaud M, Poirier G, Lavigne G, et al. Restless Legs Syndrome: scoring criteria for leg movements recorded during the suggested immobilization test. *Sleep Med.* 2001; 2(4): 317-321.

[255] Littner M, Kushida CA, Anderson WM, et al. Practice parameters for the role of actigraphy in the study of sleep and circadian rhythms: an update for 2002. *Sleep* 2003; 26(3): 337-341.

[256] Kazenwadel J, Pollmacher T, Trenkwalder C, et al. New actigraphic assessment method for periodic leg movements (PLM). *Sleep* 1995; 18(8): 689-697.

[257] Lagerlof H. [Nocturnal leg cramp is a common and painful symptom in the elderly. Underlying causes and treatment]. Lakartidningen 1999; 96(20): 2505-2506.

[258] Whiteley AM. Cramps, stiffness and restless legs. *Practitioner* 1982; 226(1368): 1085-1087.

[259] Bader G, Lavigne G. Sleep bruxism; an overview of an oromandibular sleep movement disorder. Review Article. *Sleep Med. Rev.* 2000; 4(1): 27-43.

[260] Ahlgren J, Omnell KA, Sonesson B, et al. Bruxism and hypertrophy of the masseter muscle. A clinical, morphological and functional investigation. *Pract. Otorhinolaryngol.* (Basel) 1969; 31(1): 22-29.

[261] Lavigne GJ, Rompre PH, Montplaisir JY, et al. Motor activity in sleep bruxism with concomitant jaw muscle pain. A retrospective pilot study. *Eur. J. Oral Sci.* 1997; 105(1): 92-95.

[262] Kato T, Thie NM, Montplaisir JY, et al. Bruxism and orofacial movements during sleep. *Dent. Clin. North Am.* 2001; 45(4): 657-684.

[263] Abetz L, Allen R, Follet A, et al. Evaluating the quality of life of patients with restless legs syndrome. *Clin. Ther.* 2004; 26: 925–835.

[264] Berger K, Luedemann J, Trenkwalder C, et al. Sex and the risk of restless legs syndrome in the general population. *Arch. Intern. Med.* 2004; 164: 196–202.

[265] Allen RP, Walters AS, Montplaisir J et al. Restless legs syndrome prevalence and impact. REST general population study. *Arch. Intern. Med* 2005, 165: 1286–1292.

[266] Kushida C, Martin M, Nikam P et al. Burden of restless legs syndrome on health-related quality of life. *Qual. Life Res.* 2007, 16: 617–624.

[267] Rothdach AJ, Trenkwalder C, Haberstock J, et al. Prevalence and risk factors of RLS in an elderly population: the MEMO study. Memory and Morbidity in Augsburg Elderly. *Neurology* 2000, 54: 1064–1068.

[268] Sukegawa T, Itoga M, Seno H et al. Sleep disturbances and depression in the elderly in Japan. *Psychiatry Clin. Neurosci.* 2003, 57: 265–270.

[269] Li Y, Mirzaei F, O'Reilly EJ, et al. Prospective study of restless legs syndrome and risk of depression in women. *Am. J. Epidemiol.* 2012 Aug 15; 176(4): 279-88.

[270] Ulfberg J, Nystrom B, Carter N, et al. Prevalence of restless legs syndrome among men aged 18 to 64 years: an association with somatic disease and neuropsychiatric symptoms. *Mov. Disord.* 2001, 16: 1159–1163.

[271] Ohayon MM, Roth T. Prevalence of restless legs syndrome and periodic limb movement disorder in the general population. *J. Psychosom. Res.* 2002, 53: 547–554.

[272] Winkelman JW, Finn L, Young T. Prevalence and correlates of restless legs syndrome symptoms in the Wisconsin Sleep Cohort. *Sleep Med* 2006, 7: 545–552.

[273] Winkelman JW, Shahar E, Sharief I, et al. Association of restless legs syndrome and cardiovascular disease in the Sleep Heart Health Study. *Neurology* 2008, 70: 35–42.

[274] Li Y, Walters AS, Chiuve SE, et al. Prospective study of restless legs syndrome and coronary heart disease among women. *Circulation.* 2012 Oct 2; 126(14): 1689-94.

In: Sleep Medicine
Editors: A. Del Casale, R. Brugnoli and P. Girardi

ISBN: 978-1-62808-515-0
© 2013 Nova Science Publishers, Inc.

Chapter VI

Risk Factors in Obstructive Sleep Apnea Syndrome: Cohort Analysis

F. Chéliout-Héraut[1], M. Faye[2], F. Djouadi, N. Zrek[2] and F. Bour[2]*
[1] Physiology department, Versailles University (UVSQ). France
[2] Neurophysiology Department, Gonesse Hospital. France

Abstract

Objective. The aim of this study is to evaluate the risk factors of Obstructive Sleep Apnea Syndrome (OSAS). Apneas and Hypopneas during sleep are often associated with several significant comorbidities. Epidemiologic studies have shown the high prevalence of undiagnosed obstructive sleep apnea, and even without symptoms, these cases are often associated with hypertension, cardiovascular diseases, strokes, daytime sleepiness and diminished quality of life.

Patients. 186 patients with clinical suspicion of sleep apneas/hypopneas were retrospectively studied to estimate the association between polysomnography assessed AHI and clinical affections.

Methods. All the patients have had a nocturnal polysomnography diagnosis of OSAS. The severity of OSAS was assessed through the AHI (AHI>30: severe OSAS, AHI >15 and < 30: moderate OSAS, AHI > 5 and <15: mild OSAS). All the patients have had an evaluation of their Body Mass Index (BMI), their Epworth Sleepiness Score (ESS), the presence of risk factors such as hypertension, diabetes, cardiovascular disease, ORL pathology.

Results. We observed 67% severe OSAS, 26% moderate OSAS and 6% mild OSAS. Significant predictors of higher AHI were excess body weight, daytime sleepiness, hypertension, ORL affections, cardiovascular diseases and diabetes. Treatment by CPAP was used in 88.7% of all the cases (93.6% in severe OSAS, 81.6% in moderate OSAS and 75% in mild OSAS) with a good outcome. The observance was evaluated with a technical medical home care with systematic regular home visits to adapt the CPAP

---

* Corresponding author: Dr.F.Chéliout-Héraut. Fawzia.heraut@rpc.aphp.fr Phone: 00.33.01.47.10.79.40 Fax: 00.33.01.47.10.79.43.

pressure to patients and monitor their acceptance of the machine during the first month of the treatment.

Conclusion. The major risk factors observed in our study are overweight, obesity, hypertension and nasal congestion. Several authors suggest that OSAS is associated with all these factors, but overweight and obesity constitute a very strong risk factor. This indicates the necessity of nutritional therapy in association with CPAP treatment. The good observance induces the contribution and the efficiency of a technical medical home care.

Keywords: Obstructive sleep apnea syndrome (OSAS). Sleep disorders. Obesity. Diabetes. Polysomnography. Polygraphy. CPAP treatment. Nutritional therapy

Conflicts of Interest: No conflicts of interest for all the authors.

Introduction

Comorbid factors of obstructive sleep apnoea syndrome (OSAS) are multiple and the association of risk factors such as obesity, hypertension, diabetes mellitus, cardio-vascular affections, tobacco have been largely studied [1, 2, 3, 4, 5].

The pathologies associated with OSAS are constantly increasing in Western countries, however OSAS is still today largely underestimated [6, 7]. Among the different studies, the prevalence of sleep apnea syndrome (SAS) varies between 9% and 24% [8, 9] and this pathology constitutes a real public health problem because of its multiple physiopathologic consequences such as excessive daytime sleepiness, risk factors involving road or work accidents [10], cardio-vascular complications [2, 11], cognitive disorders with decreased memory and attention, and reduction of quality of life [12]. The objective diagnosis of SAS requires nocturnal recordings which must be conducted in specifically medical and technical conditions and therefore soon become expensive and time consuming. This results in limited access to treatment in spite of a strong demand from the public. More often than not the studies concerning large populations are established only on questionnaires, to determine the clinical symptoms to prove the necessity of sleep recordings. SAS prevalence in the French population has been studied by Meslier et al [7] who have evaluated the risk factors of comorbidity in more than 4000 patients. These authors have shown the increase frequency of restlessness sleep, nocturnal awakenings, diurnal fatigability, arterial hypertension, cardiovascular affections and diabetes mellitus in patients consulting for SAS suspicion. Nevertheless, gender differences were observed with more frequent headaches among females and more snorers among males. Some authors have shown more severe degrees of OSAS in males [13] through cardio-respiratory nocturnal recordings, actimetry, body position, and snoring. In our study, the aim is to define risk factors in patients with clinical symptoms of OSAS in relation with the severity of the syndrome established through the sleep apnea index on nocturnal recordings. A second aim is to define risk factors leading to an earlier screening with nocturnal investigations in sleep lab carried out more quickly.

Ethical Considerations

All patients gave informed consent to the investigations and this work has been approved by the ethics committee of our institution. We did not cause any physical or emotional harm to our subjects and the results of our research are totally anonymous. The patients were not financially interested in the device.

Material - Method

This retrospective study concerns 186 patients: 111 males and 75 females (mean age: 54 years and 10 months). The data were obtained through the files of patients who were suspected of obstructive sleep apnea syndrome with a follow up of one year in the sleep laboratory of Gonesse Hospital (France). We have considered several parameters. On the one hand: clinical diurnal and nocturnal symptoms of OSAS, physical symptoms obtained with a pneumological and neurological examinations, the BMI, the Epworth score to evaluate excessive daytime sleepiness [14]. On the other hand, we calculated the apnea/hypopnea index (AHI) through the nocturnal polygraphic or polysomnographic recordings to establish the severity of OSAS. Last, we appreciated the comorbidity of arterial hypertension, diabetes mellitus, ORL and cardiovascular affections.

All the patients were systematically examined in a consultation dedicated specifically to sleep disorders. We excluded all the patients suffering from chronic respiratory disease (respiratory insufficiency, COBP) or chronic cardiovascular disease (cardiac insufficiency). Were also excluded all the patients suffering from chronic neurology diseases (Parkinson disease, degenerative affections, dementia...) or vascular cerebral and traumatic cerebral sequellea or restless leg syndrome and those treated with hypnotic and/or antidepressant medications.

We studied all the patients suffering from nocturnal respiratory disorders and variable diurnal consequences. Were then included all the patients with clinical suspicion of OSAS such as breathing sleep disorders (respiratory arrest, snoring) associated with excessive daytime sleepiness, fatigability, cognitive disorders.

All the patients have had a nocturnal recording to confirm the diagnosis of OSAS and its severity and a video was systematically recorded with an infrared camera. All had cardio-respiratory parameters recordings with a lower limbs EMG, and when a suspicion of paroxystical sleep disorders existed, a polysomnography was systematically recorded. Thus, out of the 186 patients, 143 had cardio-respiratory polygraphy recordings (PGV) and 43 had polysomnography recordings (PSG). In the sleep laboratory, all the patients underwent 10-hour overnight recordings (from 10 p.m to 8 a.m) for diagnosis using the Resmed system that recorded bilateral tibial EMG, EKG and the respiratory parameters which are nasal flow, thoracic and abdominal efforts (thoracic and abdominal piezo bands), oxyhemoglobin saturation (digital pulse oximetry), body position and snoring. The beginning and the end of the sleep analysis were identified with body position parameters and video. In the PSG recordings, six EEG channels (symmetrical frontal, temporal and occipital), two EOG channels and chin EMG were added to the other parameters.

BMI was calculated for all the patients. Daytime sleepiness was assessed with ESS.

The sleep stages and respiratory events from all the recordings were scored manually by the same experienced neurophysiologist. Sleep was staged according to the standard criteria. Arousals were defined according to the American Sleep Disorders Association (ASDA) guidelines [15]. Apneas/hypopneas were scored according to the American Academy of Sleep Medicine (AASM) guidelines for measurement in clinical research [16]. Apnea was defined as a complete cessation of nasal flow $\geq$ 10 seconds. Hypopnoea was defined either as a 50% reduction in respiratory airflow lasting $\geq$ 10 seconds or as a 30% reduction in respiratory airflow lasting $\geq$ 10 seconds and accompanied by a decrease of 3% from baseline in SaO2 or by an arousal. An apnea/hypopnea index (AHI) was calculated based on the number of apneas plus hypopneas per hour of sleep.

We calculated the AHI index for each patient. We considered severe OSAS patients those whose apnea index was higher than 30/h; moderate OSAS patients those whose AHI was between 15/h and 30/h; mild OSAS patients those whose AHI was between 5/h and 15/h. Daytime sleepiness was considered excessive when ESS was >10. The results were given in percentages or with a statistical analysis of mean and standard deviations. The comparison of the means was calculated through the student test (t test).

Results

Patients

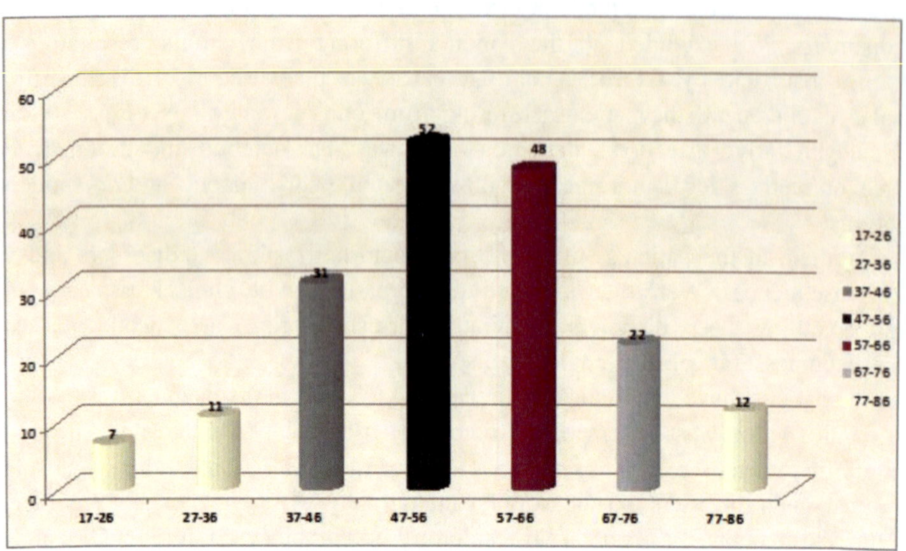

Figure 1. Distribution with the age.

The data show a different distribution according to sex with a male predominance (61% were males and 39% were females). The distribution according to age shows a mean age of 63 years and 6 months with extreme limits of 20 and 83 years (Fig 1). The more frequent age groups were between 40 and 70 years with a peak between 50 and 60 years.

The results of nocturnal sleep analysis shows that severe OSAS appears throughout PGV or PSG recordings among 125 patients out of the 186 (67%) with male predominance (83 males, mean age: 54 years and 7 months and 42 females, mean age 58 years and 3 months). Moderate OSAS is observed in 49 patients (26%) among whom 23 males (mean age 55 years and 4 months) and 26 females (mean age: 58 years and 9 months). Mild OSAS was observed in only 12 patients (6%) among whom five males (mean age: 42 years) and seven females (mean age: 54 years and 10 months).

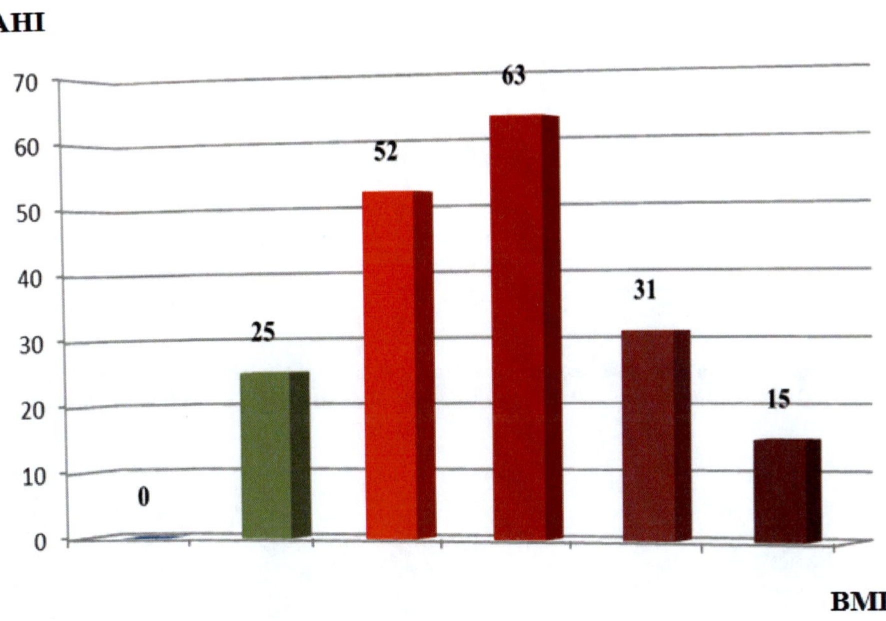

Figure 2. Relation AHI and BMI.

The calculation of BMI indicates obesity (BMI > 30) in 58.4% of the patients (Fig 2). BMI was between 25 and 29.9 in 29.8 % of the patients and a BMI< 25 was obtained in 13.8 % of the cases. Although obesity was more frequent among the males, we do not find significant difference between the sexes; however BMI is directly correlated with the severity of the OSAS (p < 0.0001).

The more common clinical symptoms (Fig 3) found in nocturnal complaints is snoring with 83.8% of the patients among whom 53% were males. "Agitated" sleep is more often observed (54.8%) than respiratory arrests (40.8%) but also more frequently among males (29%). A nyctury is indicated in 45 % of the cases among which 55 % are represented by male subjects. The diurnal complaints are marked by excessive daytime sleepiness (73.1 %), morning headaches (31.7%) and cognitive disorders (29 %). The distribution of these complaints is not differentiated between men and women; they remain more frequent in severe OSAS. The Epworth scale indicates a score above 16 in 5.2 % of the cases, between 13 and 16 in 15.7 % of the cases, between 10 and 12 in 12.2 % of the cases, but normal (under 10) in 66.6 % of the cases. The Epworth score does not show any difference between the sexes, nor does it show age-related significant differences or syndrome of apnea severity.

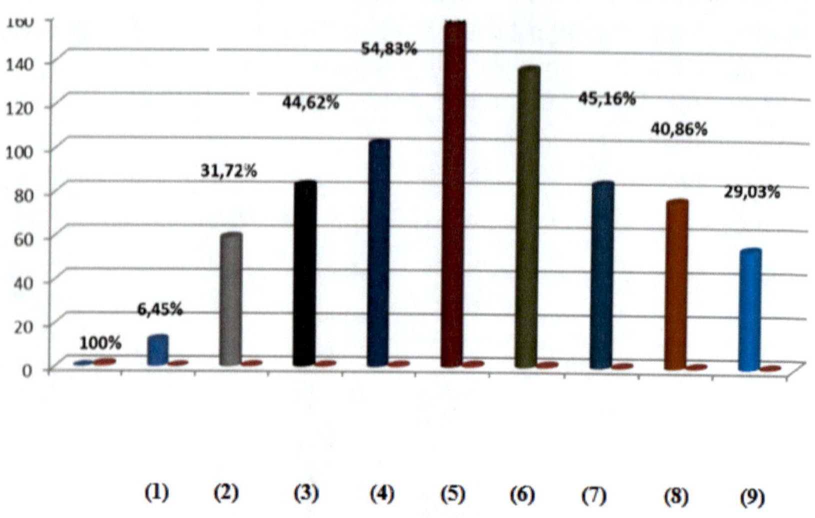

(1): Night sweat. (2): Headaches. (3): Weariness. (4): Sleep disorders. (5): Snoring. (6): Daytime sleepiness. (7): Nyctury. (8): Apneas. (9): Cognitive disorders.

Figure 3. Clinical symptomatology.

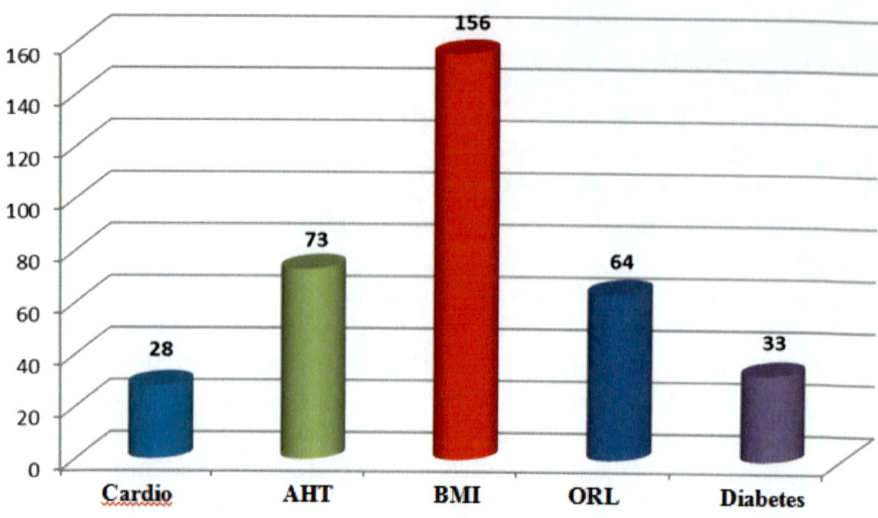

Figure 4. Comorbidity and risk factors (cardiovascular, arterial high tension, BMI, ORL affections and diabetes mellitus).

Among the pathologies found in our patients (Fig 4), the overweight, obesity and arterial high blood pressure prevail. Overweight and obesity are found in 84% of the patients. Arterial high blood pressure is observed in 39.2 % of the cases among severe cases as well as among moderated OSAS, but they are a little less frequent among mild OSAS (25 %).

The ORL affections (cranio-facial deformations, adeno-tonsillar hypertrophy, hypertrophy of the soft palate and\or lingual) are represented in 34.4 % of the cases without any man/woman distinction but with a direct connection to the severity of the OSAS (p < 0.0001).

Diabetes mellitus is found in only 17.7 % of our population. Other pathologies in particular coronary diseases and cerebral vascular accidents are found in some rare cases, essentially in severe OSAS (15 % of the cases). Addiction to smoking is found only in 10 % of the patients with severe OSAS and 12 % of the patients with moderate or mild OSAS.

In many cases we could observe an association of several pathologies, most frequently associated with overweight and arterial high pressure.

Among the patients suffering from severe or moderate apneas (93%), most cases (90%) were treated with continuous positive airway pressure (CPAP). Only 3% had to have surgical adeno-tonsyllectomy. Among the mild OSAS patients, 4% had mandibular treatment and 2% refused any kind of treatment.

Concerning the observance of the CPAP treatment, we observed that 64% of the patients used the system during five hours or so per night, 21% used it less than four hours per night, but 15% could not cope with the mask. In these last cases the mandibular treatment was used with success. The observance was evaluated with a technical medical home care with systematic home visits to adapt the CPAP pressure and to monitor its acceptance during the first month of the treatment.

All the overweight patients were put in diet. The diets were established by a nutritionist and always used in association with CPAP or mandibular treatments.

Discussion

The results of our study indicate a number of risk factors directly correlated to the severity of the obstructive sleep apnea syndrome. We note an increase of the prevalence with age with a peak between 50 and 60 years in our population and an average age of 63.5 years.

These results are in all respects in keeping with the literature as a whole [17, 18, 19, 20]. We also observed a clear male predominance of OSAS.

All the data of the literature, in particular studies of cohorts confirm this male prevalence [7, 8, 13, 21, 22, 23, 24].

So, on a longitudinal analysis (Cleveland Family Study), over a screening of five years, Redline et al [25] noticed a clear increase of the prevalence of the AHI≥15 / h in men (from 13.7 % to 23.4 %) in comparison to the women (from 5.3 % to 11.4 %).

A particular result worth noting in our population is that the moderate and mild OSAS have a quasi-identical distribution between male-female, while the number of severe OSAS cases among the male subjects is practically twice that among the female subjects.

This difference in the distribution according to the severity of OSAS indicates on the one hand, a strong prevalence of OSAS in men, but also can explain that the various clinical observed night symptoms are more frequent in males.

For some authors, this sexual differentiation has to do with hormonal factors. The prevalence of OSAS in women before the menopause and after the menopause if under hormone replacement therapy is clearly much lower than that observed after the menopause (0.6 %, 1.1 % and 5.5 %) [20, 26].

The association snoring and\or respiratory disorders associated with diurnal sleepiness which we regularly noticed in our population also constitutes a common and almost constant risk factor OSAS [7, 25, 27]. Several authors have shown the association snoring/apneas by using questionnaires during the screening OSAS consultations [28, 29].

The existence of an excessive diurnal sleepiness is also a major clinical criterion of diagnosis of OSAS, however its evaluation by the Epworth scale indicates no relation with the gravity of OSAS and as proved in numerous studies [30, 31], this subjective test cannot be considered as discriminating.

Obesity is a major factor which appears in our population: 84 % of the patients present an excess weight and 58.6 % of them are obese (BMI > 30). Obesity is recognized as major risk factor affecting at the same time the prevalence of OSAS and its evolution in time [32, 33, 34, 35].

Besides, it was shown that the risk of moderate or severe OSAS is independently associated with BMI, and with the cervical and abdominal perimeters [36] as well as with the relationship with the difference size/hip [37].

Concerning CPAP treatment, we observed a good observance in 85% of our subjects with a variation in the whole night duration between three and six hours. This result is comparable to those observed by other authors [38].

The quality of the observance is mainly linked to the efficiency of the technical medical home care during the first days of the treatment and before the return home. It also depends on the severity of OSAS and daytime sleepiness. Peppin et al [38] based their study on patients questionnaires and the number of hours they wore their masks, showing that a good compliance is observed in 65% to 80% of cases. Nevertheless some authors argued that in patients with a bad observance another treatment such as oral appliances must be proposed [39, 40]. Such situation is more often found in mild OSAS where the use of mandibular treatment can reduce the AHI and sleep fragmentation [41, 42].

Nutritional treatment constitutes a good complement to CPAP therapy in all the patients suffering from being overweight as it was suggested by other authors [43]. Some simple advice such as the necessity of reducing alcohol consumption can reduce the severity of the apneas in snoring patients [44].

Conclusion

The major risk factors observed in our study are overweight, obesity, hypertension and nasal congestion. Several authors suggest that OSAS is associated with all these factors, but overweight and obesity constitute a very strong risk factor. This indicates the necessity of nutritional therapy in association with CPAP treatment. The accurate observations induce the contribution and the efficiency of a technical medical home care.

References

[1]   Nieto FJ, Young TB, Lind BK, Shahar E, Samet JM, Redline S, D'Agostino RB, Newman AB, Lebowitz MD. Pickering TG for the Sleep Heart Health Study: Association of sleep disordered breathing, sleep apnea, and hypertension in a large community-based study. JAMA 2000; 283: 1829-36.

[2]   Peppard PE, Young T, Palta M, Skatrud J. Prospective study of the association between sleep-disordered breathing and hypertension. N Engl J Med 2000; 342: 1378-84.

[3]   Mooe T, Rabben T, Wiklund U, Franklin KA, Eriksson P. Sleep-disordered breathing in men with coronary artery disease. Chest 1996; 109: 659-63.

[4]   Shahar E, Whitney CW, Redline S, Lee ET, Newman AB, Nieto FJ, O'Connor GT, Boland LL, Schwartz JE, Samet JM. The Sleep Heart Health Study Research Group: Sleep-disordered breathing and cardio-vascular disease. Am J Respir Crit Care Med 2001; 163: 19-25.

[5]   Meslier N, Gagnadoux F, Girault P, Person C, Ouksel H, Urban T, Racineux JL. Impaired glucose-insulin metabolism in men with obstructive sleep apnea syndrome. Eur Respir J 2003; 22: 156-60.

[6]   Larsson LG, Lindberg A, Franklin KA, Lundbäck B. Gender differences in symptoms related to sleep apnea in a general population and in relation to referral to sleep clinic. Chest 2003; 124: 204-11.

[7]   Meslier N, Vol S, Balkau B, Gagnadoux F, Cailleau M, Petrella A, Racineux JL, Tichet. Prévalence des symptômes du syndrome d'apnées du sommeil. Rev Mal Respir 2007; 24 : 305-313.

[8]   Young T, Palta M, Dempsey J, Skatrud J, Weber S, Badr S. The occurrence of sleep-disordered breathing among middle-aged adults. N Engl J Med 1993; 328: 1230-1235.

[9]   Young T, Evans L, Finn L, Palta M. Estimation of the clinically diagnosed proportion of sleep apnea syndrome in middle-aged men and women. Sleep 1997; 20: 705-706.

[10]   Findley LJ, Unverzagt ME, Suratt PM. Automobile accidents involving patients with obstructive sleep apnea. Am Rev Respir Dis 1988; 138 (2): 337-340.

[11]   Hung J, Whitford EG, Parsons RW, Hillman DR. Association of sleep apnoea with myocardial infarction in men. Lancet 1990; 336 (8710): 261-264.

[12]   Flemons WW, Tsai W. Quality of life consequences of sleep-disordered breathing. J Allergy Clin Immunol 1997; 99 (2): S750-S756.

[13]   Paulino A, Damy T, Margarit L, Stoïcad M, Deswarte G , Khouri L, Vermes E, Meizels A, Hittinger L, d'Ortho MP. Prevalence of sleep-disordered breathing in a 316-patient French cohort of stable congestive heart failure. Prévalence des syndromes d'apnées du sommeil dans une cohorte française de 316 patients insuffisants cardiaques. Archives of Cardiovascular Disease 2009; 102, 169-175.

[14]   Johns MW. A new method for measuring daytime sleepiness; the Epworth Sleepiness Scale. Sleep 1991; 14: 540-545.

[15] American sleep disorders association (ASDA). EEG arousals: scoring rules and examples: a preliminary report from the Sleep Disorders Atlas Task Force of the American Sleep Disorders Association. Sleep 1992; 15 (2): 173-184.

[16] The American Association of Sleep Medicine Task Force. "Sleep-related breathing disorders in adults: recommendations for syndrome definition and measurement techniques in clinical research". Sleep 1999; 22 (5): 667-689.

[17] Krieger J. Les syndromes d'apnée du sommeil de l'adulte. Bull Eur Physiopat Resp 1986; 22 :147-186.

[18] Weitzenblum E, Racineux JL. Syndrome d'apnées obstructives du sommeil. Rev Mal Respir 1997; 6 : 322-327.

[19] Bixler EO, Vgontzas AN, Ten Have T, Tyson K, Kales A. Effects of age on sleep apnea in men: I. Prevalence and severity. Am J Respir Crit Care Med 1998; 157: 144-148.

[20] Bixler EO, Vgontzas AN, Lin HM, Ten Have T, Rein J, Vela-Bueno A, Kales A. Prevalence of sleep-disordered breathing in women: effects of gender. Am J Respir Crit Care Med 2001; 163: 608-613.

[21] Ancoli-Israel S, Kripke DF, Klauber MR, Mason WJ, Fell R, Kaplan O. Sleep-disordered breathing in community-dwelling elderly. Sleep 1991; 14: 486-495.

[22] Ancoli-Israel S, Klauber M. R, Stepnowsky C, Estline E, Chinn A, Fell R. Sleep-disordered breathing in African-American elderly. Am J Respir Crit Care Med 1995; 152, 1946–1949.

[23] Ohayon MM, Guilleminault C, Priest RG, Caulet M. Snoring and breathing pauses during sleep: telephone interview survey of a United Kingdom population sample. BMJ 1997; 314: 860-863.

[24] Duran J, Esnaola S, Rubio R, Iztueta A. Obstructive sleep apnea-hypopnea and related clinical features in a population-based sample aged 30 to 70 yr. Am J Respir Crit Care Med 2001; 163: 685-689.

[25] Redline S, Schluchter MD, Larkin EK, Tishler PV. Predictors of longitudinal change in sleep-disordered breathing in a non-clinic population. Sleep 2003; 26: 703-709.

[26] Escourrou P, Roisman GL. Epidémiologie du syndrome d'apnées-hypopnées obstructives du sommeil de l'adulte et de ses complications. Méd Sommeil 2010; 7 : 119-128.

[27] Lugaresi E, Mondini S, Zucconi M, Montagna P, Cirignotta F. Staging of heavy snorers' disease. A proposal. Bull Eur Physiopathol Respir 1983; 19: 590-594.

[28] Netzer NC, Stoohs RA, Netzer CM, Clark K, Strohl KP. Using the Berlin questionnaire to identify patients at risk for sleep apnea syndrome. Ann Inter Med 1999; 131: 485-491.

[29] Netzer NC, Hoegel JJ, Loube D, Netzer CM, Hay B, Alvarez-Sala R, Strohl KP. Prevalence of symptoms and risk of sleep apnea in primary care. Chest 2003; 124: 1406-1414.

[30] Serafini FM, MacDowell AW, Rosemurgy AS, Strait T, Murr MM. Clinical predictors of sleep apnea in patients undergoing bariatric surgery. Obes Surg 2001; 11 (1): 28-31.

[31] Nguyen AT, Baltzan MA, Small D, Wolkove N, Guillon S, Palayew M. Clinical reproducibility of the Epworth Sleepiness Scale. J Clin Sleep Med 2006; 15, 2 (2): 170-174.

[32] Strohl KP, Redline S. Recognition of obstructive sleep apnea. Am J Respir Crit Care Med 1996; 154: 279-289.

[33] Labban JP. Epidémiologie croisée de l'obésité et des troubles respiratoires du sommeil. Médecine du sommeil 2004 ; 1: 13-16.

[34] Young T, Peppard PE, Taheri S. Excess weight and sleep-disordered breathing. J Appl Physiol 2005; 99: 1592-1599.

[35] Resta O, Foschino-Barbaro MP, Legari G, Talamo S, Bonfitto P, Palumbo A, Minenna A, Giogino R, De Pergola G. Sleep related bretahing disorders, loud snoring and excessive daytime sleepiness in obese subjects. In J Obes 2000; 25: 669-675.

[36] Newman AB, Foster G, Givelber R, Nieto FJ, Redline S, Young T. Progression and regression of sleep-disordered breathing with changes in weight: the Sleep Heart Health Study. Arch Intern Med 2005; 165: 2408-2413.

[37] Tischler PV, Larkin EK, Schluchter MD, Redline S; Young T. Incidence of sleep-disordered breathing in an urban population: the relative importance of risk factors in the development of sleep-disordered breathing. JAMA 2003; 289: 2230-2237.

[38] Pépin JL, Krieger J, Rodenstein D, Cornette A, Sforza E, Delguste P, Deschaux C, Grillier V, Lévy P. Effective compliance during the first 3 months of continuous positive airway pressure: a European prospective study of 121 patients. Am J Respir Crit Care Med 1999; 160: 1124-1129.

[39] Reeves-Hoche MK, Meck R, Zwillich CW. Nasal CPAP: An objective evaluation of patient compliance. Am J Respir Crit Care Med 1994; 149: 149-154.

[40] American Sleep Disorders Association. Practice parameters for the treatment of snoring and obstructive sleep apnea with oral appliances. Sleep 1995; 18: 511-513.

[41] Ferguson KA, Ono T, Lowe AA, al-Majed S, Love LL, Fleetham JA. A short controlled trial of an adjustable oral appliance for the treatment of mild to moderate obstructive sleep apnea. Thorax 1997; 52 (4): 362-368.

[42] Powel NB, Riley RW, Troel RJ, Guilleminault C. Radiofrequency volumetric tissue reduction of the palate in subjects with sleep-disordered breathing. Chest 1998; 113: 1163-1174.

[43] Levy P, Pépin JL, Mayer P, Wuyam B, Veale D. Management of simple snoring, upper airway resistance syndrome, and moderate sleep apnea syndrome. Sleep 1996; 19 (9 Suppl): S101-110.

[44] Scanlan MF, Roebuck T, Little PJ, Redman JR, Naughton MT. Effect of moderate alcohol upon obstructive sleep apnoea. Eur Respir J 2000; 16: 909-913.

In: Sleep Medicine
Editors: A. Del Casale, R. Brugnoli and P. Girardi

ISBN: 978-1-62808-515-0
© 2013 Nova Science Publishers, Inc.

Chapter VII

Sleep Bruxism and Gastroesophageal Reflux as a Peripheral Risk Factor

Shouichi Miyawaki[1],, Takakazu Yagi[2], Kunihiro Nagayama[2],
Haruhito Ohmure[1], Kyoko Kanematsu[1] and Yoko Sakoguchi[1]*
[1]Department of Orthodontics, Field of Developmental Medicine,
Health Research Course, Kagoshima University Graduate School of Medical
and Dental Sciences, Kagoshima, Japan
[2]Department of Orthodontics, Kagoshima University Hospital, Kagoshima, Japan

Abstract

Sleep bruxism (SB) often causes sleep disturbances in sleep partners, occlusal wear, wedge-shaped defects and fracture of the teeth, prosthesis fracture, masticatory muscle discomfort upon waking, masseter muscle hypertrophy, and temporomandibular disorders (TMDs). The International Classification of Sleep Disorders 2nd edition (ICSD-2) categorizes SB as a sleep-related movement disorder. Although the clinical diagnostic criteria specified in the ICSD-2 are frequently used for diagnosis of SB, they lack accuracy. In contrast, the criteria employed for diagnosis by polysomnography (PSG) are more reliable. The prevalence of SB in adults is 8% overall and decreases with age. Although palliative therapies, such as the use of splints, counseling, and drugs, are available for patients with SB, there is no broadly accepted curative therapy. SB is more closely related to various central factors than to peripheral occlusal factors. Recent studies have proposed a multifactorial model for understanding the mechanism underlying SB. In addition, SB has recently been suggested to be caused by esophageal acid stimulation and to be related to swallowing and gastroesophageal reflux. Therefore, gastroesophageal reflux (GER) during sleep, as well as other factors, should be evaluated in future studies of SB.

---

* Corresponding Author address: Department of Orthodontics, Field of Developmental Medicine, Health Research Course, Kagoshima University Graduate School of Medical and Dental Sciences, 8-35-1 Sakuragaoka, Kagoshima City, Kagoshima 890-8544, Japan. Email: miyawaki@dent.kagoshima-u.ac.jp.

Keywords: Sleep, bruxism, gastroesophageal reflux

Introduction

Sleep bruxism (SB) is an involuntary stereotypic movement characterized by grinding, clenching, and tapping of the teeth during sleep regardless of normal oral functions, such as mastication and articulation. The International Classification of Sleep Disorders 2nd edition (ICSD-2) categorizes SB as a sleep-related movement disorder with no clear purpose. SB often causes sleep disturbances in sleep partners, occlusal wear, wedge-shaped defects of the teeth, prosthesis fracture, masticatory muscle discomfort upon waking, masseter muscle hypertrophy, and temporomandibular disorders (TMDs), which decrease the quality of life (QOL) of patients with SB and their sleep partners [1-8]. However, the mechanism underlying the pathogenesis or cause of SB is unclear. Meanwhile, rapid progress has been made in understanding the functional relationship between the oral and gastrointestinal regions, and recent reports have shed light on the significance of gastroesophageal reflux (GER) in the pathogenesis of SB [9-12].

In this review article, we first describe the definition, diagnosis, prevalence, pathology, treatment/management, and physiology of SB, including hypotheses as to its cause and details of related factors [1-8, 13-17]. We then demonstrate the relationships between SB and experimental esophageal acidification during sleep [11], sleep-related GER [9, 18, 19], and swallowing [20, 21] demonstrated by the results of previous studies from our research group and others and thereby highlight the importance of GER in the genesis of SB.

Definition

The American Academy of Orofacial Pain guidelines define bruxism as a parafunctional activity that includes nocturnal or diurnal clenching and grinding of the teeth. SB can be diagnosed only by ambulatory electromyography (EMG) or polysomnography (PSG) [22]. According to the ICSD-2, SB is an oral parafunction that includes grinding or clenching of the teeth during sleep in association with sleep arousal. SB is distinguished from diurnal bruxism. SB belongs to the simple repetitive movement disorder subcategory of the sleep-related movement disorders [1, 2, 6, 13].

Diagnosis (Clinical and Research Diagnostic Criteria)

Evaluation of SB includes assessment by a questionnaire, clinical examination, examination using an oral appliance, ambulatory EMG, and PSG. Patients are examined in a sleep laboratory. PSG is the most reliable method for evaluating SB [23]. However, PSG requires costly resources and analysis by sleep technicians and must be performed over 2 successive nights in order to remove the first-night effect from the recordings [3].

According to the clinical diagnostic criteria for SB in the ICSD-2, which are frequently used [1], SB can be diagnosed when the subjective and/or objective symptom of teeth grinding or clenching is observed along with 1 or more of the following symptoms: (1) excessive occlusal wear, (2) discomfort, lassitude, and pain of the masticatory muscles and stiff jaw or difficulty in jaw opening, and (3) masseter muscle hypertrophy determined by palpation during maximum voluntary clenching [1, 2, 6, 13, 14]. However, the disadvantages of these clinical diagnostic criteria, including poor accuracy, prompted Lavigne *et al.* to formulate a set of highly accurate research diagnostic criteria for SB that are based on PSG data including EMG with a sampling frequency of more than 128 Hz [24]. These research diagnostic criteria are obtained first by simultaneous recording of audio-video data of the head and neck along with PSG examinations including electroencephalography (EEG) from C3A2 and O2A1, electrooculography (EOG), electrocardiography (ECG), EMG from mentalis and masseter or temporalis muscles, and respiration. Next, the EMG results for the masticatory muscles are analyzed after the data are confirmed to be sleep data. The patient is diagnosed with SB if he or she meets 2 or more of the following 3 criteria: (1) more than 4 episodes of rhythmic masticatory muscle activity (RMMA) per hour, (2) more than 25 EMG bursts per hour, and (3) 1 or more teeth grinding sounds per night [6, 8, 13, 14, 25].

Prevalence

In the general population, the reported prevalence of SB as evaluated according to the ISCD-2 clinical diagnostic criteria [1] is 14–18% in children under 11 years of age, 13% in adults 18–29 years old, and 3% in elderly persons over 60 years of age [26]. The mean prevalence of SB is 8% in adults, and prevalence decreases with age because elderly persons often have too few remaining teeth to perform bruxism [2, 6, 8].

Among patients with SB who were diagnosed using on the research diagnostic criteria, the incidence of SB episodes (times per hour) was reported to be stable between days, with a coefficient of variation of 25% [4]. In contrast, the incidence of teeth grinding sounds in patients with SB varies widely between days, with a coefficient of variation of 50% [3, 8].

Pathology and Symptoms

There have been many descriptions of the pathology and symptoms of SB. Representative symptoms of SB are as follows [3, 6, 8, 13-16, 27]:
(1) Disturbance of a sleep partner's sleep due to teeth grinding sounds [3]
(2) Damage to the teeth and/or prostheses, including occlusal wear, wedge-shaped defects of the cervical regions of the teeth, hypersensitivity, and prosthesis failure [5, 8, 15, 16]

Occlusal wear refers to the state in which the enamel and dentine of the teeth are worn down by chronic contact with the teeth in the opposing jaw. Occlusal wear is usually caused by physiological movements, such as mastication of food, and progresses with age. Excessive occlusal wear of specific regions of the dentition is often observed in patients with SB. Therefore, occlusal wear is included in the clinical diagnostic criteria for SB. We must be careful to note that occlusal wear is observed in 100% of patients with SB but also in 40% of subjects without SB, i.e., occlusal wear alone is not a sufficient criterion for SB.

Wedge-shaped defects of the cervical regions of the teeth, or abfraction, are often observed in patients with SB. Abfraction is observed in the presence of excessive load on the teeth caused by SB or other movements, although to date there is no consensus regarding the mechanism by which these stimuli cause such defects.

Hypersensitivity, i.e., tooth pain due to cold or other stimuli, is often caused by occlusal wear and/or wedge-shaped defects of the teeth even when dental caries is not observed.

Patients with SB often experience recurrent detachment or destruction of prostheses after prosthetic placement. SB is considered an important cause of prosthesis failure.

(3) Damage to periodontal tissue [8, 15, 16]

Occlusal trauma and pain, alveolar bone resorption, and gingival recession are often observed in patients with SB.

(4) Masticatory muscle damage [27, 28]

SB patients often experience discomfort, lassitude, and/or pain of the masticatory muscles along with a stiff jaw upon awakening. As for occlusal wear, it is important to remember that while these symptoms are included in the clinical diagnostic criteria for SB, they are not sufficient for diagnosis [29]. If severe SB continues, masseter muscle hypertrophy [29] and addition of bone to the gonial angle may be observed. Furthermore, it has been reported that 65% of patients with SB present with tension-type headache, particularly around the region of the temporal muscles.

(5) Damage to the temporomandibular joint (TMJ) [3, 8, 15, 16, 30]

SB patients often suffer from TMD consisting of pain in the TMJ and/or masticatory muscles, TMJ sounds, jaw opening difficulty, and/or abnormal jaw movement. Many clinicians and researchers have noted this close relationship between SB and TMD. Studies of children have reported that the development of SB correlates significantly with the presence of TMD symptoms and that the rates of both TMD symptoms and parafunctions such as SB and clenching are significantly decreased by the absence of unpleasant experiences during daily life. A longitudinal study in which children and adults were followed up for 10 years found that the development of parafunctions such as SB and clenching correlated significantly with TMD symptoms. In another study of men and women over 18 years of age, bruxism increased the risk for TMD 4.2–8.4-fold. Therefore, bruxism is believed to be closely associated with TMD. However, to date, the causal relationship between bruxism and TMD remains unknown.

(6) Others [27]

Patients with SB often develop torus on the lingual surface of the mandible and the mid-palatal region and tooth indentations on the lateral portion of the tongue and the buccal mucosa.

Treatment/Management [8, 17, 27]

As the cause of SB has yet to be fully elucidated, there is no curative therapy, and only palliative treatment is available. Splint therapy is a widely used treatment that protects the teeth and can relieve pain in the muscles and TMJ. In addition to this, it has been reported that a mandibular repositioning appliance, which is used for the treatment of obstructive sleep apnea, has a superior efficacy for the management of SB than splint but many patients with SB preferred splint than mandibular repositioning appliance because of the size [17]. Surgical procedures, such as masseter muscle reduction and gonial angle plastic surgery, or injection of botulinum toxin injection can be beneficial for patients with SB with masseter muscle hypertrophy. Occlusal adjustment, psychological therapy, cognitive therapy, biofeedback therapy, physical therapy, and pharmacological therapy with muscle relaxants or antianxiety agents have also been used. However, none of these treatments has yet been accepted as a general therapy because there have been no large-scale etiological studies to validate their effects [8, 17]. In the future, randomized controlled trials of presumptive treatments for SB will be needed to elucidate which of these therapies are most effective.

Physiology

Approximately 90% of episodes of SB involve RMMA. RMMA has been reported in normal subjects who do not meet the clinical diagnostic criteria for SB of the ICSD-2 [3, 8, 15]. However, the frequency of RMMA episodes is approximately 3 times higher in patients with SB than in normal subjects, and masticatory muscle activity is approximately 40% higher in patients with SB than in normal subjects. Therefore, SB is considered to be an extreme form of RMMA, i.e., RMMA with teeth grinding sounds and higher masticatory muscle activity. RMMA has been observed mainly during light sleep (non-rapid eye movement (NREM) sleep stages 1 and 2) and often just after microarousal. Therefore, RMMA is an important physiological phenomenon for understanding the pathophysiology of SB [3, 8, 15].

The pathophysiological phenomena associated with SB occur in linear progression. First, cardiac sympathetic nervous activity increases approximately 4 minutes before the onset of SB. Then, brain activity increases approximately 4 seconds before the onset of SB, and heart rate, suprahyoid muscle activity, and respiratory rate increase 1 second before the onset of SB. Finally, the jaw-closing muscles, including the masseter and temporalis, activate and tooth grinding occurs [3]. To date, most studies have focused on the contributions of occlusion and stress to SB. However, the relationships between SB and heredity, circadian rhythms, and neurotransmitters have been recently suggested to warrant study [3, 8, 15]. More recently, we have reported a close relationship between SB and GER [9, 11].

1) Pathogenesis of SB [3, 8, 15]

Peripheral occlusal morphological abnormalities, such as malocclusion, have long been believed to be a major cause of SB. However, this theory is now almost defunct because experimental early tooth contact has been shown not to cause SB, as no occlusal contact occurs just before SB begins. At present, periodontal sensation is considered to be a factor that changes muscle activity rather than the cause of SB [3]. The central nervous system is considered to be closely involved in the etiology of SB because neurotransmitter precursors have been shown to be related to the pathogenesis of SB [31], SB occurs in conjunction with microarousal, i.e., 3–10-second periods of cortical activity [32], and psychological factors, such as emotional stress and anxiety, may also be related to SB [26, 33, 34]. In a study supporting the role of psychological factors, it has been reported that patients subjected to an experimental psychological stress task show a significant association between SB and psychological stress sensitivity, as assessed by measurement of the level of chromogranin A (CgA) in the saliva [35]. SB has also been reported to be closely related to extrinsic factors, such as selective serotonin reuptake inhibitors (SSRIs) [36], alcohol, caffeine, smoking, and late-night snacks [26, 37]. Recent research has suggested a possible genetic contribution to the etiology of SB; in a Japanese population, carriers of the C allele of HTR2A, with the single-nucleotide polymorphism rs6313 (102C>T), were at increased risk for SB (odds ratio = 4.250, 95% confidence interval: 1.599–11.297, P = 0.004) [38]. Therefore, a multifactorial etiological model for SB is favored at present [3, 8, 15].

2) Related factors

The factors other than GER that are related to the pathogenesis of SB can be summarized as follows:

(1) Sleep

SB occurs mainly during light sleep (NREM sleep stages 1 and 2), the shift to rapid eye movement (REM) sleep, and REM sleep; it rarely occurs during deep sleep (NREM sleep stages 3 and 4) [8, 15]. As previously noted, SB has been reported to occur just after natural [32] or experimental microarousal [39, 40]. Therefore, SB is closely associated with waking during sleep. On the other hand, the sleep architecture of patients with SB has been reported to be within the normal range [8, 15].

A large-scale etiological survey representing the 158 million inhabitants of the U.K., Germany, and Italy estimated to have SB based on the clinical diagnostic criteria of the ICSD-2 suggested that obstructive sleep apnea syndrome, heavy snoring, and moderate daytime sleepiness are indicators of risk for SB (odds ratio =1.3–1.8) [30]. SB has been observed in approximately 50% of patients with upper airway resistance syndrome [41], and the levels of severity of both obstructive sleep apnea and SB were reduced after the adoption of continuous positive airway pressure or an oral appliance, such as a mandibular advancement appliance (MAA) [42]. However, PSG data from patients with mild to moderate obstructive sleep apnea syndrome showed that episodes of SB were associated not with episodes of obstructive sleep apnea but rather with sleep disorder, although 40–50% of patients with obstructive sleep apnea syndrome were also diagnosed with SB [43]. Therefore, the causal relationship between obstructive sleep apnea and SB remains unclear [44].

(2) Neurotransmitters in the brain

L-dopa, a precursor of neurotransmitters in the brain, has been reported to decrease the incidence of SB [31]. However, the effect of L-dopa may not be significant, as the rate of reduction was within the variation seen between days in more than half of the patients examined [45]. Therefore, the details of the relationship between SB and L-dopa remain unknown.

(3) Lifestyle

The consumption of late-night snacks has been reported to increase the risk for SB 1.8–3.4-fold [37], and smoking, caffeine, and alcohol intake have also been reported to increase the risk for SB [8, 15, 26]. However, the mechanisms of these relationships remain unclear.

(4) Stress and psychosomatic characteristics

SB has been reported to be related to personality as well as to several psychosomatic factors, including stress, depression, anxiety, introversion, cautiousness, indifference to a particular person, inferiority complex, and worry [26, 46-50]. The aforementioned large-scale etiological survey in Europe suggested a high level of stress (odds ratio = 1.3) and anxiety (odds ratio = 1.3) to be risk indicators [26]. Another study suggested that patients with SB reacted more strongly to stress, as indicated by greater heart rate (R–R interval) variability [49]. On the other hand, it is reported that individuals with sleep disorders score higher on Minnesota Multiphasic Personality Inventory (MMPI) tests than those without, although MMPI scores did not differ significantly between patients with SB and normal volunteers [50]. According to a study which examined the relationship between the Jenkins Activity Survey (JAS) and the Life Events Scale of Holmes and Rahe in dental patients with and without SB, "Type A" behavior, rather than stress alone, was significantly associated with SB. However, the combination of stress and "Type A" behavior was also significantly associated with SB. This combination was the strongest predictor of SB [51]. Furthermore, a previous study demonstrated that bruxism-like movement occurred more frequently in laboratory rats after the induction of emotional stress using a communication box and that this movement disappeared after the administration of antianxiety agents [52].

Another animal experiment suggested a stress-reducing theory in which bruxism inhibits the development of gastric ulcers and decreases the response to autonomic nervous activity, i.e., that bruxism is performed in order to reduce stress [53]. Therefore, while the mechanism remains unknown, there is a good possibility that stress and other psychosomatic factors are related to SB [8, 15].

(5) Heritable and familial factors [54]

A large-scale etiological survey of twins suggested that most adults with SB had suffered from SB since childhood and that the concordance rate of SB was significantly higher between monozygotic twins than between dizygotic twins. These results suggest that SB may be more strongly related to heritable than to environmental factors.

(6) Body movement and sleep position [20, 55]

SB has been reported to occur more frequently in conjunction with body movement. We previously showed that SB occurred more frequently in the supine position than in other positions and occurred only rarely in the prone position.

(7) Developmental disability [56]

SB is often observed in patients with mental retardation, autism, and Down syndrome. Diagnosis and treatment are known to be difficult in such patients because of undetectable causes and difficulties during interview and examination.

(8) Swallowing

Swallowing has been observed more frequently during SB episodes, particularly during the last one-third of an episode, than at other times [20]. Swallowing movements allow the transport of a food bolus from the oral cavity to the stomach. Swallowing while awake consists of voluntary and involuntary movements, but during sleep it is an involuntary movement. The frequency of swallowing decreases during sleep to approximately one-tenth of that observed during waking [57]. The salivary flow rate is also reduced during sleep. Jaw movement and masticatory muscle activity increase the salivary flow rate over that observed at rest. Therefore, the mechanism of the onset of SB [58] can be speculated to be closely related to the initiation of swallowing and an increase in the salivary flow rate [8, 15].

3) SB and GER

(1) Commonality of factors related to SB and GER

GER is the backward flow of gastric juice from the stomach to the esophagus. It is caused mainly by transient relaxation of the lower esophageal sphincter (LES) and is observed more frequently in children than in adults [59], although GER disease (GERD), which includes esophagitis and heartburn, occurs more frequently in elderly persons than in younger persons [60]. GER is related to the swallowing of saliva in that swallowing, together with esophageal peristalsis, contributes to the clearance of acid from the esophagus after GER in healthy subjects [18, 19, 61-63]. Therefore, SB can be speculated to be closely related to the clearance of acid from the esophagus after GER through the stimulation of salivary flow and consecutive swallowing.

GER is reported to cause microarousal or temporary waking during sleep with some frequency [64]. GER is also often observed in patients with obstructive sleep apnea syndrome. The reason for this is that respiratory movement in the presence of obstruction of the upper airway produces negative pressure in the esophagus, facilitating GER [65].

GER has also been associated with neurotransmitters in the brain. The stimulated secretion of gastric juice decreases with L-dopa administration, the LES contains dopamine receptors, and GER has been reduced by the administration of dopamine receptor agonists [66].

Various lifestyle factors also appear to influence GER. The consumption of nighttime snacks within 3 hours until bedtime increases the risk for GER approximately 7.5-fold [67], and smoking is also related to increase gastric acid secretion [68]. In addition, GER is frequently associated with alcohol and caffeine intake [69].

GER is also associated with stress. Stress increases gastric acid secretion, and GERD patients under chronic stress were reported to feel pain upon even slight stimulation of the esophagus [70]. Stress is also known to inhibit serous salivary secretion [71].

Hereditary and familial factors may also contribute to GER. A large-scale twin cohort epidemiological study reported that GER may initially be more closely related to hereditary factors than to environmental factors [72].

GER can also be affected by sleep position and body movement. GER was reported to occur more frequently in the supine position than in other positions and to occur only rarely when subjects' upper bodies were elevated to 30 degrees from prone [73].

Individuals with developmental disabilities may be predisposed to GER. For example, it was reported that 14% of individuals with Down syndrome suffer from gastrointestinal disorders, and 36% of these individuals suffered from GERD [74]. In addition, 43% of individuals with Down syndrome also experience severe complications related to GERD [75]. Furthermore, patients with neuropathy, such as mental retardation, are reported to be at higher risk for gastrointestinal disease, and 77% of these patients suffer from GERD [76] that continues throughout their lifetimes [77].

As for the relationship between GER and swallowing, swallowing is known to be important in clearing acid from the esophagus after GER [57, 78]. The ability to clear acid from the esophagus is reduced when GER occurs during sleep because, as noted, the frequency of swallowing and successive peristalsis decreases considerably during normal sleep [18, 19]. GER often occurs in conjunction with microarousal or awakening during sleep and also during NREM sleep stage 2, much like SB [18, 19].

Therefore, the factors related to SB correspond almost perfectly with those related to GER. In addition to this striking pattern, the symptoms of bruxism in an adult patient with severe occlusal wear and parafunction improved after the diagnosis and treatment of GERD [79]. There thus appears to be a close relationship between the genesis of SB and GER.

(2) Evidence that esophageal acidification causes SB

After we initially hypothesized that GER is closely related to the genesis of SB, we tested this hypothesis using pH monitoring of adult participants. Patients with SB exhibited a significantly greater number of episodes of GER in the night, and most episodes of both SB and swallowing occurred during rapid decreases in pH, i.e., GER episodes. Furthermore, experimental administration of proton pump inhibitors (PPIs) significantly decreased the numbers of episodes of both SB and GER [9].

We also examined 12 healthy normal adults by PSG, including esophageal pH monitoring and EMG of the masticatory muscles. Experimental esophageal acidification during NREM sleep stage 2 significantly increased the numbers of SB episodes, EMG bursts, and tooth grinding sounds to levels comparable to those of patients with SB, and SB episodes were observed even when the acid did not reach the pharynx [11]. These results suggest the possibility that SB is stimulated by acid in the esophagus as a functional movement to increase the salivary flow rate and cause swallowing during sleep [9, 21, 80].

On the other hand, a study in which children were examined using PSG with pH monitoring found no significant temporal relationship between a decrease in esophageal pH and the onset of SB [81]. However, none of the children without SB had an esophageal pH of 4 or lower, while the pH was 4 or lower in 20% of the children with SB. Further study is needed to clarify the relationship between SB and GER in both children and adults.

Future Prospects

The cause and mechanism of the initiation of SB have not been sufficiently clarified, and as no broadly accepted curative therapy has yet been developed, palliative therapy remains the main treatment for SB [1, 2, 4, 5, 8, 17, 45]. Triple-P palliative therapy, which consists of splint therapy (Plates), counseling therapy (Pep talk), and, if the first 2 approaches are not effective, drug therapy (Pills), is considered useful at present. However, there is still no consensus regarding the overall effectiveness of this treatment for SB [23]. In keeping with our hypothesis that SB is caused by esophageal acidification, i.e., that it is due to GER, and that SB is a physiological response that promotes swallowing and increases the rate of salivary flow during sleep, we believe that several of the strategies used to cure GERD may also be curative for SB.

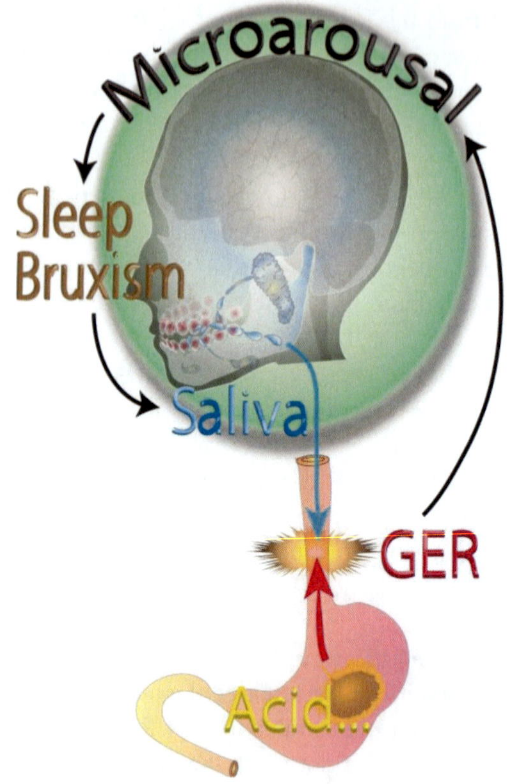

Figure. Hypothesis of SB occurrence.

According to the guidelines for treatment of GERD published by the Japanese Society of Gastroenterology [82], the purpose of treatment is to control GERD symptoms, improve QOL, and prevent various complications. The complications of GERD include anemia, bleeding, stricture of the esophagus, Barrett's esophagus, and esophageal adenocarcinoma [83]. The administration of a standard dose of a PPI is reportedly effective for curing esophagitis and maintaining a healthy state in patients with GERD, as 80–90% of patients with GERD are cured after PPI administration. Administration of H2 receptor inhibitors has also been reported to cure 40–70% of patients with GERD. However, PPIs rather than H2 receptor inhibitors are currently recommended for patients with complications of GERD [84, 85]. PPIs are used as the first-choice drug for GERD because they are reportedly more effective than H2 receptor inhibitors at improving QOL [86, 87]. Treatment approaches other than drug therapy, e.g., resting in the Fowler position (with the upper body elevated), sleeping in the left lateral decubitus position, altering the diet to reduce obesity, and moderating the intake of fatty foods, carbonated drinks, chocolate, cigarettes, and alcohol, are also recommended for GERD [82]. If both drug therapy and lifestyle changes are insufficient, patients with GERD may be treated by surgical procedures that have recently become standard, such as a laparoscopic stomach-esophagus counter current prevention operation [82].

We have shown that acid stimulation of the esophagus causes SB in healthy human volunteers [11] and that mastication induces initial gastric emptying by modulation of gastric activity [12]. These results suggest that the physiological improvement of esophageal symptoms may inhibit the onset of SB. However, randomized control trials will be necessary to determine whether treatment for GERD is also effective against SB. (Figure)

Acknowledgments

We thank Professor Gilles J. Lavigne of Montreal University, Professor Teruko Takano-Yamamoto of the Department of Orthodontics, Tohoku University, and Professor Hirohito Tsubouchi of the Department of Digestive Disease and Lifestyle-Related Disease and Professor Akio Inui of the Department of Psychosomatic Internal Medicine, Kagoshima University Graduate School of Medicine and Dentistry, for their helpful comments on our previous studies.

References

[1]   American Academy of Sleep Medicine. The international classification of sleep disorders. 2nd ed. Westchester: Diagnostic and coding manual, American Academy of Sleep Medicine; 2005.

[2]   Walters AS, Lavigne G, Hening W, Picchietti DL, Allen RP, Chokroverty S, Kushida CA, Bliwise DL, Mahowald MW, Schenck CH, Ancoli-Israel S. The scoring of movements in sleep. *J Clin Sleep Med.* 2007;15:155-167.

[3]   Lavigne GJ, Khoury S, Abe S, Yamaguchi T, Raphael K. Bruxism physiology and pathology: an overview for clinicians. *J Oral Rehabil.* 2008;35:476-494.

[4]   Lavigne GJ, Montplaisir JY. Restless legs syndrome and sleep bruxism: prevalence and association among Canadians. *Sleep.* 1994;17:739-743.

[5]   Ramfjord SP, Ash MM, eds. Occlusion. 4th ed. Philadelphia: *WB Saunders;* 1995.

[6]   Lobbezoo R, Aarab G, van der Zaag J. Chaptor 12: Definitions, Epidemiology, and Etiology of Seep Bruxism. In: Lavigne GJ, Cistulli PA, Smith MT, eds. Sleep medicine for dentists - a practical overview -, Section III: Sleep Bruxism and Movement Disorders. Chicago: *Quintessence Pub.;* 2009:95-100.

[7]   Kato T, Thie NM, Huynh N, Miyawaki S, Lavigne GJ. Topical Review: Sleep bruxism and the role of peripheral sensory influences. *J Orofac Pain.* 2003;17:191-213.

[8]   Lavigne GJ, Manzini C, Huynh NT. Sleep bruxism. In: Kryger MH, Roth T, Dement W, eds. Principles and practice of sleep medicine. Philadelphia: *WB Saunders;* 2011:1128-1139.

[9]   Miyawaki S, Tanimoto Y, Araki Y, Katayama A, Fujii A, Takano-Yamamoto T. Association

between nocturnal bruxism and gastroesophageal reflux. *Sleep.* 2003;26:888-892.

[10] Togawa R, Ohmure H, Sakaguchi K, Takada H, Oikawa K, Nagata J, Yamamoto T, Tsubouchi H, Miyawaki S. Gastroesophageal reflux symptoms in adults with skeletal Class III malocclusion examined by questionnaires. *Am J Orthod Dentofacial Orthop.* 2009;133:e1-e6.

[11] Ohmure H, Oikawa K, Kanematsu K, Saito Y, Yamamoto T, Nagahama H, Tsubouchi H, Miyawaki S. Influence of experimental esophageal acidification on sleep bruxism: A randomized trial. *J Dent Res.* 2011;90:665-671.

[12] Ohmure H, Takada K, Nagayama K, Sakiyama T, Tsubouchi H, Miyawaki S. Mastication suppresses initial gastric emptying by modulating gastric activity. *J Dent Res.* 2012;91:293-298.

[13] Kato T, Blanchet PJ. Chapter 13: Orofacial Movement Disorders in Sleep. In: Lavigne GJ, Cistulli PA, Smith MT, eds. Sleep medicine for dentists - a practical overview -, Section III: Sleep Bruxism and Movement Disorders. Chicago: *Quintessence Pub.;* 2009:101-108.

[14] Koyano K, Tsukiyama Y. Chapter 14: Clinical Approach to Diagnosis of Sleep Bruxism. In: Lavigne GJ, Cistulli PA, Smith MT, eds. Sleep medicine for dentists - a practical overview -, Section III: Sleep Bruxism and Movement Disorders. Chicago: *Quintessence Pub.;* 2009:109-116.

[15] Lavigne GJ, Tuomilehto H, Macaluso G. Chapter 15: Pathophysiology of Sleep Bruxism. In: Lavigne GJ, Cistulli PA, Smith MT, eds. Sleep medicine for dentists - a practical overview -, Section III: Sleep Bruxism and Movement Disorders. Chicago: *Quintessence Pub.;* 2009:117-124.

[16] Huynh N, Guilleminault C. Chapter 16: Sleep Bruxism in Children. In: Lavigne GJ, Cistulli PA, Smith MT, eds. Sleep medicine for dentists - a practical overview -, Section III: Sleep Bruxism and Movement Disorders. Chicago: *Quintessence Pub.;* 2009:125-132.

[17] Winocur E. Chapter 17: Management of Sleep Bruxism. In: Lavigne GJ, Cistulli PA, Smith MT, eds. Sleep medicine for dentists - a practical overview -, Section III: Sleep Bruxism and Movement Disorders. Chicago: *Quintessence Pub.;* 2009:133-144.

[18] Orr WC. Gastrointestinal physiology in relation to sleep. In: Kryger MH, Roth T, Dement W, eds. Principles and practice of sleep medicine. Philadelphia: *WB Saunders;* 2011:312-322.

[19] Orr WC. Gastrointestinal disorders. In: Kryger MH, Roth T, Dement W, eds. Principles and practice of sleep medicine. Philadelphia: *WB Saunders;* 2011:1452-1461.

[20] Miyawaki S, Lavigne GJ, Mayer P, Guitard F, Montplaisir JY, Kato T. Association between sleep bruxism, swallowing-related laryngeal movement, and sleep positions. *Sleep.* 2003;26:461-465.

[21] Miyawaki S, Katayama A, Tanimoto Y, Araki Y, Fujii A, Yashiro K, Takano-Yamamoto T. Salivary flow rates during relaxing, clenching and chewing-like movement with maxillary occlusal splints. *Am J Orthod Dentofacial Orthop.* 2004;126:367-370.

[22] De Leeu WR, ed. American Academy Orofacial Pain. Guidelines for assessment, diagnosis, and management. 4th ed. Chicago: *Quintessence Pub.;* 2008.

[23] Lobbezoo F, van der Zaag J, van Selms MK, Hamburger HL, Naeije M. Principles for the management of bruxism. *J Oral Rehabil.* 2008;35:509-523.

[24] Lavigne GJ, Rompré PH, Montplaisir JY. Sleep bruxism: validity of clinical research

diagnostic criteria in a controlled polysomnographic study. *J Dent Res.* 1996 ;75:546-552.

[25] Rompré PH, Daigle-Landry D, Guitard F, Montplaisir JY, Lavigne GJ. Identification of a sleep bruxism subgroup with a higher risk of pain. *J Dent Res.* 2007;86:837-842.

[26] Ohayon MM, Li KK, Guilleminault C. Risk factors for sleep bruxism in the general population. *Chest.* 2001;119:53-61.

[27] Koyano K, Tsukiyama Y, Ichiki R, Kuwata T. Assessment of bruxism in the clinic. *J Oral Rehabil.* 2008;35:495-508.

[28] Camparis CM, Siqueira JTT. Sleep bruxism: clinical aspects and characteristics in patients with and without chronic orofacial pain. *Oral Surg Oral Med Oral Pathol Oral Radiol Endod.* 2006;101:188-193.

[29] Bader G, Lavigne GJ. Sleep bruxism: overview of an oromandibular sleep movement disorder. *Sleep Med Rev.* 2000;4:27-43.

[30] Barbosa Tde S, Miyakoda LS, Pocztaruk Rde L, Rocha CP, Gavião MB. Temporomandibular disorders and bruxism in childhood and adolescence: Review of the literature. *Int J Pediatr Otorhinolaryngol.* 2008;72:299-314.

[31] Lobbezoo F, Lavigne GJ, Tanguay R, Montplaisir JY. The effect of catecholamine precursor L-dopa on sleep bruxism: a controlled clinical trial. *Mov Disord.* 1997;12:73-78.

[32] Kato T, Rompré P, Montplaisir JY, Sessle BJ, Lavigne GJ. Sleep bruxism: an oromotor activity secondary to micro-arousal. *J Dent Res.* 2001;80:1940-1944.

[33] Serra-Negra JM, Ramos-Jorge ML, Flores-Mendoza CE, Paiva SM, Pordeus IA. Influence of psychosocial factors on the development of sleep bruxism among children. *Int J Paediatr Dent.* 2009;19:309-317.

[34] Ferreira-Bacci Ado V, Cardoso CL, Diaz-Serrano KV. Behavioral problems and emotional stress in children with bruxism. *Braz Dent J.* 2012;23:246-251.

[35] Abekura H, Tsuboi M, Okura T, Kagawa K, Sadamori S, Akagawa Y. Association between sleep bruxism and stress sensitivity in an experimental psychological stress task. *Biomed Res.* 2011;32:395-399.

[36] Sabuncuoglu O, Ekinci O, Berkem M. Fluoxetine-induced sleep bruxism in an adolescent treated with buspirone: a case report. *Spec Care Dentist.* 2009;29:215-217.

[37] Suwa S, Takahara M, Shirakawa S, Komada Y, Sasaguri K, Onozuka M, Sato S. Sleep bruxism and its relationship to sleep habits and lifestyle of elementary school children in japan. *Sleep Biol Rhythm.* 2009;7:93-102.

[38] Abe Y, Suganuma T, Ishii M, Yamamoto G, Gunji T, Clark GT, Tachikawa T, Kiuchi Y, Igarashi Y, Baba K. Association of genetic, psychological and behavioral factors with sleep bruxism in a Japanese population. *J Sleep Res.* 2012;21:289-296.

[39] Kato T, Montplaisir JY, Guitard F, Sessle BJ, Lund JP, Lavigne GJ. Evidence that experimentally induced sleep bruxism is a consequence of transient arousal. *J Dent Res.* 2003;82:284-288.

[40] Huynh N, Kato T, Rompré PH, Okura K, Saber M, Lanfranchi PA, Montplaisir JY, Lavigne GJ. Sleep bruxism is associated to micro-arousals and an increase in cardiac sympathetic activity. *J Sleep Res.* 2006;15:339-346.

[41] Gold AR, Dipalo F, Gold MS, O'Hearn D. The symptoms and signs of upper airway resistance syndrome: a link to the functional somatic syndromes. *Chest.* 2003;123:87-95.

[42] Landry ML, Rompré PH, Manzini C, Guitard F, de Grandmont P, Lavigne GJ. Reduction of sleep bruxism using a mandibular advancement device: an experimental controlled study. *Int J Prosthodont.* 2006;19:549-556.

[43] Sjöholm TT, Lowe AA, Miyamoto K, Fleetham JA, Ryan CF. Sleep bruxism in patients with sleep-disordered breathing. *Arch Oral Biol.* 2000;45:889-896.

[44] Penzel T, Becker HF, Brandenburg U, Labunski T, Pankow W, Peter JH. Arousal in patients with gastro-oesophageal reflux and sleep apnoea. *Eur Respir J.* 1999;14:1266-1270.

[45] Lavigne GJ, Guitard F, Rompré PH, Montplaisir JY. Variability in sleep bruxism activity over time. *J Sleep Res.* 2001;10:237-244.

[46] Pierce CJ, Chrisman K, Bennett ME, Close JM. Stress, anticipatory stress, and psychologic measures related to sleep bruxism. *J Orofac Pain.* 1995;9:51-56.

[47] Fischer WF, O'toole ET. Personality characteristics of chronic bruxers. *Behav Med.* 1993;19:82-86.

[48] Manfredini D, Landi N, Romagnoli M, Bosco M. Psychic and occlusal factors in bruxers. *Aust Dent J.* 2004;49:84-89.

[49] Marthol H, Reich S, Jacke J, Lechner KH, Wichmann M, Hilz MJ. Enhanced sympathetic cardiac modulation in bruxism patients. *Clin Auton Res.* 2006;16:276-280.

[50] Harness DM, Peltier B. Comparison of MMPI scores with self-report of sleep disturbance and bruxism in the facial pain population. *Cranio.* 1992;10:70-74.

[51] Pingitore G, Chrobak V, Petrie J. The social and psychologic factors of bruxism. *J Prosthet Dent.* 1991;65:443-446.

[52] Rosales VP, Ikeda K, Hizaki K, Naruo T, Nozoe S, Ito G. Emotional stress and brux-like activity of the masseter muscle in rats. *Eur J Orthod.* 2002;24:107-117.

[53] Sato C, Sato S, Takashina H, Ishii H, Onozuka M, Sasaguri K. Bruxism affects stress responses in stressed rats. *Clin Oral Investig.* 2010;14:153-160.

[54] Hublin C, Kaprio J, Partinen M, Koskenvuo M. Sleep bruxism based on self-report in a nationwide twin cohort. *J Sleep Res.* 1998;7:61-67.

[55] Velly-Miguel AM, Montplaisir J, Rompré PH, Lund JP, Lavigne GJ. Bruxism and other orofacial movements during sleep. *J Craniomandib Disord Facial Oral Pain.* 1992;6:71-81.

[56] Dura JR, Torsell AE, Heinzerling RA, Mulick JA. Special oral concerns in people with severe and profound mental retardation. *Spec Care Dentist.* 1988;8:265-267.

[57] Lichter I, Muir RC. The pattern of swallowing during sleep. *Electroencephalogr Clin Neurophysiol.* 1975;38:427-432.

[58] Crossner CG. Salivary flow rate in children and adolescents. *Swed Dent J.* 1984;8:271-276.

[59] Poets CF. Gastroesophageal reflux: A critical review of its role in preterm infants. *Pediatrics.* 2004;113:128-132.

[60] Pilotto A. Aging and upper gastrointestinal disorders. *Best Pract Res Clin Gastroenterol.* 2004;18:73-81.

[61] Bremner RM, Hoeft SF, Costantini M, Crookes PF, Bremner CG, DeMeester TR. Pharyngeal swallowing. The major factor in clearance of esophageal reflux episodes. *Ann Surg.* 1993;3:369-370.

[62] Costa HO, Neto OM, Eckley CA. Is there a relationship between the pH and volume of saliva and esophageal pH-metry results? *Dysphagia.* 2005;20:175-181.

[63] Orr WC. The prediction of saliva swallowing frequency in humans from estimates of salivary flow rate and the volume of saliva swallowed. *Am J Med.* 2003;18:109-113.

[64] Freidin N, Fisher MJ, Taylor W, Boyd D, Surratt P, McCallum RW, Mittal RK. Sleep and nocturnal acid reflux in normal subjects and patients with reflux oesophagitis. *Gut.* 1991;32:1275-1279.

[65] Foresman BH. Sleep-related gastroesophageal reflux. *J Am Osteopath Assoc.* 2000;100:S7-S10.

[66] Caldara R, Barbieri C, Piepoli V, Borzio M, Masci E. Effect of L-dopa with and without inhibition of extra cerebral dopa decarboxylase on gastric acid secretion and gastrin release in man. *Gut.* 1985;26:1014-1017.

[67] Fujiwara Y, Machida A, Watanabe Y, Shiba M, Tominaga K, Watanabe T, Oshitani N, Higuchi K, Arakawa T. Association between dinner-to-bed time and gastro-esophageal reflux disease. *Am J Gastroenterol.* 2005;100:2633-2636.

[68] Massarrat S, Enschai F, Pittner PM. Increased gastric secretory capacity in smokers without gastrointestinal lesions. *Gut.* 1986;27:433-439.

[69] Pehl C, Pfeiffer A, Wendl B, Kaess H. The effect of decaffeination of coffee on gastro-oesophageal reflux in patients with reflux disease. *Aliment Pharmacol Ther.* 1997;11:483-486.

[70] Bradley LA, Richter JE, Pulliam TJ, Haile JM, Scarinci IC, Schan CA, Dalton CB, Salley AN. The relationship between stress and symptoms of gastroesophageal reflux: the influence of psychological factors. *Am J Gastroenterol.* 1993;88:11-19.

[71] Bergdahl M, Bergdahl J. Low unstimulated salivary flow and subjective oral dryness: association with medication, anxiety, depression, and stress. *J Dent Res.* 2000;79:1652-1658.

[72] Mohammed I, Cherkas LF, Riley SA, Spector TD, Trudgill NJ. Genetic influences in gastro-oesophageal reflux disease: a twin study. *Gut.* 2003;52:1085-1089.

[73] Meyers WF, Herbst JJ. Effectiveness of positioning therapy for gastroesophageal reflux. *Pediatrics.* 1982;69:768-772.

[74] Buchin PJ, Levy JS, Schullinger JN. Down's syndrome and the gastrointestinal tract. *J Clin Gastroenterol.* 1986;8:111-114.

[75] Hillemeier C, Buchin PJ, Gryboski J. Esophageal dysfunction in Down's syndrome. *J Pediatr Gastroenterol Nutr.* 1982;1:101-104.

[76] Del Giudice E, Staiano A, Capano G, Romano A, Florimonte L, Miele E, Ciarla C, Campanozzi A, Crisanti AF. Gastrointestinal manifestations in children with cerebral palsy. *Brain Dev.* 1999;21:307-311.

[77] Nelson SP, Chen EH, Syniar GM, Christoffel KK. Prevalence of symptoms of gastroesophageal reflux during infancy. A pediatric practice-based survey. Pediatric Practice Research Group. *Arch Pediatr Adolesc Med.* 1997;151:569-572.

[78] Brown CM, Rees WD. Review article: factors protecting the oesophagus against acid-mediated injury. *Aliment Pharmacol Ther.* 1995;9:251-262.

[79] Stephan AD. Diagnosis and dental treatment of a young adult patient with gastroesophageal reflux: a case report with 2-year follow-up. *Quintessence Int.* 2002;33:619-626.

[80] Miyawaki S, Tanimoto Y, Araki Y, Katayama A, Imai M, Takano-Yamamoto T. Relationships among nocturnal jaw muscle activities, decreased esophageal pH, and sleep positions. *Am J Orthod Dentofacial Orthop.* 2004;126:615-619.

[81] Herrera M, Valencia I, Grant M, Metroka D, Chialastri A, Kothare SV. Bruxism in children: Effect on sleep architecture and daytime cognitive performance and behavior. *Sleep.* 2006;29:1143-1148.

[82] The Japanese Society of Gastroenterology. Clinical practice guidelines about Gastroesophageal Reflux Disease (GERD). Tokyo: *NANKODO;* 2009.

[83] Katelaris PH. An evaluation of current GERD therapy: a summary and comparison of effectiveness, adverse effects and costs of drugs, surgery and endoscopic therapy. *Best Pract Res Clin Gastroenterol.* 2004;18:39-45.

[84] Jones MP. Acid suppression in gastro-oesophageal reflux disease: Why? How? How much and when? *Postgrad Med J.* 2002;78:465-468.

[85] Richter JE. Long-term management of gastroesophageal reflux disease and its complications. *Am J Gastroenterol.* 1997;92:30-34.

[86] Ofman JJ. The economic and quality-of-life impact of symptomatic gastroesophageal reflux disease. *Am J Gastroenterol.* 2003;98:S8-S14.

[87] Mathias SD, Colwell HH, Miller DP, Pasta DJ, Henning JM, Ofman JJ. Health-Related quality-of-life and quality-days incrementally gained in symptomatic nonerosive GERD patients treated with lansoprazole or ranitidine. *Dig Dis Sci.* 2001;46:2416-2423.

Part II.
Sleep Disturbance in Psychiatric Disorders

In: Sleep Medicine
Editors: A. Del Casale, R. Brugnoli and P. Girardi

ISBN: 978-1-62808-515-0
© 2013 Nova Science Publishers, Inc.

Chapter VIII

Sleep Disturbances and Related Psychopathologies

Antonio Del Casale[1], Paolo Girardi, Chiara Rapinesi,
Daniele Serata, Roberto Tatarelli and Gabriele Sani
Sapienza University, Rome
NESMOS (Neuroscience, Mental Health and Sensory Organs) Department
School of Medicine and Psychology

Abstract

Clinical and neurophysiopathological correlates of sleep disorders/disturbances often precede and predispose to psychiatric disorders or psychological distress. Sleep disturbances can constitute, for each psychiatric disorder, a genuine worsening factor and a motor for illness. For this reason, it is useful to consider clinical intervention aimed at restoring normal sleep as a preventive intervention, both on sleep alterations as well as on mental disorders and psychological distress. The mutual relationships between the patient's personal aspects, sleep habits, and manifested sleep disturbances require further clarification. This chapter will analyze the prominent clinical impact of sleep disturbances and circadian rhythm alterations in major psychiatric disorders.

Keywords: Circadian rhythm; sleep disorders; sleep disturbances; psychiatric disorders; psychological distress

---

[1] Corresponding author: Antonio Del Casale, M.D. "Sapienza" University of Rome. NESMOS (Neuroscience, Mental Health and Sensory Organs) Department, School of Medicine and Psychology. Email: antonio.delcasale@uniroma1.it.

Introduction

About 30-36% of the adult population report insomnia over a 12-month course, and about 8-16% consider it either chronic or severe. Sleep-related complaints also occur in people who do not meet criteria for psychiatric diagnoses. Insomnia, defined as subjective perceptions of inadequate or non-restorative sleep, is the most prevalent complaint. Hypersomnia is also relatively common.

Epidemiological studies have reported that sleep disturbances expressed at the first interview were strongly related to a history of a psychiatric diagnosis at that time [1-4]. In psychiatry, sleep disturbances and circadian rhythm alterations are frequent manifestations of affective and psychotic disorders and other psychiatric illnesses. Conversely, their clinical and neurophysiopathological correlates might precede and predispose to psychiatric disorders or psychological distress.

Sleep alterations and complaints can persist during phases of relative remission, for example in patients with major depressive disorder and/or alcoholism, bipolar and psychotic disorders. Their persistence or recurrence may result from inadequate treatment, individual temperament characteristics and personal aspects, subsyndromal conditions or already existing sleep structure.

Sleep disturbances are a risk factor for acute mood disorder episodes among adolescents and adults, can contribute to illness relapse, and adversely affect emotion regulation and cognitive functioning. Briefly, they can often harm general health status, and may worsen with substance use comorbidity. They may also have an impact on suicidality, although this aspect requires further study.

This evidence leads to consider sleep disturbances not only as an epiphenomenon, but also as a currently undervalued key issue of the multifactorial origin of psychiatric disorders. Scientific research focused on sleep in psychiatric disorders represents an exceptional, stimulating and interdisciplinary field across neurobiological, cognitive, behavioral, and social aspects. The knowledge gained in these areas, when associated with available powerful, easy, and low-cost innovative treatments, may have a strong positive impact on public health by reducing the length, severity, and recurrence of acute psychiatric episodes, and improve the quality of life [5].

The temporal relationship between sleep disturbance and acute psychiatric episodes may be of great importance to both clinicians and researchers. The main purpose of this chapter is to briefly illustrate how sleep disturbances and alterations constitute a risk factor for psychological distress and psychiatric illnesses, and can negatively affect most psychiatric disorders, constituting a genuine engine of illness in the context of a pathophysiological and psychopathological vicious circle.

Major Depressive and Anxiety Disorders

Recent evidence shows that the temporal alignment between the sleep-wake cycle and the circadian pacemaker affects self-assessment of mood in healthy subjects. Sleep complaints are frequent in patients with major depressive and anxiety disorders, and may be present in prodromal periods, during acute phases of disease, and even in the context of symptomatic remission.

Complaints about sleep disorders/disturbances during a first psychiatric interview is a significant risk factor for expressing depressive symptoms at the second interview [1-4].

Ford and Kamerow [4] conducted a large epidemiological study on 7954 respondents as part of the National Institute of Mental Health Epidemiologic Catchment Area study, examining at baseline and 1 year later about sleep complaints and psychiatric symptoms. They showed that, among persons without a psychiatric disorder, 17% of insomniacs and 17.5% of those with reported hypersomnia at first interview met diagnostic criteria for a psychiatric disorder during the second interview. These rates were about twice that of people free from either sleep disorders/disturbances or psychiatric illnesses at first interview [4].

Regarding the onset of new depressive episodes between the first and second interviews, Ford and Kamerow showed that depression rates were higher in subjects with insomnia (5.8%) and hypersomnia (9.1%) compared to those without sleep disturbances (1.7%). They also reported that remission of insomnia between the first and second consultations reduced the risk for depression. Moreover, reporting hypersomnia at the first interview constituted a risk factor for manifesting a depressive or anxiety disorder at the second interview, even if the same hypersomnia had remitted by this time. When hypersomnia was manifested during both meetings, it constituted a risk factor for both depression and anxiety disorders [4].

For primary care physicians, insistent or recurrent insomnia or hypersomnia complaints should be a wake-up call that can provide an opportunity to prevent the onset of a new acute psychiatric episode.

Another epidemiological study by Eaton and colleagues [6], conducted on an enlarged sample from the former database of Ford and Kamerow [4], showed that reported "sleep problems" were second only to "feelings of worthlessness and guilt" among the risk elements of a later onset of depression.

Livingston et al. [3] also reported that sleep disturbances manifested at both interviews were risk factors for depression at the second interview. A path analysis with both cross-sectional and prospective data revealed causal pathways from sleep disturbances to depression, but not from depression to insomnia [3].

Along the same line of evidence, Breslau et al. [2] reported that both total insomnia and hypersomnia in people with no history of psychiatric disorders predicted the onset of major depression, drug abuse, and dependence on nicotine. Insomnia also constituted a risk factor for anxiety disorder, while hypersomnia for alcohol abuse. The study by Breslau and colleagues [2] did not confirm the findings of Ford and Kamerow [4], indicating that the initial report of insomnia did not constitute a risk factor if it had remitted by the follow-up interview.

Breslau et al. [2] described three main risk factors for the later onset of depression: 1) psychomotor retardation or agitation; 2) suicidal ideation or behaviors represented (independent risk factors); 3) insomnia.

Perlis et al. [7] conducted a longitudinal study on 14 remitted depressed patients, showing that the factor most strongly associated with clinical relapse consisted in growing subjective sleep disturbances: the Beck Depressive Inventory (BDI) sleep item increased about 2 weeks prior to the effective and recognized relapse.

Moreover, a study by Judd and colleagues [8] reported that "insomnia" and "feeling tired all the time" were the most frequent symptoms in subjects with a subsyndromal symptomatic depression, defined as the presence of any two or more concurrent depressive symptoms with social dysfunction for most or all of the time, lasting for at least 2 weeks, occurring in the absence of the criteria for minor depression, major depression, and/or dysthymia. People with subsyndromal symptomatic depression often reported hypersomnia, which was the seventh most frequent symptom [8].

Objective sleep disturbances can predict new episodes of depression, as suggested by several polygraphic sleep studies [9,10]. Short REM sleep latency predicted later depression onset in non-affected first-degree relatives of patients with major depressive disorder [11].

Sleep disturbances also increase the risk for anxiety disorders, including post-traumatic stress disorder (PTSD) that is characterized by insomnia and nightmares, which usually appear about 6 months earlier the illness onset [12].

Bipolar Disorder

Decreased need for sleep is a major diagnostic criterion of mania, and it has important value in differential diagnosis. Switches into mania can occur with drug abuse, prescribed medications, trans-meridian travel, postpartum, bereavement, and in general in all conditions that may be associated with loss of sleep [13-19]. It is not really clear whether sleeplessness is a direct cause of the mania or a prodromal symptom of manic states. Sometimes, early manic symptoms may led to particular behaviors (e.g. drug use, hypersexuality, long journeys, overworking, etc.) that conduct in turn to sleep deprivation. Sleep deprivation procedures were associated with risks of hypomania and mania, which were, respectively, 12% and 7% [20]. Wehr [21] hypothesized that sleep deprivation is the basic proximal origin or a final common pathway of mania. He noted that all triggers of mania, including biological aspects, psychic effects, and direct disturbances of sleep schedules may be correlated with the origin of mania through sleep diminution. For Wehr's theory sleep deprivation is both a cause and a consequence of mania: self-reinforcing sleep loss perpetuates the manic state, which itself maintains sleep deprivation.

Primary sleep disorders have also been related to mania resulting from functional sleep deprivation. Specifically, obstructive sleep apnea with recurring brief arousals has been indicated as a cause of mania or treatment-resistance [22-24]. Thus, primary sleep disorders can be considered as an additional cause of functional sleep deprivation that can lead to mania, not initially integrated in Wehr's final common pathway hypothesis.

Sleep disturbances have been implicated in both the prodromal and syndromal phases of bipolar illnesses [25,26]. Sleep disturbances generally precede first bipolar disorder episodes by several years, and are also considered a risk factor for developing other mood disorders. Disordered sleep in bipolar patients often emerges during puberty and frequently remains high in individuals at high-risk [27]. Patients affected by bipolar disorder often manifest sleep complaints and, like patients with insomnia, can also be less active in the daytime, reporting more daytime sleepiness [28].

Impaired sleep can induce and predict manic episodes, and treatment of sleep disturbance is both a primary objective and measure of response in mania [29]. Moreover, maintaining adequate sleep can be considered as a goal for successful prevention of relapse in mania [29]. Depressive episodes of bipolar disorder include sleep disturbances, which may be treated with somatic therapies that target sleep and circadian rhythms. Euthymic periods may have residual insomnia that is a major vulnerability to relapses.

Patients with bipolar illnesses often manifest a circadian rhythm disorder, consisting in advanced circadian rhythm and state-dependent alterations of REM sleep latency. This has been related to evidence derived from genetic studies, which reported that clock genes have a major role in bipolar disorder, and most research has focused on polymorphisms of CLOCK and the lithium target GSK3 [30].

Confirming the close relationship between bipolar disorder and sleep abnormalities, several therapeutic agents that target disordered sleep have resulted effective in manic patients. Additionally, behavioral interventions that may improve sleep quality were useful in the treatment for mania for more than a century [31].

Briefly, sleep quality has a major role in all episodes of bipolar disorder and in euthymic periods, and a proper evaluation and management of sleep disturbances in patients with a diagnosis of bipolar disorder is crucial [29].

Schizophrenia and Other Psychoses

As is common in patients affected by mood disorders, a major tendency for patients with schizophrenia is to sleep when other people are awake. Sleep disturbances are a key symptom of this illness. Sleep-wake rhythm alterations in schizophrenia have been related to other symptoms, including cognitive impairment. This may help to direct future targeted therapeutic interventions [32].

Poor sleep quality is directly related to negative assessments of quality of life in schizophrenic patients [33]. During psychotic exacerbations, patients affected by schizophrenia can manifest periods of severe insomnia or complete sleeplessness. Moreover, severe insomnia is a common clinical feature of the prodromal phase of psychosis [34-36], and sleep disturbances such as insomnia and excessive daytime sleepiness in adolescents may predict psychotic-like experiences, which is a good predictor for psychosis [37].

Clarifications of the links between sleep disturbances and circadian rhythm disruption and schizophrenia can contribute to novel treatment approaches, which will improve health and quality of life of patients affected by schizophrenia [38].

The most frequently reported sleep disturbances in these patients, other than circadian phase abnormalities, are significant alterations in sleep continuity, rapid eye movement (REM) sleep, and slow wave sleep. Such alterations, particularly relating to REM sleep, differ from those observed in depressive episodes, although in several cases the most prominent REM abnormality may be related to current [39] or suspended [40,41] neuroleptic treatments, and tardive dyskinesia [42].

Reversal of the circadian rhythm and decreased slow-wave sleep correlate with poorer patient functioning on both the social and occupational levels; shorter REM latency is related to greater severity of psychotic symptoms, including delusions, hallucinations and thought behavior disorganizations [43].

Commonly disturbed nocturnal sleep observed in patients with chronic schizophrenia [40] is exacerbated during psychotic relapses [44]. A major problem is that although the architecture of sleep often improves with long-term neuroleptic treatment, sleep in patients affected by schizophrenia still remains fragmented, and never returns to a normal pattern [39], suggesting that such an abnormal pattern may have pathophysiologic importance. Regardless, sleep efficiency is inversely correlated with psychosis levels in patients with chronic schizophrenia [40].

Reported significant reductions in sleep continuity, prolonged sleep latency, inferior sleep efficiency, diminished total sleep, and increased waketime after sleep onset [10,45,46] are all features that worsen schizophrenic illness.

Briefly, sleep disturbances significantly correlate with clinical variables, including illness severity, frequencies of positive and negative symptoms, neurocognitive impairment, and prognosis. Prolonged sleep deprivation has been related to hallucinations and other psychotic symptoms typical of schizophrenia [47]. Several studies focused on sleep abnormalities in schizophrenia have reported that insomnia and some REM variables are related to psychotic states and positive symptoms, while deficits in slow wave sleep were correlated with negative symptoms and cognitive dysfunction (see Chapter 10).

In summary, different circadian rhythm alterations and sleep disturbances are not only a symptom of the disease, but also a factor of aggravation, in the context of a vicious cycle that worsens schizophrenia.

Conclusion

Sleep disorders and sleep disturbances are triggered and maintained by several factors, including biological and genetic elements [48-50], physical and psychological stress [51,52], organic diseases [52,53], and poor sleep hygiene [54]. Sleep disorders/disturbances are themselves associated with increased psychological stress [55] and use/abuse of psychotropic substances (e.g. nicotine, caffeine, drug abuse) (see chapter 11).

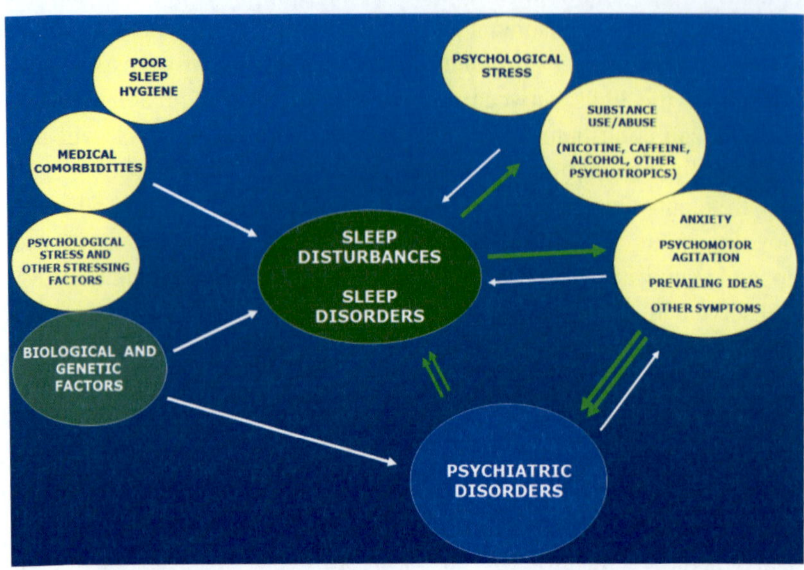

Figure 1.

In addition, sleep disorders/disturbances can increase anxiety [56], psychomotor agitation, prevailing ideas, and other psychological symptoms [55], thus constituting a risk factor or resulting in exacerbating or worsening any comorbid psychiatric disorder. In particular, such worsening may occur in cases of mania, psychosis, depression in the context of bipolar or unipolar disorders, and even in cases of anxiety disorders.

A reflection should be made with regard to some individual aspects [57-61], which can also be a trigger for sleep disturbances and in turn be affected by them. People with insomnia can manifest more frequently aspects of neuroticism, perfectionism, internalization, anxious concerns and traits. These factors may play different roles depending on the specific case. In addition, certain personality traits may affect the responses to psychoeducational and cognitive-behavioral treatments. For instance, insomniacs reporting less guardedness with a higher score on the hypomania scale of the Minnesota Multiphasic Personality Inventory [62] showed reduced psychological treatment response [57]. More longitudinal data are needed to better understand the specific role of personality traits in the etiology of insomnia and other sleep disturbances. Personality factors may have a specific causal role in the development of insomnia, but may also arise from sleep problems and their related daytime dysfunctions [57].

In conclusion, for each psychiatric disorder sleep disturbances constitute a genuine worsening factor and a motor for illness, in the context of a tangible vicious circle (see figure 1) that, if not interrupted, gradually worsens the patient's overall health and quality of life.

References

[1] Gillin JC. Are sleep disturbances risk factors for anxiety, depressive and addictive disorders? *Acta Psychiatr Scand Suppl.* 1998;393:39-43.

[2] Breslau N, Roth T, Rosenthal L, Andreski P. Sleep disturbance and psychiatric disorders: a longitudinal epidemiological study of young adults. *Biol Psychiatry.* 1996;39(6):411-8.

[3] Livingston G, Blizard B, Mann A. Does sleep disturbance predict depression in elderly people? A study in inner London. *Br J Gen Pract.* 1993;43(376):445-8.

[4] Ford DE, Kamerow DB. Epidemiologic study of sleep disturbances and psychiatric disorders. An opportunity for prevention? *JAMA.* 1989;262(11):1479-84.

[5] Harvey AG. Sleep and circadian functioning: critical mechanisms in the mood disorders? *Annu Rev Clin Psychol.* 2011;7:297-319.

[6] Eaton WW, Badawi M, Melton B. Prodromes and precursors: epidemiologic data for primary prevention of disorders with slow onset. *Am J Psychiatry.* 1995;152(7):967-72.

[7] Perlis ML, Giles DE, Buysse DJ, Tu X, Kupfer DJ. Self-reported sleep disturbance as a prodromal symptom in recurrent depression. *J Affect Disord.* 1997;42(2-3):209-12.

[8] Judd LL, Rapaport MH, Paulus MP, Brown JL. Subsyndromal symptomatic depression: a new mood disorder? *J Clin Psychiatry.* 1994;55 Suppl:18-28.

[9] Giles DE, Jarrett RB, Roffwarg HP, Rush AJ. Reduced rapid eye movement latency. A predictor of recurrence in depression. *Neuropsychopharmacology.* 1987;1(1):33-9.

[10] Kupfer DJ, Frank E, McEachran AB, Grochocinski VJ. Delta sleep ratio. A biological correlate of early recurrence in unipolar affective disorder. *Arch Gen Psychiatry.* 1990;47(12):1100-5.

[11] Giles DE, Kupfer DJ. Short REM latency: risk factor for first episode of depression (abstract). *Sleep Res.* 1994;23:197.

[12] Van Liempt S. Sleep disturbances and PTSD: a perpetual circle? *Eur J Psychotraumatol.* 2012;3. doi: 10.3402/ejpt.v3i0.19142. Epub 2012 Oct 3.

[13] Jauhar P, Weller MP. Psychiatric morbidity and time zone changes: a study of patients from Heathrow Airport. *Br J Psychiatry* 1982;140:231-235.

[14] Young DM. Psychiatric morbidity in travelers to Honolulu, Hawaii. *Compr Psychiatry.* 1995;36:224-228.

[15] Peet M, Peters S. Drug-induced mania. *Drug Saf.* 1995;12:146-153.

[16] Davenport YB, Adland ML: Postpartum psychoses in female and male bipolar manic-depressive patients. *Am J Orthopsychiatry.* 1982;52:288-297.

[17] Reich T, Winokur G:Postpartum psychoses in patients with manic depressive disease. *J Nerv Ment Dis.* 1970;151:60-68.

[18] Hollender MH, Goldin ML. Funeral mania. *J Nerv Ment Dis.* 1978;166:890-892.

[19] Rosenman SJ, Tayler H. Mania following bereavement: a case report. *Br J Psychiatry.* 1986;148:468-470.

[20] Kasper S, Wehr TA. The role of sleep and wakefulness in the genesis of depression and mania. *Encephale* 1992;18(spec no 1):45-50.

[21] Wehr TA. Sleep-loss as a possible mediator of diverse causes of mania. *Br J Psychiatry.* 1991;159:576-578.

[22] Strakowski SM, Hudson JI, Keck PE Jr, Wilson DR, Frankenburg FR, Alpert JE, Teschke GC, Tohen M. Four cases of obstructive sleep apnea associated with treatment-resistant mania. *J Clin Psychiatry.* 1991;52:156-158.

[23] Fleming JA, Fleetham JA, Taylor DR, Remick RA. A case report of obstructive sleep apnea in a patient with bipolar affective disorder. *Can J Psychiatry.* 1985;30:437-439.

[24] Blazer D. Hypersomnia in manic-depressive illness: a case of sleep apnea. *N C Med J.* 1981;42:781-782.

[25] Brill S, Penagaluri P, Roberts RJ, Gao Y, El-Mallakh RS. Sleep disturbances in euthymic bipolar patients. *Ann Clin Psychiatry.* 2011;23(2):113-6.

[26] Harvey AG. The adverse consequences of sleep disturbance in pediatric bipolar disorder: implications for intervention. *Child Adolesc Psychiatr Clin N Am.* 2009;18(2):321-38.

[27] Ritter PS, Marx C, Bauer M, Leopold K, Pfennig A. The role of disturbed sleep in the early recognition of bipolar disorder: a systematic review. *Bipolar Disord.* 2011 May;13(3):227-37. Erratum in: *Bipolar Disord.* 2011;13(4):437.

[28] St-Amand J, Provencher MD, Bélanger L, Morin CM. Sleep disturbances in bipolar disorder during remission. *J Affect Disord.* 2012 Aug 9. [Epub ahead of print]

[29] Plante DT, Winkelman JW. Sleep disturbance in bipolar disorder: therapeutic implications. *Am J Psychiatry.* 2008;165(7):830-43.

[30] Lamont EW, Legault-Coutu D, Cermakian N, Boivin DB. The role of circadian clock genes in mental disorders. *Dialogues Clin Neurosci.* 2007;9(3):333-42.

[31] Palmer HA. The value of continuous narcosis in the treatment of mental disorders. *J Ment Sci.* 1937;83:636-678.

[32] Wilson S, Argyropoulos S. Sleep in schizophrenia: time for closer attention. *Br J Psychiatry.* 2012;200(4):273-4.

[33] Ritsner M, Kurs R, Ponizovsky A, Hadjez J. Perceived quality of life in schizophrenia: relationships to sleep quality. *Qual Life Res.* 2004;13(4):783-91.

[34] Donlon PT, Blacker KH. Clinical recognition of early schizophrenic decompensation. *Dis Nerv Syst.* 1975;36(6):323-7.

[35] Kumar S, Thara R, Rajkumar S. Coping with symptoms of relapse in schizophrenia. *Eur Arch Psychiatry Neurol Sci.* 1989;239(3):213-5.

[36] Jørgensen P. Schizophrenic delusions: the detection of warning signals. *Schizophr Res.* 1998;32(1):17-22.

[37] Lee YJ, Cho SJ, Cho IH, Jang JH, Kim SJ. The relationship between psychotic-like experiences and sleep disturbances in adolescents. *Sleep Med.* 2012;13(8):1021-7.

[38] Pritchett D, Wulff K, Oliver PL, Bannerman DM, Davies KE, Harrison PJ, Peirson SN, Foster RG. Evaluating the links between schizophrenia and sleep and circadian rhythm disruption. *J Neural Transm.* 2012;119(10):1061-75.

[39] Taylor SF, Tandon R, Shipley JE, Eiser AS. Effect of neuroleptic treatment on polysomnographic measures in schizophrenia. *Biol Psychiatry.* 1991;30(9):904-12.

[40] Tandon R, Shipley JE, Taylor S, Greden JF, Eiser A, DeQuardo J, Goodson J. Electroencephalographic sleep abnormalities in schizophrenia: relationship to positive/negative symptoms and prior neuroleptic treatment. *Arch Gen Psychiatry.* 1992;49(3):185-94.

[41] Kempenaers C, Kerkhofs M, Linkowski P, Mendlewicz J. Sleep EEG variables in young schizophrenic and depressive patients. *Biol Psychiatry.* 1988;24(7):833-8.

[42] Thaker GK, Wagman AMI, Tamminga CA. Sleep polygraphy in schizophrenia: methodological issues. *Biol Psychiatry.* 1990;28(3):240-6.

[43] Krystal AD, Goforth HW, Roth T. Effects of antipsychotic medications on sleep in schizophrenia. *Int Clin Psychopharmacol.* 2008;23(3):150-60.

[44] Kupfer DJ, Wyatt RJ, Scott J, Snyder F. Sleep disturbance in acute schizophrenic patients. *Am J Psychiatry.* 1970;126:1213-23.

[45] Boivin DB. Influence of sleep-wake and circadian rhythm disturbances in psychiatric disorders. *J Psychiatry Neurosci.* 2000;25(5):446-58.

[46] Benson KL, Zarcone VP. Rapid eye movement sleep eye movements in schizophrenia and depression. *Arch Gen Psychiatry.* 1993;50:474-82.

[47] Lamont EW, Coutu DL, Cermakian N, Boivin DB. Circadian rhythms and clock genes in psychotic disorders. *Isr J Psychiatry Relat Sci.* 2010;47(1):27-35.

[48] Harvey AG, Murray G, Chandler RA, Soehner A. Sleep disturbance as transdiagnostic: consideration of neurobiological mechanisms. *Clin Psychol Rev.* 2011;31(2):225-35

[49] Sehgal A, Mignot E. Genetics of sleep and sleep disorders. *Cell.* 2011;146(2):194-207.

[50] Hamet P, Tremblay J. Genetics of the sleep-wake cycle and its disorders. *Metabolism.* 2006;55(10 Suppl 2):S7-12.

[51] Cui R, Li B, Suemaru K, Araki H. Psychological stress-induced changes in sleep patterns and their generation mechanism. *Yakugaku Zasshi.* 2008;128(3):405-11.

[52] Weinhouse GL, Schwab RJ. Sleep in the critically ill patient. *Sleep.* 2006;29(5):707-16.

[53] Barthlen GM, Stacy C. Dyssomnias, parasomnias, and sleep disorders associated with medical and psychiatric diseases. *Mt Sinai J Med.* 1994;61(2):139-59.

[54] Nino-Murcia G. Diagnosis and treatment of insomnia and risks associated with lack of treatment. *J Clin Psychiatry.* 1992;53 Suppl:43-7; discussion 48-9.

[55] Drake CL, Roehrs T, Roth T. Insomnia causes, consequences, and therapeutics: an overview. *Depress Anxiety.* 2003;18(4):163-76.

[56] Mellman TA. Sleep and anxiety disorders. *Psychiatr Clin North Am.* 2006;29(4):1047-58.

[57] Van de Laar M, Verbeek I, Pevernagie D, Aldenkamp A, Overeem S. The role of personality traits in insomnia. *Sleep Med Rev.* 2010;14(1):61-8.

[58] Sasai T, Inoue Y, Matsuura M. Do patients with rapid eye movement sleep behavior disorder have a disease-specific personality? *Parkinsonism Relat Disord.* 2012;18(5):616-8.

[59] Bassett D. Borderline personality disorder and bipolar affective disorder. Spectra or spectre? A review. *Aust N Z J Psychiatry.* 2012;46(4):327-39.

[60] Huynh C, Guilé JM, Godbout R. [Polysomnographic studies on sleep in adult borderline personality disorder]. *Presse Med.* 2012;41(2):e63-75.

[61] Kawada T. Noise and health--sleep disturbance in adults. *J Occup Health.* 2011;53(6):413-6.

[62] Hathaway SR, McKinley JC. MMPI-2 – Minnesota Multiphasic Personality Inventory-2. Firenze, *Organizzazioni Speciali:* 1997.

In: Sleep Medicine
Editors: A. Del Casale, R. Brugnoli and P. Girardi

ISBN: 978-1-62808-515-0
© 2013 Nova Science Publishers, Inc.

Chapter IX

Sleep Disturbances in Anxiety Disorders

***Chiara Rapinesi*, Antonio Del Casale, Daniele Serata
and Giovanni Manfredi***

Sapienza University, Rome, NESMOS (Neuroscience, Mental Health
and Sensory Organs) Department, School of Medicine and Psychology

Abstract

Anxiety disorders are the most frequent psychiatric disorder with a lifetime prevalence of 29% in the general population. Anxiety-related hyperarousal can often lead to persistent circadian rhythm and sleep disturbances. Patients affected by anxiety disorders, including post-traumatic stress disorder, panic disorder, obsessive compulsive disorder, generalized anxiety disorder, and phobias, often manifest sleep disturbances or complaints. Sleep disorders/disturbances are commonly associated with anxiety: impaired sleep can damage neurocognitive performance and increase daily anxiety. Restoring a correct circadian rhythm is essential and basic. The study of multiple relationships between sleep disturbances and anxiety symptoms is of considerable importance in medical practice.

Keywords: Sleep disorders; sleep disturbances; anxiety; anxiety disorders; obsessive compulsive disorder; post-traumatic stress disorder; panic disorder

Introduction

Anxiety disorders are the most frequently occurring type of psychiatric illness with a lifetime prevalence estimate of 29% in the general population [1]. They are often associated

---

* Corresponding author: Dr. Chiara Rapinesi "Sapienza" University, Rome. Email: rapinesi.chiara@libero.it.

with difficulties in initiating and maintaining sleep, and an etiopathogenetic association between anxiety-related and sleep-related symptoms is not well established [2-4].

Anxiety-related hyperarousal can often lead to persistent circadian rhythm and sleep disturbances. A large epidemiological study by Ohayon and Roth [5] reported that in 18% of cases insomnia appeared before the anxiety disorder, anxiety and insomnia manifested together in 39% of cases, and anxiety appeared before insomnia in 43% of cases.

The close relationship between anxiety and sleep disturbances is also emphasized by the official diagnostic criteria for many anxiety disorders, which incorporate sleep complaints. Another important point is the treatment of the underlying anxiety disorder, which significantly improves sleep [6,7]. In clinical practice, several patients affected by generalized anxiety disorder, panic disorder, post-traumatic stress disorder, acute stress disorder, obsessive-compulsive disorder, and social phobia refer sleep-related symptoms, the frequencies of which did not differ between sex and age: both children and adults, and men and women, can suffer from anxiety disorders with sleep-related problems. However, the type of sleep disturbances can vary by diagnostic category [8].

On the other hand, sleep disorders/disturbances are commonly associated with anxiety disorders [9]. Nightmares, insomnia, sleep apnea, and other sleep-related disturbances reduce sleep quality and/or quantity, and can result in poor concentration, anxiety, agitation, irritability, impairment of daytime functioning, or marked distress and impaired emotional coping. Poor sleep may lead to more frequent and intense negative emotions, including anger and sadness, anxiety, and mood instability. Regarding neurocognitive functioning, after disturbed sleep overnight any event may be more difficult to process and more likely to result in emotional complaints during the daytime [10]. A prospective cohort study conducted by Batterham and colleagues [11] showed that self-reported sleep disturbance significantly correlated with an increased onset-risk within 4 years not only of major depressive disorder, but also and above all of generalized anxiety disorder (GAD) and panic disorder (PD). These authors reported that the sleep disturbance effects on PD and GAD onset not correlated with personality factors, suggesting that early assessment and identification of sleep disturbances may have an important role in selective and preventive interventions in people at risk for anxiety disorders [11].

Among sleep disturbances in patients with anxiety disorders, insomnia, described as unsatisfactory sleep duration and quality, is by far the most common [7]. Insomnia may also be linked to fears for thoughts, fantasies or nightmares that occur during sleep. It can appear in different sleep stages:

1. in the early phase of sleep, resulting in the impossibility of falling asleep (*early insomnia*);

2. in the central stage of sleep, which is characterized by frequent awakenings, so that it is difficult to maintain (*middle-of-the-night, middle, or lacunar insomnia*);

3. during the latest stage of sleep, resulting in very early awakening in the morning (*late insomnia*).

Also, increased rates of cataplexy, excessive daytime sleepiness, hypnagogic and hypnopompic hallucinations, and parasomnias can be comorbid with anxiety disorders [12-14]. Isolated sleep paralysis are episodes that last from a few seconds to 1 or 2 minutes, in which the patients are unable to move or speak. These manifestations end spontaneously, or when another person touches or moves the patient. Rarely, the person has dream-like sensations or hallucinations, which can be frightening for the individual. Increased rates of isolated sleep paralysis significantly correlate with anxiety disorders, mainly panic disorder, generalized anxiety disorder, and social phobia [14].

Neurological assessment may be considered in patients affected by anxiety disorders comorbid with sleep disturbances, which can be a frequent symptom at 1 year after traumatic brain injury, often co-occurring with anxiety, depression, and pain [15].

Post-Traumatic Stress Disorder and Acute Stress Disorder

Clinical evidence

The essential feature of post-traumatic stress and acute stress disorders is the development of symptoms after the exposure to an extreme traumatic factor that caused or can result in death or serious injury or other threats to the physical integrity of the patient or other people with whom the patient has been in contact. The responses to the traumatic event in patients affected by post-traumatic stress disorder (PTSD) or acute stress disorder (ASD) include feelings of intense fear, helplessness or horror. The characteristic symptoms resulting from exposure to an extreme trauma include a constant reliving of the traumatic event, persistent avoidance of stimuli associated with the trauma, numbing of general responsiveness, and constant symptoms of increased arousal. If these symptoms are present for less than a month the diagnosis is ASD; to diagnose PTSD, symptoms must be present for more than 1 month and the disturbances must cause clinically significant distress or impairment in social, occupational or other important areas [2]. PTSD is recurrent among veterans [16], women who have suffered from sexual abuse [17,18], and persons who escaped from fire [19] or motor vehicle accidents [20] or other life-threatening catastrophic events.

These disorders commonly include sleep complaints, which correlated with two of the important clusters of symptoms included in the criteria of the Diagnostic and Statistical Manual of Mental Disorders (DSM-IV-TR) [2]: the first is the constant re-experiencing the trauma, which is commonly expressed by intrusive symptoms as recurrent distressing dreams or nightmares that can fragment sleep, decrease sleep quality, and even cause fear about going to sleep; the second is a constant hyperarousal state, perceived as difficulty in falling or staying asleep.

Nightmares and insomnia are the most common sleep-related disorders occurring in PTSD [7,16,21]. About 60% of patients affected by PTSD can experience frequent nightmares [22], and 50% of post-traumatic dreams can comprise exact replications of the traumatic events [23].

Stressful negative life events seem to be the most common precipitating factors of insomnia [24]. In fact, early and central insomnia are reported by a great number of patients with PTSD, and is interpreted as a consequence of hyperarousal. Hyperarousal in traumatized individuals correlates with the promptness to react to potentially negative events, and plays a central role in the development and maintenance of sleep disturbances. Patients with PTSD have higher rates of brief arousals from REM sleep, and sleep complaints in these patients might represent amplified perceptions of such arousals.

Patients with ASD or PTSD can also report other sleep-related anxiety symptoms, including fear of going to sleep, fear of the dark, rumination of trauma or other disturbing thoughts while lying in bed, sleep talking, sleep shouting, waking up with fear due to a nightmare, confused and disorientated wake up, and late insomnia [24,25].

Neuropathophysiology

Dysfunctional rapid-eye-movement (REM) sleep mechanisms may be involved in the neuropathology of the post-traumatic dream: in many cases, patients affected by PTSD wake up screaming and frightened [21]. PTSD patients have uniformly showed an increased rate of periodic movements in sleep during both REM and non-REM (NREM) sleep. It may also result in higher vulnerability to apnea, possibly due to alterations in mechanisms that regulate sleep, or to ventilation changes [26].

Several studies have analyzed the particular sleep architecture in patients with PTSD. A meta-analysis conducted by Kobayashi et al. [27] reported in patients affected by PTSD as compared to healthy subjects more stage 1 sleep, less slow wave sleep, and greater REM density. Breslau and colleagues [28] reported an increased number of brief arousals from REM sleep in patients with PTSD, hypothesizing that sleep complaints in PTSD might relate to augmented perceptions of brief arousals from REM sleep. Comorbid major depressive disorder (MDD) can change polysomnographic parameters. Yetkin and colleagues [29] reported that PTSD patient group with MDD experienced difficulty initiating sleep, poor sleep efficiency, reduced total sleep time, decreased slow wave sleep (SWS), and a reduced REM sleep latency. The PTSD group without any comorbid psychiatric disorders showed moderately significant disturbances of sleep continuity and decreased SWS. They did not show REM sleep abnormalities. REM sleep latency was inversely proportional to the severity of startle response. SWS inversely correlated with the severity of psychogenic amnesia.

Of note, the sleep disturbances due to nightmares increase the PTSD symptomatology. PTSD itself leads to worsened sleep fragmentation, GH hyposecretion, and increased and frequent nightmares, which may impair fear extinction and synaptic plasticity, thereby compromising recovery. Disturbed sleep represents a precipitating and perpetuating factor in PTSD symptomatology, as it creates a perpetual circle [30]. In particular, insomnia correlated with the development of additional psychological problems in veterans with PTDS, which highlights the value of longitudinal assessment, sleep disturbance monitoring, and early intervention projects [31].

The role of hypothalamic-pituitary-adrenal axis can be considered in PTSD-related sleep disturbances [30,32]: increased cortisol was negatively associated with delta sleep, which may contribute to sleep abnormalities in PTSD [32].

Briefly, PTSD in turn leads to increased sleep fragmentation, frequent nightmares, and GH hyposecretion, which can affect fear extinction and synaptic plasticity [30].

Treatments

A careful assessment of the manifested sleep disturbance is crucial to choose the best possible treatment. In any case, cognitive-behavioral therapies (CBTs) are as effective as pharmacotherapies in the short-term and more enduring in their positive effects [33]. Several patients who received CBT for PTSD-related sleep disturbances may suffer from residual difficulties, including more residual posttraumatic, depression, and anxiety symptoms, and poorer quality of mental and physical health compared to patients who did not report post-treatment sleep disturbances [34]. In short, CBT for insomnia [33,35-39], and imagery rehearsal therapies [33,38], which use techniques for rescript or alter the endings of PTSD-related nightmares during wake, can expressly treat PTSD-related insomnia and nightmares, promising new opportunities for additional benefits. Other CBTs include exposure therapies, which has been evaluated for nightmares in three contexts, including isolation, systematic desensitization, and with both relaxation and rescripting. A study of sleep-directed hypnosis as an adjunct to a cognitive-processing treatment is currently underway (NCT00725192) [38].

Pharmacotherapy is a key choice for PTSD-related sleep disturbances as an adjunct to CBT, when CBT may be unsuccessful or unavailable, or not accepted by the patient.

However, evidence-based guidelines for expressly treating PTSD-related sleep disturbances (mainly nightmares and insomnia) cannot be actually defined, considering a lack of randomized controlled trials and methodological limitations in existing studies [38,40-42].

Only a few pharmacological agents have been demonstrated to be effective for PTSD-related sleep disturbances. These include prazosin, an ⊔1-adrenergic receptor inhibiting agent [33,38,43,44], risperidone [38,40,42,45-47], olanzapine, quetiapine, and levomepromazine [38,40-42].

Evidence has suggested small effects for selective serotonin reuptake inhibitors (SSRIs) [40,42], although at least two ongoing RCTs with paroxetine among PTSD patients are including sleep outcomes (NCT00215163 and NCT00202449) [38]. Among serotonin norepinephrine reuptake inhibitors (SNRIs), duloxetine resulted effective with significant reductions in nightmares in a sample of "treatment refractory". Veterans with comorbid PTSD and major depression was recently published [48]. However, the study was uncontrolled and lacked a validated sleep-assessment, and its findings should be considered preliminary. Two trials of duloxetine for PTSD are in progress (NCT00583193, NCT00763178) [38]. Among other antidepressants, nefazodone resulted effective with significant reductions in both subjective and objective sleep disturbances in a study by Neylan and colleagues [49], but the best practice guide of the American Association for Sleep Medicine characterized these data as being insufficient [50], and do not recommend the use of nefazodone in the treatment of nightmares. Regarding anticonvulsivant agents, gabapentin and topiramate have demonstrated some efficacy on PTSD-related sleep disturbances, but the available data are insufficient to support their use in these cases [38,40,42].

In brief, despite recent pharmacological progress in the development of more specific agents for PTSD-related sleep disturbances, insomnia and nightmares may not fully resolve [33]. More investigation focused on pharmacotherapy in PTSD-related sleep disturbances is needed.

Conclusion

Nightmares and insomnia are associated with significant distress, daytime impairment, lack of sleep, and increased reactivity to emotional cues, which can compromise health and functioning of patients affected by PTSD [38].

Panic Disorder

Clinical Evidence

Panic attacks consist of sudden, unexpected, paroxystic, severe anxiety, characterized by fear of dying, going crazy or losing control. These attacks are accompanied by several physical symptoms, often cardiorespiratory, otoneurological, gastrointestinal, or autonomic. Diagnosis of panic disorder (PD) requires the manifestation of recurring panic attacks, with worrying for possible potential attacks, development of phobic avoidance, or other behavioral changes as a consequence of the attacks [2]. An epidemiological study on a nationally representative sample estimated the lifetime prevalence of PD to be 4.5% [51]. Patients with PD can also manifest agoraphobia, which is a phobia characterized by anxiety and avoidance of situations in which the environment is perceived as being difficult to escape or get help. PD-related anxiety correlated with the insidious and persistent avoidance of dissimilar situations, follow-on social impairment [2]. The prevalence of insomnia in patients with PD is about 68-93% [52], possibly correlated with anxiety, depression [53], and nocturnal panic attack [52].

Sleep disturbances, including insomnia, difficulties in falling asleep, restless sleep, increased sleep latency, middle-of-the-night insomnia, and reduced sleep efficiency are very recurrent in PD [6]. This illness is frequently comorbid with insomnia, which can exacerbate panic symptoms and contribute to PD relapses [54,55]. Nocturnal panic attacks, as daytime panic attacks, occur without obvious triggers, repetitively among 18-45% of patients affected by PD [56]. They are similar in quality, severity and length to awaken attacks, although dyspnoeic symptoms may be more common in nocturnal attacks. The majority of patients with PD clinical have manifested nocturnal panic attacks, and sleep-related panic is a major symptom for a subgroup of patients [57], with up to 18% of all attacks occurring during sleep [58]. Many patients with nocturnal panic attacks develop a conditioned fear and avoidance of sleep. This constant and intermittent sleep deprivation is an important outcome of nocturnal panic attacks [59]. PD with habitual nocturnal panic attacks is the most severe manifestation of the PD spectrum: it is characterized by more sleep disturbance, more reported current and past severe difficulties in sleep onset, with fear of not falling asleep, racing thoughts, muscular tension, sleep paralysis, sleep hallucinations, startle, restless legs, nightly waking, early morning waking and other parasomnias, non-restorative sleep, drowsiness, and weakness [60].

Moreover, patients with nocturnal panic attacks reported more frequent daytime attacks and had more somatization [61]. PD with regular nocturnal panic attacks can represent an aspecific version of PD, characterized by fearful associations with sleep and sleep-like states [62]. Schredl and colleagues [63] reported that patients with anxiety disorders showed higher occurrence of nightmares compared to controls, and higher onset of nocturnal panic attacks associated with dreams.

Nocturnal attacks should be distinguished from arousals that could be provoked by nightmares, environmental stimuli, and other sleep-related events [59]. In fact, they are often mistaken for sleep apnea, parasomnias, PTSD-related nightmares, and nocturnal epilepsy [59].

Neuropathophysiology

Insomnia is more commonly reported in patients with PD than in normal individuals [56], and impaired sleep initiation and maintenance has been confirmed by polysomnographic studies [64]. Nocturnal panic attacks generally occur during late stage 2 to early stage 3 of NREM sleep, leading to worsening of insomnia, secondary to fear of other attacks [65]. They can be distinguished from sleep terrors, which mostly occur during stage 4 sleep and from nightmares or PTSD related anxiety dreams, which generally occur during REM sleep [54,66]. Sleep panic attacks can also be differentiated from sleep apnea, which occurs during stages 1 and 2, as well as during REM sleep, and is more repetitive. They also differ from nocturnal seizures, because, unlike the latter, they do not have electroencephalographic abnormalities [62].

Individuals with PD may also have paroxysmal awakenings entering in stages 3 and 4 of NREM sleep, accompanied by tachycardia, increased respiratory rate, and cognitive and emotional symptoms [2].

Treatments

The biological etiology of PD is related to abnormalities in the function of several neurotransmitters, including serotonin (5-hydroxytyrptamine; 5-HT), noradrenaline (norepinephrine), gamma-aminobutyric acid (GABA), dopamine, and cholecystokinin [67]. Pharmacotherapeutic agents with primary action at sites within the GABA and serotonin systems resulted safe and effective in the treatment of PD [67]. Nevertheless, some patients respond to other drugs, such as tricyclic antidepressants and other antiepileptic drugs. Selective serotonin reuptake inhibitors and venlafaxine are currently considered as first-line agents for patients with panic disorder [68]. Several studies suggest the efficacy of adjunctive pharmacotherapies and combining pharmacotherapy with behavioral therapy to improve treatment response [69-72].

As our understanding of the biological etiology of PD evolves, the pharmacotherapeutic agents and strategies used in the treatment of this disorder and its sleep-related symptoms will continue to evolve as well.

Obsessive-Compulsive Disorder

Clinical Evidence

Obsessive-compulsive disorder (OCD) is a common psychiatric disorder: its one-month prevalence ranges from 0.3 to 3.1% in the general population [73]. It is characterized by clinically significant recurrent, intrusive and disturbing thoughts (obsessions) and/or repetitive stereotypic behaviors (compulsions) usually associated with anxiety or dread [2]. OCD often results in noticeable distress, social impairment, and poor occupational functioning.

As for other anxiety disorders, most patients with OCD complain of sleep-related problems, including insomnia, disrupted sleep, and sleep delay [6]. A study by Ohayon and Roth [5] reported that the majority of patients with OCD reported insomnia for at least six months. OCD-related sleep disturbances may be of different types: some patients have little or no problems, while other patients can report significant distress, particularly with initiating and maintaining sleep [54,55].

Neuropathophysiology

Few studies have examined sleep disturbances in patients with OCD, with different findings.

Rapaport et al. [74] reported a significantly decrease in total sleep time in nine inpatient children. Another study by Insel et al. [75], conducted on 14 adult inpatients with OCD compared to controls, reported in patients significantly decreased total sleep time, less stage 4 sleep, decreased REM efficiency, and shortened REM latency. In summary, investigations in both adults [75] and adolescents [74] have found a reduced total sleep duration, poor quality of sleep, more awakenings, a decrease in stage 2 sleep, and a shortened REM latency. Stage 4 sleep and slow-wave sleep were reported to be increased [74] or decreased [75].

In addition to expressing lower sleep efficiency, OCD patients compared to normal volunteers showed a concomitant increase in the number of awakenings [76].

Otherwise, a more recent study by Robinson et al. [77], conducted on 13 outpatients with pure OCD compared to 13 age- and sex-matched volunteers, showed no differences between groups on sleep latency, sleep time, minutes of movement, and sleep efficiency, suggesting that many OCD patients have essentially normal sleep EEG findings.

OCD is often comorbid with a circadian rhythm sleep disorder known as delayed sleep phase syndrome (DSPS) [78]. Patients affected by this syndrome go to bed and get up much later than normal, failing in any way to shift their sleep to an earlier time. A main outcome of this condition is daytime sleepiness, which can compromise both work and social functioning. DSPS most frequently occurs in males and youngsters, with more severe OCD symptoms [79].

The presence of long and complex rituals can result in inadequate exposure to morning, with a consequent phase delay of sleep. Social isolation, lack of activity and difficulties in conducting a regular lifestyle, which are also common manifestations of severe OCD, can worsen the problem by alterating the daily resetting of the biological clock [79]. Moreover, abnormal circadian rhythms in OCD can depend on hormonal dysregulation [80] and delayed sleep phase [78].

Treatments

Generally, a combination of pharmacotherapy with serotonin-potentiating agents and behavioral therapies is safe and effective in most patients with OCD. Drugs that inhibit serotonin reuptake have proven their efficacy in OCD [81]. A meta-analysis by Ackerman and colleagues [82] showed that clomipramine should be more effective than other drugs, but with poorer tolerance and overdose risk. SSRIs are now considered to be first-line treatment for OCD [83]. Placebo-controlled studies have reported the efficacy of paroxetine, fluoxetine, fluvoxamine, citalopram, and sertraline [84].

The importance of light and melatonin in the regulation of the sleep-wake cycle suggests a possible utilization of exogenous melatonin and/or light therapy in patients affected by OCD with sleep disturbances [85].

Conclusion

The pathophysiology of OCD may involve a possible role of abnormal circadian rhythms, with hormonal dysregulations and a delayed sleep phase. The etiology of delayed sleep phase in patients affected by OCD and its interaction with core illness symptoms remain to be investigated. Generally, several studies showed lower sleep efficiency, reduced total sleep duration, decreased stage 2 sleep, and shortened REM latency in OCD [7,85], confirming the major negative impact of this syndrome on sleep neurophysiology.

Generalized Anxiety Disorder

Clinical Evidence and Neuropathophysiology

Generalized anxiety disorder (GAD) is characterized by excessive anxiety and worry (apprehensive expectation), which occur for most of the time for at least 6 months, in respect of a number of events or activities. The individual finds it difficult to control the worry [2].

Sleep disturbances are so closely related to GAD that they are listed among DSM-IV TR diagnostic criteria: difficulty in falling or staying asleep, with a restless and unsatisfying sleep, is one of the most important symptoms addressing practitioner to diagnose this kind of illness. Patients with GAD often report insomnia as a difficulty in falling asleep and can wake up in the middle of the night in the throes of anxious rumination.

They show decreased sleep depth and continuity [7], and reduced sleep time, compared to subjects without GAD [8]. This happens both in younger individuals [86] and in older adults [87]. It has been estimated that about 60% to 70% of patients with GAD have an insomnia complaint, whose severity parallels that of the anxiety disorder [88,89] suggesting that insomnia may represent one of the core symptoms of GAD.

A recent polysomnographic study by Alfano and colleagues [90] aimed to identify clinical features linking early GAD with sleep disturbances. The authors assessed 15 children with GAD and 15 matched healthy controls, all aged 7-11 years, and non-medicated subjects. Children affected by GAD did not meet criteria for any secondary mood disorder. They showed significantly augmented sleep onset latency, and reduced latency to REM sleep compared to controls. They also manifested minor differences in the type of reduced sleep efficiency, and increased total REM sleep. These data underline some polysomnographic differences in children affected by GAD with no comorbidities [90].

The sleep disturbance mostly linked to mild-to-moderate GAD is a sleep-maintenance insomnia, and to a lesser extent a sleep-onset insomnia [91], and correlated with difficulties in concentrating and irritability during the daytime [6].

Treatments

Insomnia comorbid with mild-to-moderate GAD usually responds to psychological treatments and benzodiazepines [91]. Several other drugs appear to be effective for the often chronic and disabling GAD-related insomnia, including pregabalin [92], quetiapine [93,94], escitalopram [95], lavender [96], zolpidem extended-release [97], eszopiclone coadministered with escitalopram [98], ramelteon [99], and agomelatine [100].

It should also be considered that patients with GAD, regardless of the reason for prescription, mostly receive benzodiazepines, antidepressants and antiepileptics, while about one-third follow non-pharmacological treatment [101]. Cognitive-behavioral therapies have been shown to be effective in the treatment of insomnia in patients with GAD [102], even in older primary care patients [103], and should be considered as a first-line therapeutic strategy.

Social and Specific Phobias

The essential feature of social phobia is a marked and persistent fear that regards social or performance situations that may cause embarrassment. Exposure to social or performance situation almost invariably provokes an immediate anxiety response. Patients affected by specific phobia have a marked and persistent fear of clearly definable objects or situations, which normally create no risk. The exposition to phobic stimuli almost invariably provokes an immediate anxiety response [2].

Sleep interference may relate to anticipatory anxiety prior to a feared social event, or may occur after a person has participated in a stressful social event and is ruminating about his or her performance, or when a person has to face the object of his phobia. Persons suffering from social phobia exhibit fatigue and appear tired for no reason, as compared to control subjects [8].

In brief, Park and colleagues [104] confirmed the link between phobias and sleep disturbances, with an epidemiological study conducted to examine relationships between sleep duration with sociodemographic and health-related factors, psychiatric disorders and sleep disturbances in a nationwide sample (6.510 subjects aged 18-64 years) in Korea. This study reported strong associations between sleep duration of 5 hours or less and any mood disorder, major depressive disorder, anxiety disorder, obsessive-compulsive disorder, and social and specific phobia.

Another interesting study analyzed the link between syncope syndromes and psychiatric symptoms. Busweiler and colleagues [105] conducted this study on 54 patients with a history suggestive of one or more episodes of sleep syncope matched for age and gender to 108 patients with classical vasovagal syncope, reporting that blood-injection injury phobia is strongly associated and could be a predisposing factor or a co-existent disorder in patients with reported sleep syncope, a syndrome characterized by lifelong, intermittent but severe episodes of vasovagal syncope that may occur in the horizontal position, with distressing abdominal symptoms.

Table 1. Anxiety disorders and related sleep disturbance

Diagnosis	Clinical features	Neurophysiopathology	Treatment
POST-TRAUMATIC STRESS DISORDER AND ACUTE STRESS DISORDER	Recurrent distressing dreams or nightmares that can fragment sleep, decrease sleep quality, and even cause fear about going to sleep; 50% of post-traumatic dreams can comprise exact replications of the traumatic events; constant hyperarousal state, perceived as difficulty in falling or staying asleep	Increased rate of periodic movements in sleep during both REM and non-REM (NREM) sleep. It might also result in higher vulnerability to apnea; higher rates of brief arousals from REM sleep; more stage 1 sleep, less slow wave sleep, and greater REM density; decreased SWS; increased cortisol was negatively associated with delta sleep	Cognitive-behavioral therapies: CBT-I; Pharmacotherapies: prazosin; risperidone; olanzapine, quetiapine, levomepromazine
PANIC DISORDER	Difficulties in falling asleep, restless sleep, increased sleep latency, middle-of-the-night insomnia, and reduced sleep efficiency; nocturnal panic attacks; more severe current and past sleep onset difficulties, as racing thoughts, muscular tension, fear of not falling asleep, paralysis, startle, restless legs, sleep hallucinations, nightly waking, early morning waking, non-restorative sleep, sleepiness and fatigue when not sleepy	Nocturnal panic attacks, which are characterized by waking from sleep in a state of panic generally during late stage 2 to early stage 3 of NREM sleep; paroxysmal awakenings entering in stages 3 and 4 of NREM sleep	CBT; SSRIs and venlafaxine; tricyclic antidepressants; benzodiazepines; adequate medication dosing and adequate duration of treatment to achieve maximum improvement before discontinuing
OBSESSIVE-COMPULSIVE DISORDER	Disrupted sleep and sleep delay; reduced total sleep duration, poor quality of sleep, more awakenings, a; lower sleep efficiency and a concomitant increase in the number of awakenings; delayed sleep phase syndrome	Hormonal dysregulation; decreased stage 2 sleep and shortened REM latency	Combination of pharmacotherapy with serotonin-potentiating agents and behavioral therapy
GENERALIZED ANXIETY DISORDER	Difficulty in falling or staying asleep, with a restless and unsatisfying sleep; decreased sleep depth and continuity, reduced sleep time	Augmented sleep onset latency, and reduced latency to REM sleep	CBT; psychological treatments and benzodiazepines; other drugs: pregabalin, quetiapine, escitalopram, lavender, zolpidem extended-release, eszopiclone co-administered with escitalopram, ramelteon, and agomelatine
SOCIAL AND SPECIFIC PHOBIAS	Sleep interference may relate to anticipatory anxiety; persons suffering from social phobia exhibit fatigue and appear tired for no reason; reduced sleep duration	Blood-injection injury phobia is strongly associated and may be a predisposing factor or a co-existent disorder in patients with reported sleep syncope	CBT; benzodiazepines; serotonin-potentiating agents

Conclusion

Anxiety disorders have an estimated lifetime prevalence from 15 to 25% in the general population [106]. The high prevalence and comorbidity of anxiety and sleep problems, especially insomnia, suggest an important underlying relationship between these disorders. The sleep disturbance associated with anxiety disorders is characterized by early-, middle- or maintenance insomnia due to excessive anxiety and apprehensive expectation about one or more life circumstances. Frequent awakenings occur with or without anxiety dreams. Patients may experience ruminative thinking or acute anxiety attacks during periods of wakefulness while lying in bed, not only at sleep onset but also during awakening. They may express intense anxiety during the daytime about the inevitability of each night's poor sleep. Patients display chronic anxiety, with features that include: trembling, muscle tension, restlessness, easy fatigability, shortness of breath, palpitations, tremor, sweating, dry mouth, dizziness, keyed- up feelings, exaggerated startle response, and difficulty concentrating.

While depressed patients experience marked, albeit transient, symptomatic improvement after sleep deprivation [107,108], patients with different types of anxiety disorders report either a lack of improvement or significant worsening after the application of this method [59,109,110]. This increasing evidence indicates that anxiety disorders can be distinguished from mood disorders also on the basis of differential responses to sleep deprivation. Future studies focused on sleep will help to better distinctions between anxiety and mood disorders.

References

[1] Kessler RC, Berglund P, Demler O, Jin R, Merikangas KR, Walters EE. Lifetime prevalence and age-of-onset distributions of DSM-IV disorders in the National Comorbidity Survey Replication. Arch Gen Psychiatry. 2005;62(6):593-602. Erratum in: *Arch Gen Psychiatry*. 2005;62(7):768.

[2] American Psychiatric Association. Diagnostic and statistical manual of mental disorders: DSM-IV-TR. American Psychiatric Association. Washington, DC: 2000.

[3] Benca RM, Obermeyer WH, Thisted RA, Gillin JC. Sleep and psychiatric disorders. A meta-analysis. *Arch Gen Psychiatry*. 1992;49:651-68.

[4] Soldatos CR, Dikeos DG. An integrative approach to the management of insomnia. *Curr Opin Psychiatry*. 2003;16(Suppl. 2):93-9.

[5] Ohayon MM, Roth T. Place of chronic insomnia in the course of depressive and anxiety disorders. *Journal of Psychiatry Research*. 2003;37:9-15.

[6] Staner L. Sleep and anxiety disorders. *Dialogues Clin Neurosci*. 2003;5(3):249-58.

[7] Szelenberger W, Soldatos C. Sleep disorders in psychiatric practice. *World Psychiatry* 2005;4(3):186-90.

[8] Chase RM, Pincus DB. Sleep-related problems in children and adolescents with anxiety disorders. *Behav Sleep Med*. 2011; 9(4):224-36.

[9] Mellman TA. Sleep and anxiety disorders. *Psychiatr Clin North Am*. 2006;29(4):1047-58.

[10] Spoormaker VI, Montgomery P. Disturbed sleep in post-traumatic stress disorder: secondary symptom or core feature? *Sleep Med Rev*. 2008;12(3):169-84.

[11] Batterham PJ, Glozier N, Christensen H. Sleep disturbance, personality and the onset of depression and anxiety: Prospective cohort study. *Aust N Z J Psychiatry.* 2012;46(11):1089-98.

[12] Flosnik DL, Cortese BM, Uhde TW. Cataplexy in anxious patients: is subclinical narcolepsy underrecognized in anxiety disorders? *J Clin Psychiatry.* 2009;70(6):810-6.

[13] Yiş U, Kurul SH, Oztura I, Ecevit MC, Dirik E. Polysomnographic and long-term video electroencephalographic evaluation of cases presenting with parasomnias. *Acta Neurol Belg.* 2012 Nov 8. [Epub ahead of print].

[14] Otto MW, Simon NM, Powers M, Hinton D, Zalta AK, Pollack MH. Rates of isolated sleep paralysis in outpatients with anxiety disorders. *J Anxiety Disord.* 2006;20(5):687-93.

[15] Fogelberg DJ, Hoffman JM, Dikmen S, Temkin NR, Bell KR. Association of sleep and co-occurring psychological conditions at 1 year after traumatic brain injury. *Arch Phys Med Rehabil.* 2012;93(8):1313-8.

[16] Lewis V, Creamer M, Failla S. Is poor sleep in veterans a function of post-traumatic stress disorder? *Mil Med.* 2009;174(9):948-51.

[17] Kelly U. Intimate partner violence, physical health, posttraumatic stress disorder, depression, and quality of life in latinas. *West J Emerg Med.* 2010;11(3):247-51.

[18] Krakow B, Germain A, Warner TD, Schrader R, Koss M, Hollifield M, Tandberg D, Melendrez D, Johnston L. The relationship of sleep quality and posttraumatic stress to potential sleep disorders in sexual assault survivors with nightmares, insomnia, and PTSD. *J Trauma Stress.* 2001;14(4):647-65.

[19] Krakow B, Haynes PL, Warner TD, Santana E, Melendrez D, Johnston L, Hollifield M, Sisley BN, Koss M, Shafer L. Nightmares, insomnia, and sleep-disordered breathing in fire evacuees seeking treatment for posttraumatic sleep disturbance. *J Trauma Stress.* 2004;17(3):257-68.

[20] Kobayashi I, Sledjeski EM, Spoonster E, Fallon WF Jr, Delahanty DL. Effects of early nightmares on the development of sleep disturbances in motor vehicle accident victims. *J Trauma Stress.* 2008;21(6):548-55.

[21] Pillar G, Malhotra A, Lavie P. Post-traumatic stress disorder and sleep-what a nightmare! *Sleep Med Rev.* 2000;4(2):183-200.

[22] Berlin KL, Means MK, Edinger JD. Nightmare reduction in a Vietnam veteran using imagery rehearsal therapy. *J Clin Sleep Med.* 2010; 6(5):487-8.

[23] Wittmann L, Schredl M, Kramer M. Dreaming in posttraumatic stress disorder: A critical review of phenomenology, psychophysiology and treatment. *Psychother Psychosom.* 2007;76(1):25-39.

[24] Bader K, Schäfer V, Schenkel M, Nissen L, Schwander J. Adverse childhood experiences associated with sleep in primary insomnia. *J Sleep Res.* 2007;16(3):285-96.

[25] Harvey AG, Jones C, Schmidt DA. Sleep and posttraumatic stress disorder: a review. *Clin Psychol Rev.* 2003; 23(3):377-407.

[26] Lamarche LJ, De Koninck J. Sleep disturbance in adults with posttraumatic stress disorder: a review. *J Clin Psychiatry* 2007;68(8):1257-70.

[27] Kobayashi I, Boarts JM, Delahanty DL. Polysomnographically measured sleep abnormalities in PTSD: a meta-analytic review. *Psychophysiology.* 2007;44(4):660-9.

[28] Breslau N, Roth T, Burduvali E, Kapke A, Schultz L, Roehrs T. Sleep in lifetime posttraumatic stress disorder: a community-based polysomnographic study. *Arch Gen Psychiatry*. 2004;61(5):508-16.

[29] Yetkin S, Aydin H, Ozgen F. Polysomnography in patients with post-traumatic stress disorder. *Psychiatry Clin Neurosci*. 2010;64(3):309-17.

[30] van Liempt S. Sleep disturbances and PTSD: a perpetual circle? *Eur J Psychotraumatol*. 2012;3.

[31] Wright KM, Britt TW, Bliese PD, Adler AB, Picchioni D, Moore D. Insomnia as predictor versus outcome of PTSD and depression among Iraq combat veterans. *J Clin Psychol*. 2011;67(12):1240-58.

[32] Otte C, Lenoci M, Metzler T, Yehuda R, Marmar CR, Neylan TC. Hypothalamic-pituitary-adrenal axis activity and sleep in posttraumatic stress disorder. *Neuropsychopharmacology*. 2005;30(6):1173-80.

[33] Schoenfeld FB, Deviva JC, Manber R. Treatment of sleep disturbances in posttraumatic stress disorder: a review. *J Rehabil Res Dev*. 2012;49(5):729-52.

[34] Belleville G, Guay S, Marchand A. Persistence of sleep disturbances following cognitive-behavior therapy for posttraumatic stress disorder. *J Psychosom Res*. 2011;70(4):318-27.

[35] DeViva JC, Zayfert C, Pigeon WR, Mellman TA. Treatment of residual insomnia after CBT for PTSD: case studies. *Journal of Traumatic Stress* 2005;18,155-159.

[36] Germain A, Shear MK, Hall M, Buysse DJ. Effects of a brief behavioral treatment for PTSD-related sleep disturbances: a pilot study. *Behav Res Ther*. 2007;45(3):627-32.

[37] Krakow B, Johnston L, Melendrez D, Hollifield M, Warner TD, Chavez-Kennedy D, Herlan MJ. An open-label trial of evidence-based cognitive behavior therapy for nightmares and insomnia in crime victims with PTSD. *Am J Psychiatry*. 2001;158(12):2043-7.

[38] Nappi CM, Drummond SP, Hall JM. Treating nightmares and insomnia in posttraumatic stress disorder: a review of current evidence. *Neuropharmacology*. 2012;62(2):576-85.

[39] Swanson LM, Favorite TK, Horin E, Arnedt JT. A combined group treatment for nightmares and insomnia in combat veterans: a pilot study. *J Trauma Stress*. 2009;22:639-42.

[40] Maher MJ, Rego SA, Asnis GM. Sleep disturbances in patients with post-traumatic stress disorder: epidemiology, impact and approaches to management. *CNS Drugs*. 2006;20(7):567-90.

[41] van Liempt S, Vermetten E, Geuze E, Westenberg H. Pharmacotherapeutic treatment of nightmares and insomnia in posttraumatic stress disorder: an overview of the literature. *Ann N Y Acad Sci*. 2006;1071:502-7.

[42] van Liempt S, Vermetten E, Geuze E, Westenberg HG. Pharmacotherapy for disordered sleep in post-traumatic stress disorder: a systematic review. *Int Clin Psychopharmacol*. 2006;21(4):193-202.

[43] Kung S, Espinel Z, Lapid MI. Treatment of nightmares with prazosin: a systematic review. *Mayo Clin Proc*. 2012;87(9):890-900.

[44] Germain A, Richardson R, Moul DE, Mammen O, Haas G, Forman SD, Rode N, Begley A, Nofzinger EA. Placebo-controlled comparison of prazosin and cognitive-

behavioral treatments for sleep disturbances in US Military Veterans. *J Psychosom Res.* 2012;72(2):89-96.

[45] David D, De Faria L, Mellman TA. Adjunctive risperidone treatment and sleep symptoms in combat veterans with chronic PTSD. *Depress Anxiety.* 2006;23(8):489-91.

[46] Rothbaum BO, Killeen TK, Davidson JR, Brady KT, Connor KM, Heekin MH. Placebo-controlled trial of risperidone augmentation for selective serotonin reuptake inhibitor-resistant civilian posttraumatic stress disorder. *J Clin Psychiatry.* 2008;69(4):520-5.

[47] Kozarić-Kovacić D, Pivac N, Mück-Seler D, Rothbaum BO. Risperidone in psychotic combat-related posttraumatic stress disorder: an open trial. *J Clin Psychiatry.* 2005;66(7):922-7.

[48] Walderhaug E, Kasserman S, Aikins D, Vojvoda D, Nishimura C, Neumeister A. Effects of duloxetine in treatment-refractory men with posttraumatic stress disorder. *Pharmacopsychiatry.* 2010;43(2):45-9.

[49] Neylan TC, Lenoci M, Maglione ML, Rosenlicht NZ, Leykin Y, Metzler TJ, Schoenfeld FB, Marmar CR. The effect of nefazodone on subjective and objective sleep quality in posttraumatic stress disorder. *J Clin Psychiatry.* 2003;64(4):445-50.

[50] Aurora RN, Zak RS, Auerbach SH, Casey KR, Chowdhuri S, Karippot A, Maganti RK, Ramar K, Kristo DA, Bista SR, Lamm CI, Morgenthaler TI; Standards of Practice Committee; American Academy of Sleep Medicine. Best practice guide for the treatment of nightmare disorder in adults. *J Clin Sleep Med.* 2010;6(4):389-401.

[51] Kessler RC, Chiu WT, Jin R, Ruscio AM, Shear K, Walters EE. The epidemiology of panic attacks, panic disorder, and agoraphobia in the National Comorbidity Survey Replication. *Arch Gen Psychiatry.* 2006;63:415-424.

[52] Singareddy R, Uhde TW. Nocturnal sleep panic and depression: relationship to subjective sleep in panic disorder. *J Affect Disord.* 2009;112:262-266.

[53] Lauer CJ, Krieg JC, Garcia-Borreguero D, Ozdaglar A, Holsboer F. Panic disorder and major depression: a comparative electroencephalographic sleep study. *Psychiatry Res.* 1992;44:41-54.

[54] Uhde TW. Anxiety disorders. In: MH Kryger, T Roth, WC Dement (Eds), Principles and practice of sleep medicine. Philadelphia: W. B. Saunders Company: 2000;1123-39.

[55] Uhde TW, Cortese BM, Vedeniapin A. Anxiety and sleep problems: emerging concepts and theoretical treatment implications. *Curr Psychiatry Rep.* 2009;11:269-276.

[56] Stein MB, Chartier M, Walker JR. Sleep in nondepressed patients with panic disorder: I. Systematic assessment of subjective sleep quality and sleep disturbance. *Sleep.* 1993;16:724-726.

[57] Mellman TA, Uhde TW. Electroencephalographic sleep in panic disorder. A focus on sleep-related panic attacks. *Arch Gen Psychiatry.* 1989;46(2):178-84.

[58] Taylor CB, Sheikh J, Agras WS, Roth WT, Margraf J, Ehlers A, Maddock RJ, Gossard D. Ambulatory heart rate changes in patients with panic attacks. *Am J Psychiatry.* 1986;143(4):478-82.

[59] Craske MG, Barlow DH. Nocturnal panic: response to hyperventilation and carbon dioxide challenges. *J Abnorm Psychol.* 1990;99(3):302-7.

[60] Merritt-Davis O, Balon R. Nocturnal panic: biology, psychopathology, and its contribution to the expression of panic disorder. *Depress Anxiety.* 2003;18(4):221-7.

[61] Sloan EP, Natarajan M, Baker B, Dorian P, Mironov D, Barr A, Newman DM, Shapiro CM. Nocturnal and daytime panic attacks--comparison of sleep architecture, heart rate variability, and response to sodium lactate challenge. *Biol Psychiatry.* 1999;45(10):1313-20.

[62] Craske MG, Lang AJ, Rowe M, DeCola JP, Simmons J, Mann C, Yan-Go F, Bystritsky A. Presleep attributions about arousal during sleep: nocturnal panic. *J Abnorm Psychol* 2002;111(1):53-62.

[63] Schredl M, Kronenberg G, Nonnell P, Heuser I. Dream recall, nightmare frequency, and nocturnal panic attacks in panic disorder. *J Nerv Ment Dis.* 2001;189:559-562.

[64] Lydiard RB, Zealberg J, Laraia MT, Fossey M, Prockow V, Gross J, et al. Electroencephalography during sleep of patients with panic disorder. *J Neuropsychiatry Clin Neurosci.* 1989;1:372-376.

[65] Stein MB, Millar TW, Larsen DK, Kryger MH. Irregular breathing during sleep in patients with panic disorder. *Am J Psychiatry.* 1995;152:1168-73.

[66] Craske MG, Rowe MK. Nocturnal panic. *Clin Psychol-Sci Pr.* 1997;2,153-174.

[67] Johnson MR, Lydiard RB, Ballenger JC. Panic disorder. Pathophysiology and drug treatment. *Drugs.* 1995;49(3):328-44.

[68] Andrisano C, Chiesa A, Serretti A. Newer antidepressants and panic disorder: a meta-analysis. *Int Clin Psychopharmacol.* 2013;28(1):33-45.

[69] Davidson JR. The long-term treatment of panic disorder. *J Clin Psychiatry.* 1998;59 Suppl 8:17-21; discussion 22-3.

[70] Doyle A, Pollack MH. Long-term management of panic disorder. *J Clin Psychiatry.* 2004;65 Suppl 5:24-8.

[71] Klerman GL. Treatments for panic disorder. *J Clin Psychiatry.* 1992;53Suppl:14-9.

[72] Harden M. Cognitive behaviour therapy - incorporating therapy into general practice. *Aust Fam Physician.* 2012;41(9):668-71.

[73] Fontenelle LF, Mendlowicz MV, Versiani M. The descriptive epidemiology of obsessive-compulsive disorder. *Prog Neuropsychopharmacol Biol Psychiatry.* 2006;30(3):327-37.

[74] Rapoport J, Elkins R, Langer DH, Sceery W, Buchsbaum MS, Gillin JC, Murphy DL, Zahn TP, Lake R, Ludlow C, Mendelson W. Childhood obsessive-compulsive disorder. *Am J Psychiatry.* 1981;138(12):1545-54.

[75] Insel TR, Gillin JC, Moore A, Mendelson WB, Loewenstein RJ, Murphy DL. The sleep of patients with obsessive-compulsive disorder. *Arch Gen Psychiatry.* 1982;39:1372-77.

[76] Hohagen F, Lis S, Krieger S, Winkelmann G, Riemann D, Fritsch-Montero R, Rey E, Aldenhoff J, Berger M. Sleep EEG of patients with obsessive-compulsive disorder. *Eur Arch Psychiatry Clin Neurosci.* 1994;243(5):273-8.

[77] Robinson D, Walsleben J, Pollack S, Lerner G. Nocturnal polysomnography in obsessive-compulsive disorder. *Psychiatry Res.* 1998;80(3):257-63.

[78] Weitzman ED, Czeisler CA, Coleman RM, Spielman AJ, Zimmerman JC, Dement WC. Delayed sleep phase syndrome: a chronobiological disorder with sleep-onset insomnia. *Arch Gen Psychiatry.* 1981;38:737-46.

[79] Turner J, Drummond LM, Mukhopadhyay S, Ghodse H, White S, Pillay A, Fineberg NA. A prospective study of delayed sleep phase syndrome in patients with severe resistant obsessive-compulsive disorder. *World Psychiatry.* 2007;6(2):108-11.

[80] Monteleone P, Catapano F, Del Buono G, Maj M. Circadian rhythms of melatonin, cortisol and prolactin in patients with obsessive-compulsive disorder. *Acta Psychiatr Scand.* 1994;89:411-15.

[81] Ellingrod VL. Pharmacotherapy of primary obsessive-compulsive disorder: review of the literature. *Pharmacotherapy.* 1998;18(5):936-60.

[82] Ackerman DL, Greenland S. Multivariate meta-analysis of controlled drug studies for obsessive compulsive disorder. *J Clin Psychopharmacol.* 2002;22:309-17.

[83] Goodman WK. Obsessive-compulsive disorder diagnosis and treatment. *J Clin Psychiatry.* 1999;60(suppl 6):16-20.

[84] Bourin M, Lambert O. Pharmacotherapy of anxious disorders. *Hum Psychopharmacol Clin Exp.* 2002;17:383-400.

[85] Lange KW, Lange KM, Hauser J, Tucha L, Tucha O. Circadian rhythms in obsessive-compulsive disorder. *J Neural Transm.* 2012;119(10):1077-83.

[86] Alfano CA, Pina AA, Zerr AA, Villalta IK. Pre-sleep arousal and sleep problems of anxiety-disordered youth. *Child Psychiatry Hum Dev.* 2010;41(2):156-67.

[87] Brenes GA, Miller ME, Stanley MA, Williamson JD, Knudson M, McCall WV. Insomnia in older adults with generalized anxiety disorder. *Am J Geriatr Psychiatry.* 2009;17(6):465-72.

[88] Anderson DJ, Noyes R, Crowe RR. A comparison of panic disorder and generalized anxiety disorder. *Am J Psychiatry.* 1984;141:572-575.

[89] Hoehn-Saric R, McLeod DR. Generalised anxiety disorder in adulthood. In: Hersen M, Last CG, eds. Handbook of Child and Adult Psychopathology: A Longitudinal Perspective. New York, NY, *Pergamon Press:* 1990;247-260.

[90] Alfano CA, Reynolds K, Scott N, Dahl RE, Mellman TA. Polysomnographic sleep patterns of non-depressed, non-medicated children with generalized anxiety disorder. *J Affect Disord.* 2012 Sep 28. [Epub ahead of print].

[91] Monti JM, Monti D. Sleep disturbance in generalized anxiety disorder and its treatment. *Sleep Med Rev.* 2000;4(3):263-276.

[92] Holsboer-Trachsler E, Prieto R. Effects of pregabalin on sleep in generalized anxiety disorder. *Int J Neuropsychopharmacol.* 2012 Sep 25:1-12. [Epub ahead of print].

[93] Endicott J, Svedsäter H, Locklear JC. Effects of once-daily extended release quetiapine fumarate on patient-reported outcomes in patients with generalized anxiety disorder. *Neuropsychiatr Dis Treat.* 2012;8:301-11.

[94] Khan A, Joyce M, Atkinson S, Eggens I, Baldytcheva I, Eriksson H. A randomized, double-blind study of once-daily extended release quetiapine fumarate (quetiapine XR) monotherapy in patients with generalized anxiety disorder. *J Clin Psychopharmacol.* 2011;31(4):418-28.

[95] Stein DJ, Lopez AG. Effects of escitalopram on sleep problems in patients with major depression or generalized anxiety disorder. *Adv Ther.* 2011;28(11):1021-37.

[96] Woelk H, Schläfke S. A multi-center, double-blind, randomised study of the Lavender oil preparation Silexan in comparison to Lorazepam for generalized anxiety disorder. *Phytomedicine* 2010;17(2):94-9.

[97] Fava M, Asnis GM, Shrivastava R, Lydiard B, Bastani B, Sheehan D, Roth T. Zolpidem extended-release improves sleep and next-day symptoms in comorbid insomnia and generalized anxiety disorder. *J Clin Psychopharmacol.* 2009;29(3):222-30.

[98] Pollack M, Kinrys G, Krystal A, McCall WV, Roth T, Schaefer K, Rubens R, Roach J, Huang H, Krishnan R. Eszopiclone coadministered with escitalopram in patients with insomnia and comorbid generalized anxiety disorder. *Arch Gen Psychiatry.* 2008;65(5):551-62.

[99] Gross PK, Nourse R, Wasser TE. Ramelteon for insomnia symptoms in a community sample of adults with generalized anxiety disorder: an open label study. *J Clin Sleep Med.* 2009;5(1):28-33.

[100] Stein DJ, Ahokas AA, de Bodinat C. Effiacy of agomelatine in generalized anxiety disorder: a randomized, double-blind, placebo-controlled study. *J Clin Psychopharmacol.* 2008;28(5):561-6.

[101] García-Campayo J, Caballero F, Perez M, López V. Prevalence and Clinical Features of newly diagnosed Generalized Anxiety Disorder patients in Spanish Primary Care Settings: The GADAP study. *Actas Esp Psiquiatr.* 2012;40(3):105-13.

[102] Bélanger L, Morin CM, Langlois F, Ladouceur R. Insomnia and generalized anxiety disorder: effects of cognitive behavior therapy for gad on insomnia symptoms. *J Anxiety Disord.* 2004;18(4):561-71.

[103] Bush AL, Armento ME, Weiss BJ, Rhoades HM, Novy DM, Wilson NL, Kunik ME, Stanley MA. The Pittsburgh Sleep Quality Index in older primary care patients with generalized anxiety disorder: Psychometrics and outcomes following cognitive behavioral therapy. *Psychiatry Res.* 2012;199(1):24-30.

[104] Park S, Cho MJ, Chang SM, Bae JN, Jeon HJ, Cho SJ, Kim BS, Chung IW, Ahn JH, Lee HW, Hong JP. Relationships of sleep duration with sociodemographic and health-related factors, psychiatric disorders and sleep disturbances in a community sample of Korean adults. *J Sleep Res.* 2010;19(4):567-77.

[105] Busweiler L, Jardine DL, Frampton CM, Wieling W. Sleep syncope: important clinical associations with phobia and vagotonia. *Sleep Med.* 2010;11(9):929-33.

[106] Kessler RC, McGonagle KA, Zhao S, Nelson CB, Hughes M, Eshleman S, Wittchen HU, Kendler KS. Lifetime and 12-month prevalence of DSM-III-R psychiatric disorders in the United States. Results from the National Comorbidity Survey. *Arch Gen Psychiatry.* 1994;51(1):8-19.

[107] Papadimitriou GN, Christodoulou GN, Katsougianni K, Stefanis CN. Therapy and prevention of affective illness by total sleep deprivation. *J Affect Disord.* 1993;27:107-16.

[108] Wu JC, Bunney WE. The biological basis of an antidepressant response to sleep deprivation and relapse: Review and hypothesis. *Am J Psychiatry.* 1990;147:14-21.

[109] Joffe RT, Swinson RP. Total sleep deprivation in patients with obsessive-compulsive disorder. *Acta Psychiatr Scand.* 1988;77(4):483-7.

[110] Labbate LA, Johnson MR, Lydiard RB, Brawman-Mintzer O, Emmanuel N, Crawford M, Kapp R, Ballenger JC. Sleep Deprivation in social phobia and generalized anxiety disorder. *Biol Psychiatry.* 1998;43(11):840-2.

In: Sleep Medicine
Editors: A. Del Casale, R. Brugnoli and P. Girardi

ISBN: 978-1-62808-515-0
© 2013 Nova Science Publishers, Inc.

Chapter X

Sleep Disturbance in Mood Disorders

Lidia Petrone, Stefano Porcelli and Alessandro Serretti[*]
Department of Biomedical and NeuroMotor Sciences,
University of Bologna, Bologna, Italy

Abstract

Our world is characterized by daily and seasonal rhythms in light intensity, ambient temperature and humidity. To adapt to these rhythms, most organisms, including humans, developed rhythms in almost every aspect of their biology, ranging from gene expression, physiology, cognitive functions and activity rest patterns. In mood disorders, several abnormalities in circadian rhythms as well as sleep disturbances have been repeatedly reported. It has been hypothesized that depressed patients may have a greater predisposition to adapt poorly to environmental challenges. Particularly, the stress-diathesis model hypothesized that several factors increase individual risk for the development of a fragile circadian system, which predisposes to the development of mood disorders. Here, we report on several abnormalities found in these diseases and the pathophysiological theories developed in the last decades to explain the relationship between circadian rhythms and mood disorders. In addition, we review the effects of antidepressant treatment on sleep and briefly report on strategies to improve sleep quality and insomnia associated with mood disorders.

Keywords: Mood Disorders, Depression, Mania, Sleep disturbances, Circadian Rhythms

1. Introduction

We live in a rhythmic world. The rotation of earth on its axis and around the sun causes daily and seasonal rhythms in light intensity, temperature and. To optimally adapt to these

---

[*] Corresponding author: Prof. Alessandro Serretti, Institute of Psychiatry, University of Bologna, Italy. Email: alessandro.serretti@unibo.it.

rhythms most organisms, including humans, developed rhythms in almost every aspect of their biology, ranging from gene expression (expression levels of approximately 15% of the genes in our body show daily rhythms), physiology (e.g. hearth rate, metabolism, hormone secretion), cognitive functions (e.g. learning, memory) and activity rest patterns. As a part of the adaptations to a rhythmic world, virtually all species studied to date have developed an internal circadian timing system composed of a master clock, which in mammals is located in the suprachiasmatic nucleus and subsidiary clocks in nearly every body cell. This internal timing system allows the individual to prepare itself, rather than respond, to the changing environment, to choose the right time for a given response or activity without being easily mislead by minor environmental changes and to assure that a temporal order between internal processes and between them and the environment maximizes performance. A disruption of the circadian clock or activity during the abnormal part of the daily cycle (shift-work, jet-lag) may result in misalignment between the internal circadian clock and the activity pattern which may have adverse consequences such as metabolic syndrome, obesity and insomnia, as well as other psychological and mental disorders.

Humans have developed to be active during the daytime. Thus, our mental ability and energy levels are highest during daylight hours, when we engage in exercise and social interactions, and our metabolism and physiology are adapted to this. During the night, when activity levels drop, core body temperature falls and reaches its nadir, while cortisol levels rise before awakening. There are cyclic changes in the level of sleep (as shown by electroencephalogram changes) with hormonal release, such as the release of growth hormone, linked to specific phases of the regular sleep cycle. These rhythmic changes in metabolism and psychological activity are under the control of a circadian clock as stated above; this ensures that our body is attuned to the level of mental and physical activity associated with a particular time of day or night. When free of external environmental clues, the amplitude of our daily rhythm is longer than the 24-hour day-night cycle as demonstrated in experiments when individuals were placed in temporal isolation or in conditions of permanent darkness. When our sleep-cycle is out of phase with the day-night cycle, we can experience dysphoria, poor functioning and increased health risks.

Table 1.

Proximal Factors	
Biological	Seasonal Maturation/aging hormonal status Internal dysregulation associated with physical illness or primary sleep disorders
Psychological	Change in temporal order (e.g. shift work) Social rhythm disruption (SDR) events (e.g. major life events involving separation or death)
Distal factors	
Biological	Genetics Perinatal factors Circadian rhythm (CR) pacemaker characteristics (e.g. abnormal period)
Psychological	Developmental (e.g. repetitive early life stress) Increased sensitization to negative life events and/or personality style (e.g. high neuroticism, learned helplessness)

In mood disorders, several abnormalities in circadian rhythms (CRs) as well as sleep disturbances have been repeatedly reported. To explain these findings, it has been hypothesized that depressed patients may have a greater predisposition to adapt poorly to environmental challenges. Indeed, the stress-diathesis model hypothesized that biological factors increase individual risk for the development of a fragile circadian system. Psychological vulnerabilities are also implicated, such as an altered intensity of cognitive, affective and behavioural responses to environmental cues because of hypersensitivity to certain types of stimuli (and/or reduced sensitivity to other cues). In particular, Hallonquist [1] and Leonhardt [2] identified biological and psychological factors that may predispose to (distal factors) or precipitate (proximal factors) circadian dysregulation in affective disorders (Table 1).

1.1. Circadian Rhythms: Human Circadian Pacemaker, Sleep Cycle and Sleep Study

1.1.1. Human Circadian Pacemaker

The human circadian pacemaker or "clock" is located in the suprachiasmatic nucleus of the anterior hypothalamus. This regulates the key circadian rhythmic changes such as cortisol and thyroid hormone levels and core body temperature. The pacemaker is governed by a set of genes that operate through a series of feedback mechanisms with a regular cycle of about 24 hours. The main gene that affects both the persistence and period of circadian rhythms is the *Clock* gene (*Circadian Locomotor Output Cycles Kaput*), which encodes a basic helix-loop-helix-PAS transcription factor. CLOCK functions as an essential activator of downstream elements in the pathway critical to the generation of circadian rhythms, as demonstrated by animal studies. In particular, in drosophila the newly synthesized Clock protein (CLK) stays in the cytoplasm in a hypophosphorylated state before entering the nucleus. Once in the nucleus, CLK is localized in nuclear foci and is later redistributed homogeneously. Here, the CYCLE protein (CYC) (also known as dBMAL for the BMAL1 orthologue in mammals) dimerizes with CLK via their respective PAS domains. This dimer then recruits the co-activator CREB-binding protein (CBP) and is further phosphorylated. Once phosphorylated, this CLK-CYC complex binds to the E-box elements of the promoters of period (*per*) and timeless (*tim*) via its bHLH domain, causing the stimulation of gene expression of *per* and *tim*. A large molar excess of period (PER) and timeless (TIM) proteins causes formation of the PER-TIM heterodimer which prevents the CLK-CYC heterodimer from binding to the E-boxes of *per* and *tim*, acting as internal feedback signal. Further, CLK is hyperphosphorylated when double-time (DBT) kinase interacts with the CLK-CYC complex in a PER reliant manner, destabilizing both CLK and PER, leading to the degradation of both proteins. Hypophosphorylated CLK then accumulates, binds to the E-boxes of *per* and *tim* and activates their transcription once again. This cycle of post-translational phosphorylation suggest that temporal phosphorylation of CLK helps the timing mechanism of the circadian clock. A similar model is found in other mammalians, including humans. The circadian pacemaker has to be resynchronized regularly to compensate for the slightly longer than 24 hour cycle of the "endogenous" circadian rhythm. This synchronization to the external environment is mediated through the retinohypothalamic tract.

1.1.2. Sleep Cycle

Although the precise function of sleep is still unknown, decades of research strongly demonstrated that sleep has a vital role in central nervous system (CNS) restoration, memory consolidation and affect regulation. Sleep is a natural periodic state of rest for the mind and body, in which the eyes usually close, and consciousness is completely or partly lost, so that there is a decrease in bodily movement or external stimuli. Table 2 shows the usual sleep cycle, which is normally repeated four times during the night. The average length of the first sleep cycle is around 90 minutes and lasts for about 100–120 minutes from the second to the fourth cycle. The last sleep cycle is usually the longest. The organization of NREM and REM sleep also changes with each cycle. There is a predominance of SWS during the first two sleep cycles and a predominance of REM sleep in the last two cycles. SWS (N3) is rare to non-existent in the last cycle, while REM sleep is the longest.

Table 2.

	Stage	Duration	EEG	Frequency	Description	
NREM (synchronized) 75-80%	I (3-8%)	1-7 min	Alpha activity	2–7 Hz	Stage between sleep and wakefulness (seen at sleep onset). Muscles are active, eyes roll slowly opening and closing moderately.	Light stage of sleep (can be interrupted by wakefulness) (N1 and N2)
	II (45-55%)	10-25 min	Theta activity	12-14 Hz	Harder to wake the sleeper. Alpha waves are interrupted by abrupt activity called sleep spindles and K-complex.	
	III (15/20%) IV (15-20%)	20-40 min	Delta activity	0,5-3,5 Hz	scored when a moderate amount (20–50% of an epoch) of high-amplitude (75 mV or greater) slow-wave EEG activity is observed.	Deeper stages of sleep (N3) SWS (slow wave sleep)
			Delta activity		defined by a predominance (greater than 50% of an epoch) of high-amplitude, slow-wave activity.	
A brief switch to stage 2 may precede the occurrence of REM sleep.						
REM (desynchronized) 20-25%	tonic	4-8 min			scored epoch consists only of the REM sleep EEG and muscle atonia.	
	phasic				muscle atonia is interrupted by bursts of muscle tone. These twitches and bursts of eye movements are called phasic events, occurring on a background of tonic muscle inhibition. Abnormalities in heart and breath frequencies Variability in blood pressure	

At the broadest levels, there is a seasonal tendency for longer and deeper sleep in winter and a circadian propensity for the onset of sleep (i.e. after dark and after midday). Onset of sleep is promoted by a surge in secretion of the pineal hormone melatonin (after the onset of darkness). Sleep onset is followed by the nocturnal surge in GH secretion, which occurs within the first 90 minutes of sleep onset. A reduction of core body temperature and diurnally low levels of cortisol secretion further promote the maintenance of sleep. Orchestrated across each 24-hour period is an oscillating, 90-minute, infraradian cycle defined by rapid eye movement (REM) sleep. Within each cycle, there is a characteristic progression from light to deeper levels of sleep (defined by different types of EEG activity), culminating in the paradoxical central activation of REM sleep, during which most of night-time dreaming occurs. An 8-hour night of sleep thus typically includes four or five cycles consisting of non-rapid eye movement (NREM) sleep and REM sleep. The propensity for deep sleep is greatest within the first 3 hours after sleep onset. REM sleep periods, by contrast, tend to become longer and more intense as the night of sleep progresses.

Prefrontal cortical metabolism is normally decreased during NREM sleep, a time of physical and metabolic rest. The frontal cortex is essentially off-line during deep sleep, and the characteristic rhythm of brain activity consists of slow (delta) desynchronized waves of thalamocortical origin. REM sleep, in contrast, is characterized by fast, low-amplitude electrical activity and increased glucose metabolism in the limbic system. REMs are under the direct control of cholinergic neurons in the pons, which are tonically inhibited by the reticular activating system (predominately by histaminergic and noradrenergic neurotransmission) during wakefulness. During sleep, inhibitory 5-HT projections from the dorsal raphe nuclei phasically suppress REM. Pharmacological manipulations that increase central cholinergic activity lighten sleep and increase phasic REM activity. Dietary depletion of 5-HT and exogenous administration of glucocorticoids can similarly increase phasic REM indices. Injections of CRH and ingestion of potent noradrenergic agonists decrease total sleep time, reduce slow wave sleep and suppress REM sleep.

1.3. Sleep Studies

Table 3.

Polysomnography (PSG)	PSG is a comprehensive recording of the biophysiological changes that occur during sleep, including brain (EEG), eye movements (EOG), muscle activity or skeletal muscle activation (EMG) and heart rhythm (ECG) during sleep. Oximetry measures breathing functions such as respiratory airflow. It also records the flow of air through the mouth and nose, snoring, body muscle movements, and chest and belly movements.
Multiple sleep latency test (MSLT)	It measures how long it takes the patient to fall asleep several times in one day. It also determines whether REM sleep occurs upon falling asleep.
Actigraphy	Generally watch-shaped and worn on the wrist of the non-dominant arm. Useful for determining sleep patterns and CR and may be worn for several weeks at a time. Patient remains mobile. It is used to clinically evaluate insomnia, circadian rhythm sleep disorders, excessive sleepiness and restless legs syndrome. It is also used to assess the effectiveness of pharmacologic, behavioural, phototherapeutic or chronotherapeutic treatments for these disorders.
Maintenance of wakefulness test (MWT)	This test measures whether you can stay awake during a time when you are normally awake.

During the last years a number of tests have been developed for the investigation the CRs, such as 24-hour cortisol secretion and the dexamethasone suppression test. Moreover, several non-invasive markers of CR disruption can be measured in clinical practice, such as actigraphic recording of sleep–wake cycle, sleep phase profiles, self-reported ratings of sleep pattern and sleep efficiency (Table 3). Obviously, in affective disorders such measures should be associated with concurrent monitoring of mood states (including diurnal variation), concentration patterns and/or activity levels and behaviour using self-rated daily diaries (hand-written or electronic).

2. Circadian Rhythms and Sleep Disturbances in Major Depressive Disorder

Major depressive disorder (MDD), or unipolar depression, is a serious mental illness and is a common condition associated with increased rates of disability, morbidity and mortality. Diagnosis is often complex because of the absence of biological markers as well as for the broad clinical variability present in depressed patients. Indeed, until now, diagnosis of depression is necessarily psychopathological and clinical, according to well defined criteria such as those in the Diagnostic and Statistical Manual of Mental Disorders IV Text Revised (DSM IV TR) or those proposed by the International Classification of Diseases 10 (ICD-10).

As stated above, several lines of evidence have clearly demonstrated a relationship between depression and CRs. Patients suffering from depression complain of sleep disruptions mainly consistent with symptoms of insomnia (prolonged sleep latency, frequent nocturnal awakenings and early morning awakening), which are part of the core complaints of depression. Indeed, sleep disturbances are described by up to 90% of patients with a major depressive episode and can be confirmed by PSG study. Furthermore, a growing body of evidence has suggested a potential causal role of insomnia in the development of depression in patients who have no previous history of MDD and in predicting relapse in patients with MDD in remission [3]. In particular, chronic insomnia may increase the individual's risk of developing depression by five-fold compared to the general population [4]. Thus, disturbed sleep might be involved, at least partially, in the onset and course of depression as well as in response to treatment. However, there is considerable heterogeneity in the nature of the sleep disturbance among patients. For example, among the subtypes of depression identify by DSM IV TR, melancholic and atypical depression show different CR abnormalities, which in turn give different sleep disturbances. In particular, melancholic depression is characterized by a worsening of symptoms in the morning hours and early-morning waking. In contrast, atypical depression is characterized by excessive sleep or sleepiness (hypersomnia). However, since these two particular subtypes of depression are relevant in both clinical and research situations, this issue is better addressed in a further specific paragraph.

The most consistent circadian alterations that have been described in MDD patients include changes in daily mood variation, brain activity, core body temperature, hormone secretion (such as altered 24-hour secretion patterns for cortisol, prolactin, TSH, and melatonin), sleep-wake cycle, motor activity and seasonal mood variation [5].

More in detail, sleep and PSG studies demonstrate changes in CRs, particularly to the sleep architecture that indicates a "phase advance" of such rhythms, and specifically in the temperature nadir and cortisol levels, which occur earlier in the night. Sleep architecture in depressed patients also reflects this "phase advance". Indeed, depressed patients show a premature loss of deep sleep (Slow Wave Sleep, SWS) associated with an increase in nocturnal arousal. The latter is reflected by four types of disturbances often observed in such patients: an increase in nocturnal awakenings, a reduction in total sleep time, increased phasic REM sleep and increased core body temperature. The combination of increased REM "drive" and decreased SWS results in a significant reduction in the first period of NREM sleep, a phenomenon referred to as reduced REM latency. Further, PSG shows a decrease in the percentage of stage 2 sleep, while rapid eye movement sleep is increased. Thus, the patterning of REM sleep periods is characterized by reduced REM latency and increased REM density (i.e. an increased number of eye movements during the REM period). Interestingly, high-risk studies investigating unaffected relatives of patients with MDD demonstrated that REM density changes are already present before the onset of the disorder, and may predict its development. Furthermore, the results of family and twin studies suggest that these related abnormalities are partly heritable. Consistent with the expected behaviour of a heritable trait, reduced REM latency and deficits of SWS typically persist after recovery of a depressive episode. Finally, REM sleep alterations often persist beyond the clinical episode and are thus believed to increase vulnerability to relapse or recurrence, and in general may have a negative effect on treatment response.

2.1. Neuroimaging Correlates of Sleep Disturbances in Mood Disorders

The above-stated abnormalities also showed several correlates in brain-imaging studies. Particularly, depressed patients showed an increased global cerebral metabolism during the first non-REM sleep period (¼ REM latency). Instead, from waking to REM sleep, activation in the anterior paralimbic structures has been observed. Additionally, activation in bilateral dorsolateral prefrontal, left premotor, primary sensorimotor, and left parietal cortices, as well as in the midbrain reticular formation, has been described. On these bases, it has been hypothesized that altered function of limbic/anterior paralimbic and prefrontal circuits in depression is accentuated during the REM sleep state and that this may be related to affective dysregulation.

The investigation of functional neuro-anatomical correlates of sleep in depressed patients evidenced that REM density positively correlates with regional metabolic rate bilaterally. REM density appears to negatively correlate with the relative regional cerebral metabolic rate in areas corresponding bilaterally to lateral occipital cortex, cuneus, temporal cortices and parahippocampal gyrus. It has been hypothesized that since temporal and occipital cortices showed hyper-metabolism during REM sleep in depressed patients compared with healthy controls, REM density might be an indirect correlate of metabolic activity in these areas [6].

Recently, McNamara et al. [7] suggested that one mechanism that directly reflects the pathophysiologic pattern of hyperactive paralimbic/ventromedial prefrontal cortex (vmPFC) and hypoactive dorsomedial prefrontal cortex (dPFC) in mood disorders might be "REM-hyperactivation or -disinhibition" driven. This neurometabolic activation/hypoactivation exactly characterizes normal REM-related brain activation/deactivation patterns throughout the sleep cycle. Several times per night, REM sleep selectively and intensively activates paralimbic/vmPFC systems and down-regulates dPFC systems. This pattern of vmPFC overactivation and dPFC hypoactivation naturally occurs only in REM sleep. Taken as a whole, these findings indicate that the neuronal processes underlying sleep differ between brain regions in depression and that REM sleep dysregulations might be an indirect correlate of temporal and occipital cortices showing hypermetabolism in depressed patients. Nonetheless, this hypothesis needs further investigation.

3. Pathophysiology of Circadian Rhytms Abnormalities in Major Depression Disorder

Even if the connections between CRs and MDD have now been established, the exact mechanisms underlying the specific biology of these interactions is still not fully clarified [8]. Several theories and models have been developed in the last decades to explain this relationship. Roughly, these theories can be divided into those viewing the observed changes in sleep as a consequence or reflection of some basic underlying mechanism involved in the pathogenesis of MDD (e.g. the cholinergic/aminergic hypothesis) and other models ascribing a more independent role for sleep dysregulation in the aetiology/pathophysiology of MDD (e.g. the REM sleep deprivation/ontogeny model).

3.1. Cholinergic/Aminergic Imbalance Model

This hypothesis is based on observations that organophosphate poisoning, which leads to an inhibition of acetylcholinesterase and therefore elevates acetylcholine levels throughout the brain and body, provokes depression-like symptoms in humans. This theory, at the time it was published, was seen as an extension and improvement over the classical monoamine deficiency theory, which had primarily postulated that depression is causally linked to a decreased production of CNS serotonin, noradrenalin and dopamine.

Introducing an (im-)balance model between different neurotransmitters seemed to overcome some caveats of the monoamine hypothesis and was also more appealing from a neurobiological point of view. There are several lines of evidence to support the involvement of central cholinergic neurotransmission in the regulation of mood, REM sleep and pathophysiology of affective disorders. Some studies have shown how cholinomimetics, probably via muscarinic receptors, induce depression-like symptoms such as anhedonia and anergia in healthy volunteers.

Supersensitive responses of several parameters to an acute cholinergic challenge have been described in affective disorders, including: 1. increased anergia and anhedonia and full-blown depression, even in the euthymic interval; 2. increased secretion of adrenocorticotropic hormone (ACTH), cortisol and endorphin; 3. dramatic shortening of REM sleep latency.

Thus, both the spontaneous hypercortisolism and reduced REM sleep latency frequently observed in depression may be provoked through overactivity of central nervous cholinergic neurotransmission. Independently from observations in depression, the temporal dynamics of the neuronal activity triggering REM sleep (REM-on cholinergic activity) and inhibiting REM sleep (REM-off aminergic activity) were described in cats, and later in humans. These data indicated that cholinergic neurons in the brainstem are mainly responsible for triggering and maintaining REM sleep, whereas noradrenergic and serotonergic neurons, mainly in the locus coeruleus and the dorsal raphe, were identified as REM-off neurons being mainly active during non-REM sleep ("reciprocal interaction model of non-REM/REM sleep regulation"). These animal data thus confirmed that a disinhibition of REM sleep might result from an altered balance between cholinergic and aminergic neurotransmission at the brainstem level. In the meantime, there is an on-going debate whether the response of the REM sleep system to a cholinergic stimulus is a trait or a status marker of depression. Important in that context are findings revealing that healthy relatives of depressed patients show a more pronounced REM sleep response to a cholinergic stimulus than general population and, furthermore, those subjects with an excessive REM sleep response seem to have a higher risk of developing MDD [9,10]. Some recent studies report significant antidepressant responses to the antimuscarinic compound scopolamine in depressed patients, but the antidepressant effect is dose-dependent. The potential antidepressant property of anticholinergic is probably related to a specific muscarinic receptor subtype and needs further studies, considering the lack of other anticholinergic drugs with an antidepressant effect [11-13].

The cholinergic and aminergic imbalance hypothesis of affective disorders, as formulated initially, still seems to have its merits and relationships to basic neurobiological knowledge about REM sleep regulation and is convincing with respect to REM sleep changes in depression. Unfortunately, experimental work in humans testing the impact of cholinomimetics on sleep is expensive and time consuming, and this may be one reason why the exciting results of an increased sensitivity of the REM sleep system to a cholinergic stimulus even in healthy first-degree relatives of depressed patients have not been further studied. This finding is among the very few empirical hints strongly suggesting that a given biological abnormality (following a cholinergic challenge) is present long before the onset of the disorder itself.

3.2. The Two-Process Model of Sleep-Wake Regulation and the "S-Deficiency" Model

Several years ago, Borbely proposed a general model of sleep-wake regulation based on the assumption that sleep is dependent on two processes: a homeostatic process "S" and a circadian process "C" [14]. According to this model, the interaction between the homeostatic sleep drive and a circadian process determines sleep propensity. This model also attempts to explain REM and non-REM sleep dysregulation in depression. The author assumed a deficiency of process "S" in depressed patients, as reflected by the observed reduction in SWS during night-time sleep in depression. He hypothesized that as a consequence of reduced SWS, particularly during the first phase of non-REM sleep, REM sleep may occur earlier. The model also postulates that measures of phasic REM activity are inversely related to process "S", suggesting that process "S" can be regarded as exerting an inhibitory influence on phasic REM activity. In contrast, Knowles et al. suggested that REM sleep is strongly influenced by circadian processes and its own intrinsic homeostatic properties, while process "S" might play only a relatively minor role in its regulation [15]. According to this model, the antidepressant effect of sleep deprivation was attributed to the increased level of process "S", attained by prolonging wakefulness. Nonetheless, after the first night of sleep after sleep deprivation these positive effects usually disappear.

Conflicting evidence to this model came from several studies that did not confirm a reduction of SWS in depressed patients. A recent meta-analysis of PSG studies of depressed patients [16] revealed that differences in effect size between depressed patients and healthy sleepers were far greater for REM latency and REM density compared to SWS, suggesting an independence of REM sleep findings from SWS regulation. Therefore, at present, the two process model, at least in its application to explain REM sleep changes, is seriously challenged by empirical evidence.

3.3. Circadian Rhythm Abnormalities and REM Sleep Dysregulation: The "Phase-Advance" Hypothesis

In 1975, Papousek [17] integrated rhythm disturbances in mood disorders within a framework of CR regulation: phase advance of CRs was proposed to account for abnormalities of REM sleep in depression. Later on, it was hypothesized that in depression the rhythm of the central pacemaker driving REM sleep, temperature and cortisol, was abnormally advanced relative to the rhythm of the "weak" oscillator that controls sleep onset. Findings indicative of advanced circadian phase such as early morning awakenings and shortened REM latency in patients with depression compared to non-depressed subjects were thought to confirm these assumptions. The finding that advancing main sleep episodes in depressed patients to the afternoon, thereby reducing the mismatch between sleep onset and REM onset, was associated with improvements in mood further supported this hypothesis [18,19]. In addition, complex modulation of sleep-wake cycle and circadian phase can modulate mood in healthy subjects, which lasts between 1.5 and 2 days. However, this procedure is also considered to be too strenuous for clinically depressed patients. On the other hand, other evidence supporting this hypothesis come from molecular/genetic studies on clock genes. Indeed, polymorphisms in the CRs genes - CLOCK, BMAL1, Period 3 (Per 3) and TIMELESS - have been associated with an increased susceptibility to mood disorders. Single nucleotide polymorphisms and haplotypes in several circadian genes have been observed among those displaying certain circadian phenotypes, including impaired mood in the evening, insomnia in mania and early, middle or late insomnia in depression. However, despite these interesting preliminary findings, the molecular and genetic features underlying this hypothesis need further clarification.

3.4. Basal Sleep-Wake Regulation and REM Sleep Abnormalities: The Hypocretin Hypothesis

Orexin (also known as hypocretin) is a hypothalamic neuropeptide that contributes to stabilize the transition from wake to sleep and vice versa. Studies indicate that sleep-wake switching and vice versa depend on the interaction of cell groups that cause arousal with other nuclei that induce sleep, a mechanism called the "flip-flop switch". This switch may help to produce distinct transitions between discrete behavioural states, but it is not necessarily stable. The orexinergic neurons in the lateral hypothalamus may help stabilize this system by exciting arousal regions during wakefulness, preventing unwanted transitions between wakefulness and sleep. The importance of this stabilizing role is clear in narcolepsy, in which an absence or dysfunction of the orexin neurons causes numerous, unintended transitions in and out of sleep and allows fragments of REM sleep to intrude into wakefulness or to initiate sleep with REM sleep.

This phenomenon of starting sleep with REM sleep has been termed SOREM (¼ sleep onset REM period) and can also be observed, though less frequently, in depressed patients. The shortening of REM latency in depression typically refers to a change in REM latency from on average 70-90 min characterizing healthy sleep to mean values of 50-60 min in depressed patients. Accordingly, it has been suggested that understanding the pathways that underlie the regulation of sleep and wakefulness may provide important insights into how cognitive and emotional systems interact with basic homeostatic and circadian drives for sleep. In fact, major targets of orexin-containing fibres include the locus coeruleus and the raphe nucleus, areas that play important roles in the regulation of mood and sleep. Because of the observed REM sleep alterations, especially shortened REM sleep latency, it has been suggested that there might be a reduction in orexin secretion in depression. Consistently, a defect in the lateral hypothalamus, including the orexin neurons, has been described in an animal model of depression [20]. During the 10 years since the discovery of orexin, the list of their physiologic implications has extended from their primary roles in the sleep-wake cycle and feeding to the control of stress, and mental disorders such as panic, anxiety and depression. This different set of functions is consistent with the localization of orexin neurons in the lateral hypothalamus, a major integrating centre of sensory inputs and emotional processes, and their widespread excitatory projections throughout the brain.

Animal studies have produced a growing body of evidence supporting this hypothesis and suggest that dysfunction of the orexin system might be involved in both the pathophysiology of MDD and in REM sleep alterations [21,22].

3.5. REM Sleep Deprivation/Ontogeny Model

Vogel et al. [23] suggested that an excess production of REM sleep might be involved causally in the aetiology and pathophysiology of depression. Consistently, these authors demonstrated that selective REM sleep deprivation by awakenings over a period of 2-3 weeks exerts an antidepressant effect comparable to antidepressant drugs in depressed patients. Unfortunately, these early studies on the effects of REM sleep deprivation on mood were not replicated in further, independent, studies. On the other hand, the observation that most of the effective antidepressant drugs suppress REM sleep supports this hypothesis, although some notable exceptions among antidepressant drugs can be found.

More recently, Vogel et al. [24] revisited this idea based on studies that ascribe an important role of brain maturation on REM sleep. This line of thinking assumes that the ontogeny of REM sleep in humans (with very high amounts of REM sleep prenatally, after birth and in the first year of life) is indicative of a developmental process that may be altered in humans predisposed to MDD, and thus it may account for the life-long REM sleep abnormalities observed in the disorder. In particular, the REM sleep-ontogeny hypothesis proposes that alterations in REM sleep provide an endogenous source of activation, which may be critical for CNS maturation, and thus might lead to depression in later life. This proposal led to a series of experiments examining the role of REM sleep in brain development. During the CNS maturational processes in the late prenatal and neonatal periods, a large percentage of time is spent in REM sleep (up to 50% of all sleep in the first two weeks of life), characterized by endogenous, intense, generalized neuronal firing in most areas of the brain. The intensity of phasic neuronal activity during REM sleep is high in early development and diminishes as brain maturation is completed. Additionally, studies of REM sleep deprivation in animal models have provided consistent support for the role of REM sleep in brain maturation, as a suppression of REM sleep was capable of disrupting the aforementioned maturational processes. Other recent studies indicate that mechanisms of synaptic plasticity, which are important for brain development, remain susceptible to the effects of REM sleep deprivation in the adolescent rat [25]. Moreover, REM sleep deprived animals have a reduced brain size and display increased hyperactivity, anxiety, attention and learning difficulties and increased voluntary alcohol consumption. While environmental enrichment has been shown to enhance cortical maturation, this effect is abolished in rats that underwent prior REM sleep deprivation [26]. Interestingly, Vogel et al. [24] described that adult rats subjected to an animal model mimicking endogenous depression had the same distinctive REM sleep characteristics as healthy neonatal rats (i.e. displayed high amounts of REM sleep). This similarity suggests that an underdeveloped, relatively weak, REM sleep inhibitory process may account for the REM sleep abnormalities observed in depression.

Accordingly, Vogel et al. [24] hypothesized that the ontogeny of REM sleep may suggest an altered CNS developmental process in humans predisposed to MDD, which may account for the lifelong REM sleep abnormalities observed in the disorder. Despite these intriguing findings, the hypothesis of a role of REM sleep for CNS development needs to be investigated more intensively. Interestingly, evidence from research in insomnia delivers additional data for this hypothesis. Particularly, PGS studies showed that primary insomnia is characterized by a decreased percentage of REM sleep and increased EEG arousals during REM sleep. Riemann et al. [27] recently speculated about REM sleep instability as a new pathway for insomnia and depression.

Based on this observation, the "REM instability" hypothesis was advanced: modest REM sleep reduction and fragmentation increases arousals and awakenings in patients with chronic insomnia and is associated with the experience of stress. Consistent with this, enhanced arousal during REM sleep might be partly perceived and memorized as wake and could result in the experience of disrupted and non-restorative sleep. With respect to the relationship with depression, this hypothesis suggests that the chronic fragmentation of REM sleep in insomnia might interfere with basal processes of emotion regulation and with the underlying network functioning in a limbic and paralimbic system. With persistence of the insomnia, at some point a REM sleep rebound (as seen by shortened REM latency and increased REM density) might occur, which would facilitate the development of a depressive episode. This kind of reasoning is supported by a recent meta-analysis demonstrating that insomnia is an early and independent risk factor for the development of depression [28]. In summary, this line of thinking brings together ontogenetic data from REM sleep regulation, which clearly revealed high amounts of this sleep stage in early developmental periods in mammals, with REM sleep abnormalities observed in adult depression and evidence from insomnia research.

3.6. Stress, Brain Plasticity and REM Sleep: The "Allostatic Load" Hypothesis

The stress system represents an essential alarm system that is activated by internal and environmental stimuli, such as lack of information, loss of control, unpredictability or psychosocial overload. The stress system is subject to allostasis, i.e. by the adaptive response of the organism to internal and external stressful agents essential to the development of the optimal individual homeostatic capability. These adaptive changes are produced by (neuro)chemical mediators, such as catecholamine, glucocorticoids and cytokines that act on specific receptors localized in different organs.

In addition to the physiological role of stress, stress "overload" is one of the most important causes of disease in western countries. Chronic stress leads to receptor desensitization and tissue damage, generating a state termed "allostatic load". The latter has been demonstrated to have far-reaching consequences, such as insomnia, depression and cardiovascular disease [29,30].

In this context, the study of bi-directional interactions between sleep and stress represents a crucial research field for preclinical medicine. Chronic sleep disruption can be regarded as both a stress result and a physiological stressor per se, since it impairs brain functions. In particular, it increases sympathetic tone, blood pressure and evening cortisol levels, and it also raises blood levels of pro-inflammatory cytokines, insulin and glucose. Experimental studies in rats have shown that chronic sleep curtailment gradually leads to neurobiological and neuroendocrine changes similar to those found in depression [31]. Preclinical studies demonstrate that chronically disrupted and restricted sleep can also interfere with hippocampal neurogenesis and may contribute to depression and other stress-related mental disorders. The mechanisms by which sleep loss affects different aspects of adult neurogenesis are still unknown. It has been proposed that adverse effects of sleep disruption may be mediated by the stress system and glucocorticoids. However, a number of studies clearly showed that prolonged sleep loss can inhibit hippocampal neurogenesis independent of adrenal stress hormones. These effects of sleep loss may endanger hippocampal integrity, thereby leading to cognitive dysfunction and contributing to the development of mood disorders. Furthermore, exposure to chronic stress causes alterations in REM sleep, such as an increase of: 1) the duration of the first REM period; 2) the density of eye movements; and 3) an increase of the total REM sleep duration. Animal models suggest that changes in REM sleep included increases in the duration of and transitions into REM sleep and a reduced latency to the onset of the first REM period. These sleep abnormalities, in particular the decrease in REM latency, are consistent with those reported in depression [32].

The REM sleep changes seem essential to link sleep both with stress and psychopathology. As mentioned above, short REM latency and increased REM density seem to be sustained by a central cholinergic hyperactivity, either absolute or relative. Recent evidence indicates that pontine cholinergic REM-on cells are tonically activated during sleep by neuronal groups belonging to the amygdaloid complex. This structure, which during wakefulness plays a key role in the modulation of emotional responses, such as fear, anxiety or stress, is overactivated in wakefulness and in the sleep of depressed patients. The hyperactivation of the amygdaloid complex and REM sleep alterations, sustained by HPA axis activation, thus seem to contribute to some depressive symptoms, such as insomnia, negative emotional memory consolidation and depressive mood. The "allostatic load" hypothesis allows us to establish a connection between genetic predisposition and environment or stressful situations, and REM sleep alterations supposedly mark the transition between eu-stress and di-stress. In particular, the role of REM sleep in emotional memory consolidation may explain the reinforcement of negative stimuli even unconsciously. On the other hand, some subjects react to stress without involvement of the HPA axis, and thus this theory does not seem to be appropriate for this kind of population. For this type of sub-population, depressive outcome could be sustained by completely different mechanisms.

4. Clinical Correlates in MDD of REM Abnormalities

4.1. Cognition and REM Sleep

In 1986, Giles et al. [33] showed a correlation between REM sleep alterations in depression and some clinical features of depressive symptoms. Among so-called "endogenous" depressive symptoms, anhedonia, unreactive mood and appetite loss were reported to be related to short REM latency in depressed patients.

The additional finding that both selective REM sleep deprivation and total sleep deprivation provide immediate, though only temporary, relief for some patients with mood disorders supported the claim that REM sleep plays a role in the genesis of at least some clinical symptoms of depression. A role of REM sleep in overnight regulation of negative mood has also been recently suggested . REM sleep related indices, such as REM density, have been strongly correlated with neurocognitive distortions in depression such as self-aggression, suicidal ideation, rumination and difficulties in concentration. More recently, McNamara and colleagues explored the possibility that REM sleep physiology might differentially impact the neurocognitive symptoms of depression including executive cognitive dysfunction and distorted evaluative appraisals of self, unpleasant dream content and biased emotional memory processing [7]. The authors hypothesized that REM sleep physiology significantly contributes to the production of these cognitive distortions in depressed patients. They found a significant reduction in positive ratings and a significant increase in negative ratings of self after awakenings from REM sleep, but not non-REM sleep in depressed/anxious patients, demonstrating an impact of REM sleep on the cognitive appraisal of the self-concept. Moreover, the dream-self was rated as negative relative to both a significant other and daytime-self after REM sleep awakenings. These are important clinical findings as both REM sleep-related indices and poor self-concept predict mood dysfunction and suicidal ideation and attempts. Greater production of emotionally negative memories after REM sleep awakenings was also found. Negative memories were retrieved more quickly after REM sleep awakenings vs. non-REM sleep awakenings or wake conditions. Dreams from REM sleep contained greater amounts of negative emotion and aggression than did sleep dreams. These results suggest that REM sleep itself may significantly contribute/reinforce cognitive distortions typical for mood disorder.

4.2. Emotion Regulation and REM Sleep

Until recently, the impact of sleep dysregulation on affective and emotional regulation has received only limited attention. Nevertheless, a number of recent studies offer an emerging understanding for the critical role of sleep in regulating emotional brain function. Sleep might play an important role in both affective reactivity and emotional information processing. In particular, insomnia, which is a common feature of depression, is associated with altered subjectively reported emotional reactivity. Furthermore, both conditions of sleep loss and deprivation continue to be associated with maladaptive emotional regulation, leading to exaggerated neural and behavioural reactivity to negative, aversive experiences. Sleep loss has been shown to amplify negative emotional consequences of disruptive daytime events, while blunting the positive benefit associated with rewarding activities.

To date, numerous investigations have begun to test a selective REM-dependent hypothesis of affective human memory consolidation based on the consideration that both sleep and emotion modulate processes of memory consolidation. The actual model of sleep-dependent emotional memory processing is the "sleep to forget and sleep to remember" hypothesis [34]. When formed, a newly encoded "emotional-memory" is created in a milieu of high adrenergic tone, which results in an associated affective "blanket." With multiple iterations of sleep, particularly REM sleep, memory contained within the affective experience strengthens overnight(s) resulting in improved memory for the event; the autonomic tone "enveloped" around the memory becomes gradually ameliorated, leading to emotional forgetting. The neuroanatomical, neurophysiological and neurochemical conditions of REM sleep might offer a unique biological state in which to achieve both a balanced neural potentiation of the informational core of emotional experiences, the memory, and also depotentiate and ultimately ameliorate the autonomic arousing load originally acquired at the time of learning the emotion. Neurochemically, levels of limbic and forebrain acetylcholine (ACh) are markedly elevated during REM sleep. Considering the known importance of ACh in the long-term consolidation of emotional learning, the pro-cholinergic REM sleep state may result in a selective facilitation of affective memories, similar to that reported using experimental manipulations of ACh. Thus, one of the most intriguing hypotheses of emotional brain processing is the "REM sleep hypothesis of emotional memory processing" that ascribes a crucial role of REM sleep in the affective modulation of human brain function. This model predicts that a pathological increase in REM, as seen in depression [35,36], may disproportionately amplify the strength of negative memories, so much that it would create a perceived autobiographical history dominated by an excess of negative memories.

5. Impact of Antidepressant Treatment on Sleep

A consistent body of evidence supports the effectiveness of antidepressant drugs in depression. Nonetheless, these treatments do not seem to fully address the problem of sleep disturbances in mood disorders. In fact, persistent insomnia is one of the most common residual symptoms in depressed patients with incomplete remission. This is a relevant problem because of a direct impact on the patient's quality of life, and residual insomnia confers a greater risk of subsequent depressive episode.

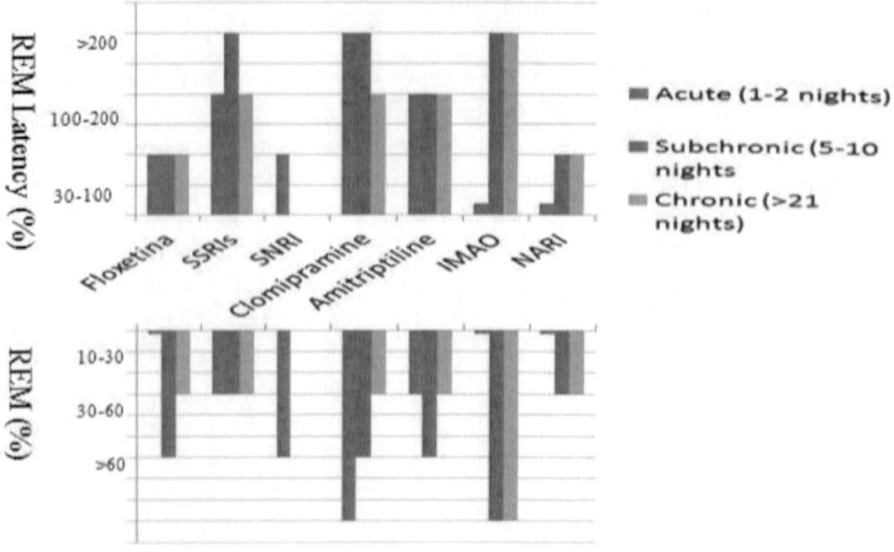

Adapted from Palagini et al. [38].

Figure 1.

Antidepressant drugs exert an effect on sleep architecture that varies over time and tends to ameliorate the sleep disturbances of depression. Almost all antidepressants inhibit REM sleep, thus delaying the onset and reducing the amount of REM sleep [37]. The REM sleep suppressing effects of TCAs are dose-dependent and consist of a drastic reduction in the overall amount of REM sleep, followed by REM sleep rebound after abrupt drug discontinuation, a phenomenon which has been described for all antidepressant substances that possess an initial strong REM sleep suppression. This REM sleep rebound may be related to a rebound increase in cholinergic neurotransmission, especially for those substances (such as TCAs) that have a strong anticholinergic effect. REM sleep suppression following the administration of the older, irreversible MAOI phenelzine is profound, with a total suppression of REM sleep during the first week of treatment. An important recent finding is that the REM sleep suppression by phenelzine can be reversed by rapid tryptophan depletion, suggesting that these effects on sleep are mediated through an enhancement of serotonin transmission. Interestingly, the reversible MAOI moclobemide shows a lower REM sleep suppression, although a rebound increase of REM sleep after drug discontinuation is observed for this antidepressant class as well. Similar to TCAs and IMAO, the REM sleep suppressing effects described for both SSRIs and SNRIs are dose-related and consist in a strong reduction in the overall amount of REM sleep during the entire night, including a delay of the first REM period. REM sleep suppression after SSRI administration is probably mediated via an increase of serotoninergic tone. Other antidepressants that act through different mechanisms (e.g. mianserin, mirtazapine, trazodone and nefazodone) less strongly suppress REM sleep. On the other hand, some studies have suggested that antidepressant treatments may even impair physiological sleep regulation and sleep continuity. Some authors suggested that the effects on sleep patterns are specific for each antidepressant drug, as suggested, for example, by a study on trimipramine. Figure 1 summarizes the effects of antidepressants on REM sleep (duration and latency).

Literature data suggest that the same neurotransmitter systems which regulate mood, motivation and energy may be modified in depression and contribute to sleep disturbance [39]. Indeed, some neurotransmitter systems have been implicated in the maintenance of wakefulness, the initiation and maintenance of sleep and the transitions, within sleep, from one phase to another. In particular, the serotonin system seems to play a major role in the regulation of sleep patterns, as stated above. Additionally, serotonergic neurons play a main role in modulation of onset and maintenance of sleep. Furthermore, the complexity of the serotonin system allows the accurate regulation of the circadian rhythm sustaining the sleep-wakefulness turnover, as well as its adaptation to environmental changes. Therefore, it is not surprising that treatment with SSRIs modify this subtle mechanism, often leading to persistent sleep disturbances such as insomnia and daytime somnolence. Corroborating clinical data, PSG studies often demonstrate that SSRI therapy is associated with substantial fragmentation of sleep, suppression of REM sleep, prolonged sleep latency and reduced total sleep time. Along these lines, insomnia during the use of fluoxetine represented one of the most common side effects, and fluoxetine has been shown to reduce REM sleep. Paradoxically, daytime somnolence has frequently been reported. PSG studies have shown that paroxetine, sertraline, citalopram and escitalopram show similar adverse effects on sleep, although less pronounced. Overall, SSRIs appear to cause insomnia in 10-20% of depressed patients through suppression of REM sleep, with a dose-dependent effect.

The exact mechanisms at the basis of this relevant side effect are unclear. In experimental conditions, blockage of 5-HT synthesis caused long-lasting insomnia, as well as the depletion of 5-HT by reserpine administration. On the other hand, the precursors of 5-HT biosynthesis, L-tryptophan and 5-hydroxytryptophan, seem to promote the onset of sleep. Within the system sustaining sleep-wakefulness cycle, 5-HT receptors seem to exert different functions in the complex regulation and promotion of wakefulness and sleep. In particular, 5-HT1A and 5-HT1B seem to have an inhibitory action on REM sleep, while 5-HT2 receptors (A, B and C subtypes) can be considered excitatory. It is believed that 5HT2 receptor stimulation is subjacent to insomnia and sleep architecture alterations related to SSRIs. For this reason, 5HT2 blockers such as trazodone improve insomnia and ameliorate sleep structure. Consistent with this, PSG studies in patients treated with trazodone showed increased SWS during the first half of the night. Long-term treatment showed increased sleep duration in stage 2, reduced sleep latency, increased delta sleep and reduced REM latency. Therefore, 5HT2-blocker antidepressants may be a good option to treat depressed patients with relevant insomnia.

6. Treatment of Comorbid Insomnia and Depression

Successful treatment of patients with comorbid insomnia and depression requires attention to both conditions. Depressed patients with sleep disturbance have significantly worse prognosis in relation to remission rates and the likelihood of complete and sustained recovery. Moreover, continued insomnia following antidepressant therapy is related to a higher risk of relapse [40].

There is general consensus in considering insomnia as a comorbid disorder of depression instead of a simple depressive symptom when sleep disturbances become associated with distress and impairment of functioning in significant domains, and criteria for the diagnosis of insomnia are met. In this case, insomnia may also impair the response to antidepressant drugs. Indeed, the most part of currently available antidepressants and hypnotic medications do not improve SWS, a target for improving both depression and insomnia. However, some antidepressants such as trazodone and nefazodone are effective in restructuring sleep architecture, and are good options for simultaneously reducing depression and insomnia in patients with concomitant conditions. The effects of these antidepressants on sleep (i.e. enhancement of SWS and minimal suppression of REM sleep) are thought to be due to the combination of the weak inhibition of reuptake and the blockade of 5-HT2 receptors. Nonetheless, trazodone also exerts inhibitory proprieties on alpha-1 adrenoreceptors and histamine H1 receptors, which may account, at least partially, for its positive effects on sleep. Another therapeutic option for insomnia in depression is mirtazapine, which has potent sleep-promoting effects. It acts through the inhibition of the presynaptic alpha-2 autoreceptors, which increases NE and 5-HT transmissions, and the block of both 5-HT2 and 5-HT3 postsynaptic receptors, as well as the block of histamine-H1 receptors.

Deeper non-REM sleep (i.e. SWS) is very important for maintaining homeostasis and is related to restorative sleep and well-being. Nonetheless, as stated above, some of the current available antidepressant drugs may worsen insomnia and, thus, impair full recovery from depression. Therefore, in the last years several drugs have been tested and developed for the management of depression and insomnia symptoms simultaneously. In this field, 5-HT2 receptor antagonists are among the most promising drugs. Ritanserin, a potent 5-HT2 antagonist, have been shown to significantly improve SWS and sleep quality in major depression; similar drugs under development include eplivanserin and volinanserin. Other drugs under development combine blockade of 5-HT2 receptors with other pharmacological targets for the treatment of insomnia. From this line of research the newer antidepressant agomelatin has emerged, which is a melatonin receptor agonist and 5-HT2 antagonist. Consistent with its theoretical features, the drug has both antidepressant and hypnotic effects.

7. Circadian Rhythms in Major Depressive Disorder Research

7.1. To Distinguish Different Biological Substrates: The Example of Melancholic and Atypical Depression

Recently, research has emphasized the importance of establishing biological subtypes of depression with treatment specificity and prognostic value. PSG measures, among other biological markers, may be suitable for this aim. In particular, several differences in the sleep patterns have been identified between two depression subtypes, which are known to have robust biological differences: melancholic and atypical depression subtypes.

Melancholic depression tends to be associated with high activity of the HPA and NA systems, as well as the amygdala, and seems to involve 5-HT1A receptor dysfunction (exacerbated by feedback from the HPA axis). Conversely, atypical depression is associated with reduced HPA activity, owing to a strong inhibitory response to cortisol and hypoactivity of NA and 5-HT systems. These biological differences seem to have an impact on treatment response of these two depression subtypes. Indeed, in people with melancholic depression tricyclic antidepressants (TCAs) and serotonin and norepinephrine reuptake inhibitors (SNRIs) are more effective than selective serotonin reuptake inhibitors (SSRIs); furthermore, melancholic depression appears to response better to electroconvulsive therapy (ECT), while it responds poorly to psychotherapy. On the other hand, atypical depression tends to respond better to MAOIs than to TCAs or SSRIs; it also appears to respond well to cognitive-behavioural therapy.

Recently, Antonijevic [41] identified specific differences in the sleep patterns of melancholic and atypical depression. In particular, only patients affected by melancholic depression showed the typical sleep pattern of depression described above, i.e. low sleep efficiency, NREM deficiency and increased REM pressure. This result is consistent with the strong links among HPA overactivity, CNS hyperarousal and monoamine–ACh imbalance. In contrast, patients affected by the atypical subtype did not show the typical depressive sleep pattern. Instead, they showed reduced delta wave production in the first NREM sleep period, which may be due to diminished 5-HT activity. Furthermore, literature data suggest that the atypical subtype is associated with hypersomnia, which may be a consequence of reduced HPA activity.

Clinically, the sleep pattern of atypical depression is characterized by increased TST, significant nocturnal insomnia, frequent daytime napping and excessive daytime sleepiness. Unfortunately, literature data on hypersomnia in depression is still lacking, partly because different diagnostic systems place different importance on sleep features in the diagnosis of depression. Moreover, as well as several other sleep measures, the study of hypersomnia also suffers from a lack of a consistent definition across different research centres. Even if sleep measures may have potential utility to differentiate melancholic from atypical depression, at present sleep study is not routinely used in clinical practice with this aim, although this differentiation could lead to clinical advantages. Indeed, about 30% of depressed patients are purely melancholic, while 12% are purely atypical, accounting for 42% of depressed patients. The remaining 58% of depressed patients fail to match either of these two subtypes, suggesting the need for further identification of other depressive subtypes with strong biological correlates. From this point of view, sleep measures may also be useful to help detect new depressive subtypes, together with other biological and psychopathological measures.

In conclusion, these data suggest that the study of sleep with modern digital recordings and mathematical analysis may be of even greater benefit in diagnosing depression. Furthermore, it may be useful to provide a distinction of different depression subtypes sustained by different physiopathological mechanisms.

7.2. Sleep Abnormalities as Major Depressive Disorder Endophenotypes

Endophenotypes are thought to represent a bridge between the involved genes and overt, measurable behavioural abnormalities; as such, they also represent relatively elementary functional phenomena of any behaviour and are encountered in mental disorders where they may help identify the responsible gene(s). Endophenotypes should fulfil the following specific criteria: a) the marker must be specifically associated with the illness in the general population; b) state-independent stability over time, observable in partial or complete remission; c) heritability, associated with genetic variance; d) familial association should segregate with illness within families; e) co-segregation should be observed at a higher rate among unaffected family members compared to the general population.

Recently, the REM sleep disinhibition of depression was suggested to be a good candidate for an endophenotype of depression [42,43]. Indeed, REM sleep dysregulation in depression shows state independent stability over time, which is also observable in partial or complete remission (especially REM density).

In many patients, changes in REM sleep persist despite full clinical remission, and seem to be associated with an increased risk of relapse. REM sleep dysregulation in depression shows heritability, associated with genetic variance. High-risk studies in relatives supported the existence of a genetic influence on depression, sleep and its regulation. Sleep studies in relatives of depressed subjects, including healthy monozygotic and dizygotic twin pairs, found a greater concordance of sleep patterns among monozygotic twins than dizygotic twins. Giles et al. [44,45] investigated the PSG parameters in first-degree relatives of unipolar patients, classifying these probands according to the presence or absence of a reduced REM latency in the index patient. In the "short REM latency" group, they found sleep-EEG alterations similar to those of depressed patients regardless of a personal history of depression. Moreover, the prevalence of psychiatric illness, especially depression, was very high among relatives with reduced REM latency and was almost three times greater than for those with normal REM latency. In a subsequent investigation, parents and probands of unipolar depressed patients were evaluated for lifetime history of psychiatric disorders and for their sleep-EEG profile [46]. Shortened REM latency was found to be familial and was associated with an increased risk of major depression beyond the "normal" familial risk. Sitaram and Gillin [47] applied the cholinergic REM induction test to a sample of depressed patients and their relatives, and observed a much faster induction of REM sleep in relatives with a lifetime diagnosis of depression compared to relatives without such a diagnosis. Thus, although not unequivocal, the bulk of the evidence suggests that altered REM sleep parameters, especially increased REM density, may constitute an endophenotype for depression. While the identification of vulnerability genes for depression is still an open field, endophenotypes, such as REM sleep changes, can decisively help in the search by reducing the phenotypic heterogeneity of MDD.

8. Circadian Rhythms and Sleep Disturbances in Bipolar Disorder

Bipolar disorder (BD) is a severe recurrent psychiatric condition, with a detrimental effect on quality of life and socioeconomic status. BD is common and has a lifetime morbid risk of approximately 1%. The characteristic feature of BD is the occurrence of one or more (hypo)manic or mixed (manic/depressive) episodes, interspersed with major depressive episodes. BD is a complex multi-factorial disorder with the implication of psychological, physiological, genetic and environmental factors. Altered rhythmicity of circadian functions during mania and depression (changes in mood, appetite, sleep, energy, etc.) has long been demonstrated. More recently, the persistence of abnormal CRs during euthymic periods has also been shown in BD patients. To date, the aetiological determinants of BD remain poorly understood. The growing literature investigating circadian genes, chronotypes and circadian physiological processes in BD strongly suggests that chronobiology may help in clarifying the mechanisms underlying this disorder.

The current understanding of the sleep-wake rhythm posits that it is the product of the combined influences of a circadian oscillation and a homeostatic sleep drive, which act reciprocally to govern sleep onset and maintenance. Given the interaction between sleep and circadian processes, it is difficult to discuss one separately from the other, particularly in BD patients, a population in which disruption of both sleep and circadian rhythms are well-documented [48]. Indeed, a growing body of evidence support the involvement of disrupted biological rhythms in the cyclicity of BD.

Clinically, BD patients have been found to sleep less efficiently and hold more dysfunctional and anxious beliefs regarding their sleep when compared with healthy controls. In addition, studies using actimetry have found the sleep of remitted BD patients to be more variable both in length [49] and longer [50], and characterized by less wake time. Finally, accumulating evidence suggests that alterations in sleep are not only an epiphenomenon of the disease process, but that the two are deeply intertwined [50].

In particular, it has been hypothesized that CNS abnormalities found in BD patients may also alter "free-running" rhythms, cycles that are not entrained to the 24-hour day/night cycle, which may desynchronize other CRs, adversely affecting mood. This hypothesis is also supported by an animal model of a genetically fast biological clock in rats missing the tau gene, which have behavioural characteristics roughly analogous to manic-depressive symptoms [51].

Thus, CR abnormalities seem to be trait markers of BD and may represent biomarkers of the disorder. Finally, a dysfunctional regulation of sleep has been postulated to be a vulnerability factor, and there is considerable evidence that disturbed sleep during adolescence conveys a long-term risk for the development of the disorder [52].

8.1. Circadian Rhythms and Sleep Disturbances in BD During Depressive Episodes

Overall, studies on sleep in bipolar depression found similar abnormalities in unipolar and bipolar depression. Nonetheless, some data suggest that BD patients may have more early morning awakenings and greater total REM density than MDD patients. Expert opinions suggest that hypersomnia is more indicative of BD than unipolar depression [53]. Nonetheless, a study that investigated hypersomnolence in BD patients during depression using the Multiple Sleep Latency Test failed to find evidence of excessive daytime sleepiness. This result suggests that BD hypersomnolence may be reflective of anergia/fatigue rather than true excessive sleepiness, as observed in primary sleep disorders [54]. On the other hand, the larger effectiveness of sleep deprivation as an antidepressant treatment in BD depression compared to MDD depression suggests the existence of some biological difference in the CR systems of these patients [55,56]. Unfortunately, this strategy and the difference between unipolar and bipolar depression have not been thoroughly investigated, not only because of the frequent relapse rate observed in the first studies after sleep recovery [57], but also due to the dominance of other areas of research in mood disorder field, such as pharmacotherapy, neurochemistry and genetics.

8.2. Circadian Rhythms and Sleep Disturbances in BD During Manic Episodes

Clinically, the relevance of sleep in BD, and in particular in manic episodes, has been recognized since the first studies in this field. Several clinical observations support the fundamental role of sleep in several aspects of this phase of the disease. Moreover, PSG studies show sleep disturbances during the manic state, such as shorted total sleep time, increased time awake in bed and a shortened REM latency.

More in detail, the relationship between sleep and mania involves the following aspects:

1. Decreased need of sleep is a fundamental marker of the manic state;
2. Sleep deprivation may cause mania and, thus, may be an etiological agent for mania;
3. Total sleep time is a predictor of future manic episodes;
4. Total sleep time may be a marker of treatment response in mania.

8.2.1. Decreased Need of Sleep as a Marker of Mania

Decreased need of sleep is one of the seven diagnostic criteria of the DSM-IV TR for BD mania. This symptom may be detrimental in differential diagnosis, since the ability to maintain energy without sufficient sleep is seen in few other disorders. Although manic patients experience this decreased need of sleep, they still require at least few hours of sleep to sustain life; indeed, Bell et al. in the middle of the 19th century documented several cases of florid mania characterized by nearly no sleep that typically ended fatally for patients. In modern times, manic patients are unlikely to die consequent to prolonged sleeplessness during treatment, thanks to improvement in manic treatments. Furthermore, the majority of manic patients, despite prolonged sleeplessness, ultimately have a physiological need for sleep.

8.2.2. Sleep Reduction as a Trigger for the Manic Phase

Several triggers in the genesis of mania have been identified. Several reports have described switches to mania following various triggers, such as drug abuse, prescribed drugs, transmeridian travel, postpartum status, bereavement, etc. However, all these triggers seem to finally result in sleep loss. Thus, it is still unclear whether sleeplessness was the final trigger for mania or if it is only a prodromal symptom of the condition. In addition, in some cases, early manic symptoms may have spurred the behaviour (e.g. drug abuse, travel, etc.) which then produced sleep deprivation. Taking into account these observations, Wehr et al. hypothesized that sleep deprivation is the fundamental proximal cause, or the "final common pathway", of mania [58]. Indeed, it has been observed that all the triggers of mania, including biological causes (drugs, hormones, withdrawal, etc.), psychic effects (separation, bereavement, etc.) and direct disturbances of sleep schedules (from newborn infants, shift work, travel, etc.) may be related to the genesis of mania through sleep reduction. Furthermore, this theory posits that sleep deprivation is both a cause and a consequence of mania, and thus mutually self-reinforcing sleep loss perpetuates the manic state. Although prospective testing of this hypothesis is logistically complicated by the fact that sleep deprivation is both a cause and an early symptom of mania, cases of bipolar in patients who switch to mania after sleep deprivation have often been reported, supporting the final common pathway hypothesis.

On the other hand, studies on the antidepressant effect of sleep deprivation in unipolar and bipolar depression provide clearer evidence of the potential causal, or "switching", proprieties of sleep deprivation. A previous review [57] reported that 29% of BD depressed patients and 25% of unspecified depressed patients become hypomanic after one night of total sleep deprivation. Unfortunately, the majority of studies included in that review were conducted on both BD and MDD patients, and were not designed to detect mania, allowing only post-hoc analyses. Thus, these limitations may have therefore modified the results. In fact, a more recent study by Colombo et al. analyzed data from 206 patients who received total sleep deprivation as treatment for BD depression (often associated with pharmacological treatments intended to extend the duration of antidepressant response); it was found that switch into hypomania and mania occurred in only 5.8% and 4.9%, respectively, of the sample [59]. However, to better understand this issue, it would be necessary to test the sleep deprivation effects on euthymic BD patients, which are theoretically at greater risk of switch than depressed ones. Unfortunately, these types of studies are lacking because of their potentially deleterious effects on patients. However, studies focused on primary sleep disorders, such as obstructive sleep apnoea syndrome, suggested that these disorders may also lead to mania in BD patients. Thus, these data support the "final common pathway" hypothesis.

8.2.3. Sleep Time as a Predictor of Manic Episodes

To date, only a few studies have been investigated the role of sleep duration as a predictive factor for further affective episodes. These studies, overall, suggest that the majority of BD patients (about 77%) experienced sleep disturbances prior to a manic episode [60]. This finding is used in the psycho-educational approach, which teaches patients that insomnia is one of the early symptoms of manic relapse. Insomnia should be used to seek early treatment, and thus avoid the complete development of a manic episode.

Other authors have approached this issue from another prospective: they hypothesized that stressful life events associated with social rhythm disruption (particularly sleep deprivation) could be commonly observed in prodromal periods prior to an affective episode. A study by Malkoff-Schwarts et al. showed that social rhythm disruption was observed in about two-thirds of manic prodromal periods [61]. Thus, disruption of the daily rhythm may often occur before a manic episode in BD patients. However, it is still not possible to infer a cause-and-effect relationship between sleep disruption stemming from social rhythm disruption and subsequent mania.

8.2.4. Sleep Time as a Marker of Treatment Response in Mania

Some authors have suggested that improved sleep in the in-patient setting may be a predictor of positive outcome, even if a causal relationship has not yet been demonstrated. Nonetheless, clinical experience suggests than sedation alone is valuable in managing manic behaviours, supporting the importance of improving sleep in these patients. In this regard, the use of sedative-hypnotics is widespread in routine clinical treatment of manic patients.

Nonetheless, it is still unclear whether sleep induced by sedative/hypnotic drugs only masks manic symptoms or actually reverses the underlying process responsible for mania.

Interestingly, historical treatments suggest that forced extended sleep improves symptomatology, as demonstrated by the "rest cure" (i.e. patients were forced to stay in bed) developed my Weir Mitchell in the 19th century, which was used in several neuropsychiatric disorders. Indeed, this treatment, although it did not directly increase the total sleep time, appeared to reduce the variability of sleep durations, which is thought to be the mechanism accountable for its positive clinical effects. More recently, other behavioural treatments have been applied in mania treatment, often as add-on therapy. One such treatment that was found to be effective in improving the pharmacological treatment of mania is the so-called "dark therapy". It consists of adding 14 hours of enforced darkness to the treatment regimen of hospitalized manic patients. According to nursing observation of sleep duration, manic patients treated with enforced darkness had more sleep than controls and they improved faster and needed lower doses of antimanic drugs [62]. The improvements seen with "rest cure" and "dark therapy" may occur through circadian manipulation, since light is the primary *zeitgeber* (time-giver) of the circadian clock. Thus, patients may improve thanks to this manipulation, which may occur without a clear improvement of the sleep-time per se.

8.3. Circadian Rhythms and Sleep Disturbances in BD During Euthymia

Modern classification systems fail to accurately capture the pathology of the euthymic state in BD. Indeed, BD is characterized by a relative high frequency of sub-syndromal inter-episode symptoms. Thus, it not surprising that sleep in BD patients may continue to be disturbed during euthymia. Unfortunately, only few studies investigated the quality of sleep in BD during this phase of the disease with objective instruments, such as PSG. The few studies available on this issue show that euthymic BD patients have a higher arousal [63] and increased REM density and percentage, as well as increased sensitivity to the REM-latency-reducing effect of arecoline (an acetylcholine agonist) [64]. More recently, Millar et al. [49], using sleep diaries and actigraphy, found that remitted BD patients had greater sleep onset latency, increased sleep duration and more night-to-night variability of sleep patterns. Another actigraphy study by Jones et al. found greater variability of activity patterns among days in BD patients compared to healthy subjects, while no difference was detected concerning sleep parameters. However, these parameters were calculated from actigraphic measures, which may underestimate sleep latency and waking after sleep onset and overestimate sleep efficiency [65]. Indeed, another study by Harvey et al. which examined both actigraphy and sleep data, showed that remitted BD patients exhibited diminished sleep efficiency, increased anxiety and fear about poor sleep, decreased daytime activity levels and a tendency to misperceive sleep [50].

Thus, although there are a limited number of studies, BD patients seem to exhibit sleep disturbances even in the euthymic phases. These data support the relevance of impairment in sleep and circadian rhythms in the pathophysiology of BD. On the other hand, impaired sleep may represent vulnerability to relapse into pathological phases of illness. Therefore, sleep disturbances during euthymic phases may represent a potential therapeutic target to avoid relapses or at least reduce their frequency [66].

9. Pathophysiology of Circadian Rhytms Abnormalities in Bipolar Disorder

Several studies have investigated the biological correlates of the CR abnormalities observed in BD patients. Several lines of data supports the relevance of circadian gene expression in key "mood related" brain regions and outside the CNS. These genes form peripheral clocks that respond to CNS signals or function independently in response to certain stimuli. For example, circadian activity rhythms in rodents can be entrained to daytime methamphetamine injections, even in CNS damaged animals. This treatment shifts the expression of the period genes in striatal regions in a way that matches the shift in activity rhythms. Interestingly, a study by Ogden [67] found that the mood stabilizer valproic acid decreased the expression of the circadian genes CK1δ and Cry2 in the amygdale, a region of the brain associated with emotional behaviour and fear. These changes were prevented by concomitant treatment with methamphetamine, which was given to induce manic-like symptoms, suggesting that these changes may be involved in the treatment of mania. Therefore, mood stabilizer treatment may involve a change in rhythms in the amygdale, at least partially. Furthermore, some studies found that treatment with fluoxetine altered the expression of the Clock and Baml1 genes in the mouse hippocampus. In addition, other studies suggest that Clock functions to regulate the expression of other circadian genes and several genes involved in dopaminergic transmission in the ventral tegmental area (VTA), including the rate-limiting enzyme in dopamine synthesis tyrosine hydroxylase. Clock mutated mice show an increase in dopaminergic activity in the VTA that correlates with their manic-like behaviour (i.e. hyperactivity, increase in reward value for sucrose, cocaine, and brain stimulation; a decrease in measures of depression-like behaviour). Furthermore, when a functional Clock protein was expressed specifically in the VTA using virus-mediated gene transfer, at least a portion of their manic behaviour could be rescued [68]. Therefore, these studies suggest that proper Clock expression in VTA is important for the regulation of dopaminergic activity and, at least, for some of the behaviour associated with mania. However, further studies are required to better clarify this issue, since it is still unclear if the manic-like phenotypes of the Clock mutant mice are due to the loss of Clock function in the VTA or other brain regions.

Consistent with animal and clinical studies, human genetic investigations also support the involvement of circadian genes in the pathophysiology of BD, which has been strongly linked to variations in Clock and Bmal1. A single-nucleotide polymorphism (SNP) in the 3'-flanking region of the Clock gene in BP patients was associated with a higher recurrence rate of bipolar episodes, as well as with greater insomnia and decreased need of sleep in bipolar patients [69]. In addition, haplotypes and SNPs in the Bmal1 gene were found to be associated with the disorder itself [70]. Recently, it has also been hypothesized that the connection between BD and CRs may be mediated by an epigenetic mechanism, such as the phosphorylation of multiple circadian genes by the glycogen synthase kinase 3 beta (GSK3β), which is inhibited by lithium, the gold standard among mood stabilizers. Lastly, GSK3β seems to phosphorylate the PER2, CRY2 and Rev-erbα genes leading to the proper regulation of circadian rhythms. Lithium inhibition of GSK3β activity results in a promotion of a long circadian period, accountable for its therapeutic effects, at least partially [51].

10. Treatment of Comorbid Insomnia and Bipolar Diosrder

10.1. Pharmacotherapy for Insomnia in BD

Several drugs are used empirically for the treatment of insomnia in BD, such as benzodiazepines, z-drugs, sedating antidepressants, sedating antipsychotics, mood stabilizers/anticonvulsants and melatonin receptor agonists. Here, we briefly discuss the pros and cons of these medications in the context of BD, with the caveat that no medication has been specifically approved for management of insomnia in BD.

10.1.1. Benzodiazepine

Benzodiazepines (BDZ), long considered first-line therapy for insomnia, offer several benefits in this field, such as known efficacy, high tolerability and wide range of half-life and potency. Interestingly, one review by Sachs et al. [71] suggested that in BD patients clonazepam may be effective in addition to other antipsychotics as add-on therapy to lithium in maintenance treatment. However, two additional studies failed to replicate this result [71,72]. On the other hand, the potential for abuse, tolerance, withdrawal, daytime sedation and motor/cognitive impairment is often a limiting factor in the use of BDZ, particularly in BD patients because of their higher tendency to abuse compared to the general population.

10.1.2. Z-Drugs

Z-Drugs (i.e. zolpidem, zaleplon and eszopiclone) are similar to traditional BDZ concerning their mechanism of action. Indeed, they act through stimulation of the γ-aminobutyric acid (GABA) receptor, but are more specific for GABA-A receptors, which contain their target, i.e. α-1 subunits. All these drugs have short to intermediate half-life, and thus do not cause daytime sedation. Additionally, despite their potential for tolerance and withdrawal, there is evidence that non-nightly use over 8-12 weeks is not associated with such sequelae, and extended use (up to 6 months) does not cause tolerance or rebound insomnia on discontinuation [73]. Although Z-drugs are largely used clinically as hypnotics in BD insomnia, to the best of our knowledge there are no studies investigating their effectiveness as adjunctive medications in the management of BD.

10.1.3. Sedating Antidepressants

At present, sedating antidepressants at low dosages are among the most widely-used drugs to treat chronic insomnia. Their use in the treatment of insomnia increased dramatically since the early 1990s, probably because of concerns about long-term use of BDZ and Z-drugs (including label restrictions on duration of use), and widespread use of SSRIs in depression treatment (which, in contrast to older antidepressants, are not sedating and may in fact be alerting). Nonetheless, in BD, trazodone as well as other old sedating antidepressants such as TCAs are known to have the capacity to induce mania. Paradoxically, these antidepressants seem to induce mania more frequently than SSRIs, despite their positive effects on sleep [74,75]. Therefore, these drugs should be avoided in the treatment of BD patients or, at least, their use requires special attention.

10.1.4. Mood Stabilizers/Anticonvulsants

Some anticonvulsants approved for the treatment of BD as mood stabilizers also show sedative effects. Among these, there are two of the most effective mood stabilizers available: valproic acid and carbamazepine. Unfortunately, to the best of our knowledge no study has specifically investigated their effects on sleep in BD. Thus, it is not possible to distinguish whether their sedative effects are implicated in the effectiveness observed in the treatment of BD. Nonetheless, studies on other anticonvulsants (e.g. gabapentin, topiramate, tiagabine), which are not approved for the treatment of BD because of their ineffectiveness, may provide some suggestions on this issue. Indeed, in daily clinical practice these drugs are sometimes used off-label as hypnotics in BD patients. However, there is little evidence supporting this strategy in BD. One study suggested that gabapentin can improve subjective sleep quality, decrease light sleep, and increase REM sleep and SWS [76]. Nonetheless, overall these drugs seem to be less effective than BDZ and Z-drugs in the treatment of insomnia, and their side effects (cognitive impairment, daytime sedation, etc.) should be considered before prescribing them as hypnotics in BD.

10.1.5. Sedating Antipsychotics

Antipsychotics, particularly second-generation antipsychotics (SGAs), are often used as adjunctive or primary agents in BD treatment. SGAs are also used in BD with the aim of improving sleep because of their effectiveness demonstrated by their widespread use off-label in resistant insomnia. However, the use of an antipsychotic solely as a hypnotic is controversial, since they have a propensity to cause metabolic abnormalities and weight gain, daytime sedation and extra-pyramidal symptoms. In clinical practice, the most used antipsychotic as a sedative-hypnotic is quetiapine, typically at low doses (25-100 mg/day). This strategy seems to be effective in increasing total sleep time and improving subjective sleep quality in healthy subjects [77]. In BD, quetiapine is used in all phases of the disorder, and it may be a good option to treat insomnia in these patients. Nonetheless, clinicians should be cautious in using quetiapine or other antipsychotics for the treatment of insomnia in BD patients since these drugs may induce or worsen sleep-related movement disorders, such as restless legs syndrome and periodic limb movements of sleep, which may in turn diminishes the quality of sleep. Thus, when clinicians do choose this strategy, they should pay careful attention to tolerability.

10.1.6. Melatonin Receptor Agonists

Another pharmacological approach to improve sleep in BD patients is the use of agents with melatonin receptor agonist activity. Melatonin is a neuro-hormone secreted by the pineal gland in a circadian fashion under conditions of darkness, whereas light inhibits its secretion. Theoretically, it exerts its effects through interactions with the supra-chiasmatic nucleus, i.e. the site of the circadian pacemaker. Melatonin is a relative poor hypnotic, but it seems to influence sleep patterns through its effects on phase-shifting the circadian rhythm. Although melatonin has shown some promise in treatment-refractory mania in rapid-cycling patients, its efficacy has not been thoroughly studied in maintenance treatment of BD, and further investigations are required to test its effectiveness in this area. More recently, a new antidepressant with a peculiar receptor profile has been introduced in clinical practice, namely agomelatine. This antidepressant is a norepinephrine and dopamine disinhibitor drug, acting as a 5-HT2C/2B serotonin receptor antagonist and MT1/MT2 melatonin receptor agonist. In MDD, it has been shown to improve sleep, and it has been hypothesized that it may have benefits in BD depression. However, to date, only preliminary studies are available suggesting the effectiveness of this drug in BD depression [78]. Interestingly, it seems to improve sleep in BD patients, and thus it might be useful in maintenance treatment of BD. Nonetheless, further investigations are needed to better investigate its therapeutic proprieties in BD and its capacity to induce mania.

10.2. Psychotherapy for Insomnia in BD

First line psychotherapy for insomnia is cognitive-behavioural therapy for insomnia (CBT-I). The efficacy of CBT-I in primary insomnia is well established and is comparable in efficacy to pharmacotherapy. Strategies of CBT-I can include sleep restriction therapy, sleep hygiene education, stimulus control therapy and relaxation training. Unfortunately, there are no studies specifically focused on CBT-I in bipolar insomnia, and thus their effectiveness in this population is not yet clear. Nonetheless, these strategies are safe and have no side effects. Therefore, they may be applied in clinical practice to BD patients, except for sleep restriction therapy, since it may induce mania through sleep deprivation [79]. Management of insomnia in BD patients using CBT-I may be also complicated by the fact that BD patients often complain of difficulty arising in the morning, and they can have mild hypomanic symptoms that intensify over the course of the day, potentially disrupting their ability to sleep at night or adhere to prescribed CBT-I interventions.

Psychotherapies used successfully in the treatment of BD often utilize psychoeducational components that emphasize the identification of prodromal symptoms (e.g. sleep disturbances) and the importance of life-style regularity, including stabilization of sleep-wake rhythms. Even interpersonal and social rhythm therapy, which is based on the notion that management of life stressors that disrupt patterns (e.g. social patterns, sleep-wake patterns) seems to improve outcomes in BD, prolonging euthymic phases and reducing affective relapse [80,81].

10.3. Sleep Deprivation in BD Depression

Although sleep deprivation has been demonstrated to have an antidepressant effect in bipolar depression, its clinical utility as mono-therapy is limited by the rate of depression relapse after sleep recovery. Various pharmacological approaches have been studied as potential augmentation strategies to improve or extend the antidepressant effect of sleep deprivation. Several reports have demonstrated that lithium treatment may improve response to sleep deprivation and sustain remission in both unipolar and bipolar depressed patients [82,83]. In addition to pharmacological approaches, manipulation of the circadian system has also been used to maintain the antidepressant effects of sleep deprivation in bipolar patients. In particular, bright light in the morning seems to sustain an antidepressant response to sleep deprivation in bipolar patients. Furthermore, phase advance (e.g., moving the sleep period several hours earlier than usual) of the sleep period after sleep deprivation has been shown to sustain the antidepressant effects of sleep deprivation in both unipolar and bipolar depressed patients [84,85].

Despite data suggesting that sleep deprivation may be effective in bipolar depression, the American Psychiatric Association guidelines for the treatment of BD lists it as a novel approach. This is appropriate given the limited data comparing it with conventional treatments, concern about switching patients into mania, the logistical difficulties of sleep deprivation on inpatient psychiatric units and the high rate of depressive relapse after sleep recovery.

11. Sleep Disturbances and Suicide

Suicide is a leading cause of death, particularly among young adults. Attempted suicides are believed to far exceed the number of suicides. Therefore, suicidal behaviours represent a relevant public health problem, with far reaching personal and societal consequences. Improvements in the identification of risk factors for suicidal behaviour are thus a fundamental step to manage this complex behaviour and, consequently, to reduce the number of suicides and suicide attempts.

A growing body of evidence suggests a relationship between sleep and suicidal behaviour. Unfortunately, the majority of studies investigating this link were conducted on depressed patients, and it is therefore hard to distinguish the role of insomnia in determination of the suicidal behaviour and from the role of MDD itself. Nonetheless, some suggestions could be drawn from studies available to date. A review by McCall et al. concluded that insomnia is the most common sleep disturbance associated with suicidal ideations or attempts [86], although the main studies included were conducted on depressed patients. In a sample of depressed patients, Fawcett et al. found that symptoms of global insomnia were more severe among those who completed suicide within a 13-month period [87]. Agargun et al. found a relationship between suicidality, depression and sleep complaints [88]. These authors also reported that nightmares were more common among suicidal individuals than in non-suicidal ones [89-91]. Moreover, electroencephalographic sleep studies showed that subjects with a history of suicide attempts have lower sleep efficiency, longer sleep latency and fewer late-night delta counts. Suicidal patients further showed shorter REM sleep latency, higher REM percentage and a more negative dream-like quality of REM [92]. Thus, taken overall, these data suggest poor sleep quality is present in suicidal subjects.

Despite the observed relationship between sleep and suicide, it is still unclear how these two constructs relate to one another after controlling for depressive symptoms. Indeed, several reports investigated only MDD patients [88,89], while others showed an effect of depressive symptomatology on this association [93]. In facts, mood regulation factors may play a primary role in the relationship between sleep and suicide. Sleep may, for example, fail to provide an emotional refuge for distressed individuals or frequent nightmares may exacerbate feelings of ineffectiveness; in addition, poor sleep quality may disrupt within-sleep mood regulation processes. This explanation is supported by research conducted in depressed patients. For example, Cartwright et al. found that patients who reported more affectively negative dreams early in the night were more likely to achieve remission within one year compared to patients who reported more negative dreams at the end of the night [94].

Additionally, suicidal patients showed a more negative dream-like quality of REM [92]. Taken together, these data suggest that dream content and within-sleep mood regulation processes may play a significant role in the association between sleep and suicidality.

The association between sleep disturbances and suicidal behaviours may be due to a common neurobiological basis of these two conditions. In this regard, the serotonin system seems to play a relevant role in both suicide and regulation of sleep. In particular, serotonin release appears to be highest during waking states, reduced during SWS and lowest during REM sleep. It has been recently hypothesized that serotonin release during waking states drives the homeostatic regulation of SWS and, thus, serotonergic dysfunction is believed to promote wakefulness.

Sleep is a complex behavioural phenomenon, driven by circadian and homeostatic sleep factors. Sleep and suicidal behaviours may be influenced by various time cues, which have received little attention in research. However, several reports have shown a diurnal variation in the timing of self-injurious behaviour and complete suicide, although the results are often conflicting. Interestingly, it has been reported that there is a difference across different age groups as subjects who deliberate self-harm in the morning are more likely to be older in age. On the other hand, for completed suicides the suicide peaks are reported both in the morning and evening, independently of age. Nonetheless, additional research is needed to clarify whether suicidal behaviours are a function of clock time, and if so whether this relationship is associated with sleep, the light-dark cycle and a dysregulated mood state, or if diurnal variation in suicidal behaviours may be explained only by social factors.

Even if a precise relationship has not emerged between sleep and suicide from a physiopathological point of view, quality of sleep may represent a prognostic factor in suicidal patients. In depression, insomnia may be considered a clinical indicator of higher suicidal risk. Consistent with these data, the Substance Abuse and Mental Health Services Administration (SAMSHA) lists sleep problems, and more specifically significant changes in sleep, among the top 10 warning signs for suicide. Nonetheless, further research is needed to better clarify the relationship between suicide and sleep to give to clinicians definitive results that can be beneficial for the daily clinical prevention of suicidal behaviours.

References

[1]   Hallonquist JD, Goldberg MA, Brandes JS. Affective disorders and circadian rhythms. *Can J Psychiatry*. 1986;31(3):259-72.

[2]   Leonhardt G, Wirz-Justice A, Krauchi K, Graw P, Wunder D, Haug HJ. Long-term follow-up of depression in seasonal affective disorder. *Compr Psychiatry*. 1994;35(6):457-64.

[3]   Riemann D. Insomnia and comorbid psychiatric disorders. *Sleep Med.* 2007;8 Suppl 4:S15-20.

[4]   Neckelmann D, Mykletun A, Dahl AA. Chronic insomnia as a risk factor for developing anxiety and depression. *Sleep*. 2007;30(7):873-80.

[5]   Monteleone P, Martiadis V, Maj M. Circadian rhythms and treatment implications in depression. *Prog Neuropsychopharmacol Biol Psychiatry*. 2011;35(7):1569-74.

[6]   Nofzinger EA, Buysse DJ, Germain A, Carter C, Luna B, Price JC, et al. Increased activation of anterior paralimbic and executive cortex from waking to rapid eye movement sleep in depression. *Arch Gen Psychiatry*. 2004;61(7):695-702.

[7]   McNamara P, Auerbach S, Johnson P, Harris E, Doros G. Impact of REM sleep on distortions of self-concept, mood and memory in depressed/anxious participants. *J Affect Disord*. 2010;122(3):198-207.

[8]   Kronfeld-Schor N, Einat H. Circadian rhythms and depression: human psychopathology and animal models. *Neuropharmacology*. 2012;62(1):101-14.

[9]   Schreiber W, Lauer CJ, Krumrey K, Holsboer F, Krieg JC. Cholinergic REM sleep induction test in subjects at high risk for psychiatric disorders. *Biol Psychiatry*. 1992;32(1):79-90.

[10]   Lauer CJ, Modell S, Schreiber W, Krieg JC, Holsboer F. Prediction of the development of a first major depressive episode with a rapid eye movement sleep induction test using the cholinergic agonist RS 86. *Journal of clinical psychopharmacology*. 2004;24(3):356-7.

[11]   Furey ML, Drevets WC. Antidepressant efficacy of the antimuscarinic drug scopolamine: a randomized, placebo-controlled clinical trial. *Arch Gen Psychiatry*. 2006;63(10):1121-9.

[12]   Janowsky DS. Serendipity strikes again: scopolamine as an antidepressant agent in bipolar depressed patients. *Curr Psychiatry Rep*. 2011;13(6):443-5.

[13]   Howland RH. The antidepressant effects of anticholinergic drugs. *J Psychosoc Nurs Ment Health Serv*. 2009;47(6):17-20.

[14]   Borbely AA. The S-deficiency hypothesis of depression and the two-process model of sleep regulation. *Pharmacopsychiatry*. 1987;20(1):23-9.

[15]   Knowles JB, Coulter M, Wahnon S, Reitz W, MacLean AW. Variation in process S: effects on sleep continuity and architecture. *Sleep*. 1990;13(2):97-107.

[16]   Pillai V, Kalmbach DA, Ciesla JA. A meta-analysis of electroencephalographic sleep in depression: evidence for genetic biomarkers. *Biol Psychiatry*. 2011;70(10):912-9.

[17]   Papousek M. [Chronobiological aspects of cyclothymia (author's transl)]. Fortschr Neurol Psychiatr Grenzgeb. 1975;43(8):381-440. *Chronobiologische Aspekte der Zyklothymie*.

[18]   Wehr TA, Wirz-Justice A, Goodwin FK, Duncan W, Gillin JC. Phase advance of the circadian sleep-wake cycle as an antidepressant. *Science*. 1979;206(4419):710-3.

[19]   Sack RL, Lewy AJ, White DM, Singer CM, Fireman MJ, Vandiver R. Morning vs evening light treatment for winter depression. Evidence that the therapeutic effects of light are mediated by circadian phase shifts. *Arch Gen Psychiatry*. 1990;47(4):343-51.

[20]   Bonnavion P, de Lecea L. Hypocretins in the control of sleep and wakefulness. *Curr Neurol Neurosci Rep*. 2010;10(3):174-9.

[21]   Nollet M, Gaillard P, Minier F, Tanti A, Belzung C, Leman S. Activation of orexin neurons in dorsomedial/perifornical hypothalamus and antidepressant reversal in a rodent model of depression. *Neuropharmacology*. 2011;61(1-2):336-46.

[22]   von der Goltz C, Koopmann A, Dinter C, Richter A, Grosshans M, Fink T, et al. Involvement of orexin in the regulation of stress, depression and reward in alcohol dependence. *Horm Behav*. 2011;60(5):644-50.

[23]   Vogel GW, McAbee R, Barker K, Thurmond A. Endogenous depression improvement and REM pressure. *Arch Gen Psychiatry*. 1977;34(1):96-7.

[24]   Vogel GW, Feng P, Kinney GG. Ontogeny of REM sleep in rats: possible implications for endogenous depression. *Physiol Behav.* 2000;68(4):453-61.

[25]   Shaffery JP, Lopez J, Bissette G, Roffwarg HP. Rapid eye movement sleep deprivation in post-critical period, adolescent rats alters the balance between inhibitory and excitatory mechanisms in visual cortex. *Neurosci Lett.* 2006;393(2-3):131-5.

[26]   Mirmiran M, Scholtens J, van de Poll NE, Uylings HB, van der Gugten J, Boer GJ. Effects of experimental suppression of active (REM) sleep during early development upon adult brain and behavior in the rat. *Brain Res.* 1983;283(2-3):277-86.

[27]   Riemann D, Spiegelhalder K, Nissen C, Hirscher V, Baglioni C, Feige B. REM sleep instability--a new pathway for insomnia? *Pharmacopsychiatry.* 2012;45(5):167-76.

[28]   Baglioni C, Battagliese G, Feige B, Spiegelhalder K, Nissen C, Voderholzer U, et al. Insomnia as a predictor of depression: a meta-analytic evaluation of longitudinal epidemiological studies. *J Affect Disord.* 2011;135(1-3):10-9.

[29]   McEwen BS, Stellar E. Stress and the individual. Mechanisms leading to disease. *Arch Intern Med.* 1993;153(18):2093-101.

[30]   McEwen BS. Sleep deprivation as a neurobiologic and physiologic stressor: Allostasis and allostatic load. *Metabolism.* 2006;55(10 Suppl 2):S20-3.

[31]   Novati A, Roman V, Cetin T, Hagewoud R, den Boer JA, Luiten PG, et al. Chronically restricted sleep leads to depression-like changes in neurotransmitter receptor sensitivity and neuroendocrine stress reactivity in rats. *Sleep.* 2008;31(11):1579-85.

[32]   Cheeta S, Ruigt G, van Proosdij J, Willner P. Changes in sleep architecture following chronic mild stress. *Biol Psychiatry.* 1997;41(4):419-27.

[33]   Giles DE, Roffwarg HP, Schlesser MA, Rush AJ. Which endogenous depressive symptoms relate to REM latency reduction? *Biol Psychiatry.* 1986;21(5-6):473-82.

[34]   Saletin JM, Goldstein AN, Walker MP. The role of sleep in directed forgetting and remembering of human memories. *Cereb Cortex.* 2011;21(11):2534-41.

[35]   Tsuno N, Besset A, Ritchie K. Sleep and depression. *J Clin Psychiatry.* 2005;66(10):1254-69.

[36]   Armitage R, Hoffmann R, Trivedi M, Rush AJ. Slow-wave activity in NREM sleep: sex and age effects in depressed outpatients and healthy controls. *Psychiatry Res.* 2000;95(3):201-13.

[37]   Riemann D, Berger M, Voderholzer U. Sleep and depression--results from psychobiological studies: an overview. *Biol Psychol.* 2001;57(1-3):67-103.

[38]   Palagini L, Baglioni C, Ciapparelli A, Gemignani A, Riemann D. REM sleep dysregulation in depression: State of the art. *Sleep medicine reviews.* 2013.

[39]   Santos Moraes WA, Burke PR, Coutinho PL, Guilleminault C, Bittencourt AG, Tufik S, et al. Sedative antidepressants and insomnia. *Rev Bras Psiquiatr.* 2011;33(1):91-5.

[40]   Reynolds CF, 3rd, Frank E, Houck PR, Mazumdar S, Dew MA, Cornes C, et al. Which elderly patients with remitted depression remain well with continued interpersonal psychotherapy after discontinuation of antidepressant medication? *Am J Psychiatry.* 1997;154(7):958-62. Epub 1997/07/01.

[41]   Antonijevic I. HPA axis and sleep: identifying subtypes of major depression. *Stress.* 2008;11(1):15-27.

[42]   Hasler G, Drevets WC, Manji HK, Charney DS. Discovering endophenotypes for major depression. *Neuropsychopharmacology.* 2004;29(10):1765-81.

[43] Modell S, Lauer CJ. Rapid eye movement (REM) sleep: an endophenotype for depression. *Curr Psychiatry Rep.* 2007;9(6):480-5.

[44] Giles DE, Biggs MM, Rush AJ, Roffwarg HP. Risk factors in families of unipolar depression. I. Psychiatric illness and reduced REM latency. *J Affect Disord.* 1988;14(1):51-9.

[45] Giles DE, Kupfer DJ, Roffwarg HP, Rush AJ, Biggs MM, Etzel BA. Polysomnographic parameters in first-degree relatives of unipolar probands. *Psychiatry Res.* 1989;27(2):127-36.

[46] Kupfer DJ. REM latency: a psychobiologic marker for primary depressive disease. *Biol Psychiatry.* 1976;11(2):159-74.

[47] Sitaram N, Gillin JC. Development and use of pharmacological probes of the CNS in man: evidence of cholinergic abnormality in primary affective illness. *Biol Psychiatry.* 1980;15(6):925-55.

[48] Wehr TA, Sack D, Rosenthal N, Duncan W, Gillin JC. Circadian rhythm disturbances in manic-depressive illness. *Fed Proc.* 1983;42(11):2809-14.

[49] Millar A, Espie CA, Scott J. The sleep of remitted bipolar outpatients: a controlled naturalistic study using actigraphy. *J Affect Disord.* 2004;80(2-3):145-53.

[50] Harvey AG, Schmidt DA, Scarna A, Semler CN, Goodwin GM. Sleep-related functioning in euthymic patients with bipolar disorder, patients with insomnia, and subjects without sleep problems. *Am J Psychiatry.* 2005;162(1):50-7.

[51] Lowrey PL, Takahashi JS. Genetics of circadian rhythms in Mammalian model organisms. *Adv Genet.* 2011;74:175-230.

[52] Ritter PS, Marx C, Bauer M, Leopold K, Pfennig A. The role of disturbed sleep in the early recognition of bipolar disorder: a systematic review. *Bipolar Disord.* 2011;13(3):227-37.

[53] Bowden CL. A different depression: clinical distinctions between bipolar and unipolar depression. *J Affect Disord.* 2005;84(2-3):117-25.

[54] Nofzinger EA, Thase ME, Reynolds CF, 3rd, Himmelhoch JM, Mallinger A, Houck P, et al. Hypersomnia in bipolar depression: a comparison with narcolepsy using the multiple sleep latency test. *Am J Psychiatry.* 1991;148(9):1177-81.

[55] Szuba MP, Baxter LR, Jr., Fairbanks LA, Guze BH, Schwartz JM. Effects of partial sleep deprivation on the diurnal variation of mood and motor activity in major depression. *Biol Psychiatry.* 1991;30(8):817-29.

[56] Barbini B, Colombo C, Benedetti F, Campori E, Bellodi L, Smeraldi E. The unipolar-bipolar dichotomy and the response to sleep deprivation. *Psychiatry Res.* 1998;79(1):43-50.

[57] Wu JC, Bunney WE. The biological basis of an antidepressant response to sleep deprivation and relapse: review and hypothesis. *Am J Psychiatry.* 1990;147(1):14-21.

[58] Wehr TA, Sack DA, Rosenthal NE. Sleep reduction as a final common pathway in the genesis of mania. *Am J Psychiatry.* 1987;144(2):201-4.

[59] Colombo C, Benedetti F, Barbini B, Campori E, Smeraldi E. Rate of switch from depression into mania after therapeutic sleep deprivation in bipolar depression. *Psychiatry Res.* 1999;86(3):267-70.

[60] Jackson A, Cavanagh J, Scott J. A systematic review of manic and depressive prodromes. *J Affect Disord.* 2003;74(3):209-17.

[61] Malkoff-Schwartz S, Frank E, Anderson B, Sherrill JT, Siegel L, Patterson D, et al. Stressful life events and social rhythm disruption in the onset of manic and depressive bipolar episodes: a preliminary investigation. *Arch Gen Psychiatry.* 1998;55(8):702-7.

[62] Barbini B, Benedetti F, Colombo C, Dotoli D, Bernasconi A, Cigala-Fulgosi M, et al. Dark therapy for mania: a pilot study. *Bipolar Disord.* 2005;7(1):98-101.

[63] Knowles JB, Cairns J, MacLean AW, Delva N, Prowse A, Waldron J, et al. The sleep of remitted bipolar depressives: comparison with sex and age-matched controls. *Can J Psychiatry.* 1986;31(4):295-8.

[64] Sitaram N, Nurnberger JI, Jr., Gershon ES, Gillin JC. Cholinergic regulation of mood and REM sleep: potential model and marker of vulnerability to affective disorder. *Am J Psychiatry.* 1982;139(5):571-6.

[65] Jones SH, Hare DJ, Evershed K. Actigraphic assessment of circadian activity and sleep patterns in bipolar disorder. *Bipolar Disord.* 2005;7(2):176-86.

[66] Sylvia LG, Dupuy JM, Ostacher MJ, Cowperthwait CM, Hay AC, Sachs GS, et al. Sleep disturbance in euthymic bipolar patients. *J Psychopharmacol.* 2012;26(8):1108-12.

[67] Ogden CA, Rich ME, Schork NJ, Paulus MP, Geyer MA, Lohr JB, et al. Candidate genes, pathways and mechanisms for bipolar (manic-depressive) and related disorders: an expanded convergent functional genomics approach. *Mol Psychiatry.* 2004;9(11):1007-29.

[68] McClung CA, Sidiropoulou K, Vitaterna M, Takahashi JS, White FJ, Cooper DC, et al. Regulation of dopaminergic transmission and cocaine reward by the Clock gene. *Proc Natl Acad Sci U S A.* 2005;102(26):9377-81.

[69] Serretti A, Cusin C, Benedetti F, Mandelli L, Pirovano A, Zanardi R, et al. Insomnia improvement during antidepressant treatment and CLOCK gene polymorphism. *Am J Med Genet B Neuropsychiatr Genet.* 2005;137B(1):36-9.

[70] Mansour HA, Wood J, Logue T, Chowdari KV, Dayal M, Kupfer DJ, et al. Association study of eight circadian genes with bipolar I disorder, schizoaffective disorder and schizophrenia. *Genes Brain Behav.* 2006;5(2):150-7.

[71] Sachs GS, Rosenbaum JF, Jones L. Adjunctive clonazepam for maintenance treatment of bipolar affective disorder. *Journal of clinical psychopharmacology.* 1990;10(1):42-7.

[72] Winkler D, Willeit M, Wolf R, Stamenkovic M, Tauscher J, Pjrek E, et al. Clonazepam in the long-term treatment of patients with unipolar depression, bipolar and schizoaffective disorder. *Eur Neuropsychopharmacol.* 2003;13(2):129-34.

[73] Krystal AD, Walsh JK, Laska E, Caron J, Amato DA, Wessel TC, et al. Sustained efficacy of eszopiclone over 6 months of nightly treatment: results of a randomized, double-blind, placebo-controlled study in adults with chronic insomnia. *Sleep.* 2003;26(7):793-9.

[74] Peet M. Induction of mania with selective serotonin re-uptake inhibitors and tricyclic antidepressants. *Br J Psychiatry.* 1994;164(4):549-50.

[75] Terao T. Comparison of manic switch onset during fluoxetine and trazodone treatment. *Biol Psychiatry.* 1993;33(6):477-8.

[76] Foldvary-Schaefer N, De Leon Sanchez I, Karafa M, Mascha E, Dinner D, Morris HH. Gabapentin increases slow-wave sleep in normal adults. *Epilepsia.* 2002;43(12):1493-7.

[77] Cohrs S, Rodenbeck A, Guan Z, Pohlmann K, Jordan W, Meier A, et al. Sleep-promoting properties of quetiapine in healthy subjects. *Psychopharmacology* (Berl). 2004;174(3):421-9.

[78] Fornaro M, McCarthy MJ, De Berardis D, De Pasquale C, Tabaton M, Martino M, et al. Adjunctive agomelatine therapy in the treatment of acute bipolar II depression: a preliminary open label study. *Neuropsychiatric disease and treatment*. 2013;9:243-51.

[79] Smith MT, Huang MI, Manber R. Cognitive behavior therapy for chronic insomnia occurring within the context of medical and psychiatric disorders. *Clin Psychol Rev*. 2005;25(5):559-92.

[80] Frank E, Swartz HA, Kupfer DJ. Interpersonal and social rhythm therapy: managing the chaos of bipolar disorder. *Biol Psychiatry*. 2000;48(6):593-604.

[81] Frank E, Kupfer DJ, Thase ME, Mallinger AG, Swartz HA, Fagiolini AM, et al. Two-year outcomes for interpersonal and social rhythm therapy in individuals with bipolar I disorder. *Arch Gen Psychiatry*. 2005;62(9):996-1004.

[82] Baxter LR, Jr., Liston EH, Schwartz JM, Altshuler LL, Wilkins JN, Richeimer S, et al. Prolongation of the antidepressant response to partial sleep deprivation by lithium. *Psychiatry Res*. 1986;19(1):17-23.

[83] Benedetti F, Colombo C, Barbini B, Campori E, Smeraldi E. Ongoing lithium treatment prevents relapse after total sleep deprivation. *Journal of clinical psychopharmacology*. 1999;19(3):240-5.

[84] Berger M, Vollmann J, Hohagen F, Konig A, Lohner H, Voderholzer U, et al. Sleep deprivation combined with consecutive sleep phase advance as a fast-acting therapy in depression: an open pilot trial in medicated and unmedicated patients. *Am J Psychiatry*. 1997;154(6):870-2.

[85] Benedetti F, Barbini B, Campori E, Fulgosi MC, Pontiggia A, Colombo C. Sleep phase advance and lithium to sustain the antidepressant effect of total sleep deprivation in bipolar depression: new findings supporting the internal coincidence model? *J Psychiatr Res*. 2001;35(6):323-9.

[86] McCall WV, Blocker JN, D'Agostino R, Jr., Kimball J, Boggs N, Lasater B, et al. Insomnia severity is an indicator of suicidal ideation during a depression clinical trial. *Sleep Med*. 2010;11(9):822-7.

[87] Fawcett J, Scheftner WA, Fogg L, Clark DC, Young MA, Hedeker D, et al. Time-related predictors of suicide in major affective disorder. *Am J Psychiatry*. 1990;147(9):1189-94.

[88] Agargun MY, Kara H, Solmaz M. Sleep disturbances and suicidal behavior in patients with major depression. *J Clin Psychiatry*. 1997;58(6):249-51.

[89] Agargun MY, Kara H, Solmaz M. Subjective sleep quality and suicidality in patients with major depression. *J Psychiatr Res*. 1997;31(3):377-81.

[90] Agargun MY, Cilli AS, Kara H, Tarhan N, Kincir F, Oz H. Repetitive and frightening dreams and suicidal behavior in patients with major depression. *Compr Psychiatry*. 1998;39(4):198-202.

[91] Agargun MY, Besiroglu L, Cilli AS, Gulec M, Aydin A, Inci R, et al. Nightmares, suicide attempts, and melancholic features in patients with unipolar major depression. *J Affect Disord*. 2007;98(3):267-70.

[92] Agargun MY, Cartwright R. REM sleep, dream variables and suicidality in depressed patients. *Psychiatry Res*. 2003;119(1-2):33-9.

[93] Krakow B, Artar A, Warner TD, Melendrez D, Johnston L, Hollifield M, et al. Sleep disorder, depression, and suicidality in female sexual assault survivors. *Crisis.* 2000;21(4):163-70.

[94] Cartwright R, Young MA, Mercer P, Bears M. Role of REM sleep and dream variables in the prediction of remission from depression. *Psychiatry Res.* 1998;80(3):249-55.

In: Sleep Medicine
Editors: A. Del Casale, R. Brugnoli and P. Girardi

ISBN: 978-1-62808-515-0
© 2013 Nova Science Publishers, Inc.

Chapter XI

Sleep Disturbance in Schizophrenia

Roberto Brugnoli, [*] *Simone Pallottino and Paolo Girardi*
Sapienza University, NESMOS (Neuroscience, Mental Health and Sensory Organs)
Department, School of Medicine and Psychology, Rome, Italy

Abstract

Schizophrenia can be considered a neurodevelopmental disorder resulting from a complex interplay between multiple susceptibility genes and environmental factors. This illness shows a heterogeneous patchwork of three classes of psychopathological alterations: positive symptoms, negative symptoms and cognitive impairment.

Eventually, schizophrenia leads to significant sleep disturbance, even if this is seldom reported as predominant complaint and physicians often overlook it.

The aim of the present chapter is to review the existing literature on sleep disorders in schizophrenia, describe sleep features in different phases of the disease and the effect of antipsychotic drugs on sleep patterns and architecture. Practical advice is also offered for the treatment of sleep disturbance in patients with schizophrenia.

Keywords: Schizophrenia, Psychosis, Sleep disturbance, Sleep disorders, Antipsychotic drugs

Introduction

Schizophrenia is perhaps the most devastating neuropsychiatric illness, and affects up to 1% of world's population, with similar prevalence rates among different countries, sexes and cultural groups [1]. The illness tends to develop between the ages of 16 and 30 years and mostly persists throughout the patient's lifetime [2]. Prognosis greatly improved over the last decades. Indeed, the advent of antipsychotic drugs dramatically changed patients' outcome:

---

[*] Corresponding Author. E-mail: roberto.brugnoli@uniroma1.it.

while patients once experienced frequent hospitalizations, nowadays this is uncommon. Moreover with new therapeutic approaches, like cognitive remediation therapy, it is now possible to improve several neurocognitive areas eventually leading to improved social functioning [3].

Despite global efforts for the understanding of the pathophysiology underlying schizophrenia and its aetiology, the disease is still enigmatic. In thepresent view, schizophrenia is seen as a neurodevelopmental disorder resulting from a complex interplay between multiple susceptibility genes and environmental factors [4]. This view is in line with the extreme clinical variability of schizophrenia. Indeed, schizophrenia is a heterogeneous patchwork of three classes of psychopathological alterations: positive symptoms, negative symptoms and cognitive impairment. Positive symptoms include delusions, hallucinations (false perceptions) and thought disorganization. Negative symptoms refer to the loss of motivation and emotional vibrancy. Cognitive impairment, now believed to represent the fundamental defining symptom of schizophrenia, includesdeficits in attention, executive functions and specific forms of memory (particularly working memory). In addition, many patients may experience concomitant mood symptoms including depression and anxiety that may contribute to the 10% lifetime incidence of suicide in schizophrenia [5]. Eventually, schizophrenia leads to significant sleep disturbance, even if this isseldom reported as predominant complaint and physicians often overlook it.

Subjective Reports

Patients affected by schizophrenia commonly complain of difficulties falling asleep, problems in staying asleep and impaired sleep quality. This impairment of subjective sleep quality in schizophrenia patients parallels the severity reported by patients with primary insomnia or major depression [6]. Moreover, it has been shown that poor sleep quality is directly related to negative assessments of quality of life in patients with schizophrenia [7]. During the active state of psychosis, sleep disturbances in schizophrenia patients can range from a period of complete sleeplessness to severe insomnia. Not surprisingly, severe insomnia experienced as difficulty initiating and maintaining sleep is a common clinical feature of the prodromal phase before developing manifest psychotic symptomatology [8-10].

Treatment with antipsychotic drugs (APD) improves the severity of sleep disturbances in schizophrenia. Nevertheless, even among patientswho are clinically stable and in treatment with APD, sleep disturbance remainsa common complaint. In addition, APD treated patients have a higher risk to develop circadian rhythm disruption, resulting in daytime sleep and night wakefulness, compared to community individuals [11].

Lately, the relevance of sleep disturbances in psychosis has been further highlighted by two cross-sectional studies. In their study, Mattai and co-workers [12], showed that among patients affected by childhood onset schizophrenia, a particularly severe form psychosis of the young, poor sleepers (< 6 hours slept per night) hadsignificantly higher scores in clinical scales assessing positive (SAPS) and negative symptoms (SANS) compared to their good sleeper counterparts (> 6 hours slept per night). Moreover, Lee and colleagues [13] showed that sleep disturbancesin adolescentssuch asinsomnia and excessive daytime sleepiness are able to predict psychotic-like experiences, which is a good clinical predictor for psychosis.

There are few studies that have systematically evaluated the prevalence of sleep disturbance in schizophrenia. Interestingly, an early study on recently admitted psychiatric patients found that 83% of patients with acute schizophrenia versus 47% of patients with chronic psychosis had at least one type of sleep disturbances between difficulty in falling asleep, early morning awakening, night awakening, impaired sleep quality and increased time in bed [14]. Subsequent studies found that some type of sleep disturbance wasexperienced by 30-55% of mostly APD treated patients with schizophrenia [15-17].

EEG Studies

The high prevalence of sleep disturbances and theirpossible relationship to the pathophysiology of schizophrenia has inspired a large number of experimental sleep studies. The introduction of EEG and the international standardization of scoring rules for polysomnographic recordings provided researchers a powerful tool to directly evaluate schizophrenic brain dynamics with objective measures.

In order to discriminate the effects of schizophrenia itself from those of antipsychotic drugs, several studies have been conducted in drug-free schizophrenic patients, either at their first psychotic episode or after pharmacological wash-out, versus healthy controls. Chouinard and colleagues [18], with their meta-analysis, effectively summarized the best available studies: 20 studies, published between 1973 and 2000, were selected, providing a population of 652 individuals: 321 patients with schizophrenia and 331 healthy subjects. The main analysis found that schizophrenic patients have an increasedsleep latency (SL) and decreased total sleep time (TST) and sleep efficacy (SE) compared to healthy controls, further confirming subjective reports from patients.

No significant differences were found in any of the other variables: total awake time (TAT), percentage of stage 2 and stage 4, slow sleep waves (SWS), REM percentage, REM density and REM latency. Nevertheless, a closer look at the data showed that some differences could have been missed due tothe presence of moderating factors. Moreover, the specificity report, a measure that indicates the variance not explained by sample error, was very high for eachvariable that did not reach statistical significance. Indeed, despite rigorous selection criteria, Chouinard et al. reported that a very heterogeneous population had been investigated, including patients in different phases of illness (chronic, sub-chronic, sub-acute and acute) and different disease subtypes (paranoid, residual, undifferentiated, catatonic and disorganized).

To provide a more definite picture of sleep disturbances in schizophrenia, herein we briefly report on studies according to clinical phase (acute vs. chronic) andtheir medication status (never medicated vs. previously medicated).

Never-medicated patients showed increases in TAT and SL and reductions in TST and SE when compared with controls [19-23]. In the same studies, no differences were found for eitherS4 sleep time orREM sleep duration, but REM sleep latency was greatly decreased in schizophrenia patients in two different studies [19, 21].

Compared with controls, previously-treated schizophrenia patients showed increased TAT and decreased TST and SE. Moreover, stage 4 sleep was reduced in the majority of studies[24-26], but it was not possible to establish a correlation between this reduction and the length of the wash-out period before the EEG recording. REM latency was shortened in 5studies but unchanged in 4studies in which the wash-out time ranged from 3 to 4 weeks [21, 24-25], possibly indicating thisreduction was the result of antipsychotic treatment.

The sleep disturbance inschizophrenia patients that were either never medicated or previously treated with antipsychoticsshowed no major differences, and was characterized by sleep-onset and sleep maintaining insomnia. Moreover, the majority of studies found a decrease in S4 sleep and REM latency, and no differences in REM time.

To date, few studies have included exclusively schizophrenics experiencing their first episode or an acute relapse of disease. In this regard, the study by Poulin and co-workersis the mostinformative due toits strict criteria [27]. The study included first-episode drug naïve schizophrenia patients (most of whomwere successfully diagnosed with paranoid type) and healthy subjects as a control group. Relative to controls, schizophrenia patients showed increases in sleep latency and decreases in Stage 4 sleep time and REM latency. No differences were found between the two groups for TST, SE, S2 time orSWS. However, it should be noted that previous studies found a decrease in TST in schizophrenia patients during the acute phase of illness [22-23].

There are a large number of studies that have analysed the sleep of schizophrenics during the chronic phase of the disease [19, 21, 26, 28, 29]. Compared with control individuals, most studies found a reduction in TST in schizophrenia patients relative to controls. Moreover, reductions in S4 sleep and REM latency were also observed in some studies. Nevertheless, chronic patients could also have high inter-individual variability due to differences in disease subtype, age, illness duration and other clinical variable. For this reason, Yang and Winkelman [30] recruited a relatively homogeneous (diagnostically) group of patients with schizophrenia (undifferentiated type, clinically stable, withdrawn from routine medication for the time of the study) and a control group. Relative to controls, patients with schizophrenia showed important sleep alterations in different sleep continuity measures (SL and SE) and specific sleep stages (S2 time, S4 time, SWS and REM density), some of which had never been described in previous studies.

The available evidence suggests that sleep onset and sleep maintenance are impaired in schizophrenia patients irrespective of the phase of disease or length of pharmacological wash-out period before polysomnographic recording. Moreover, the clinical phase does not seem to influence either stage 4 sleep orREM variables.

Although stage 4 sleep has been found unchanged in many studies, there is a growing body of evidence supporting its relevance in schizophrenia. Indeed, with the recent implementation of more rigorous inclusion criteria and polysomnographic recording procedures, newer studies have consistently shown areduction in stage 4 sleep relative to control individuals [27, 30]. Moreover, a recent study found a reduction in SWS in schizophrenic patients and, to a lesser extent, intheir first-degree relativescompared with healthy controls [31]. This study suggests that SWS could be a trait rather than a state marker in schizophrenia, but more studies are needed to support this hypothesis.

More recently, Ferrarelli and co-workers focused their attention on sleep spindles [32]. These are synchronous oscillation in the range of stage 2 sleep. Implementing a high frequency EEG recording, they were able to show that schizophrenia patients have a deficit in sleep spindles compared to healthy controls.

Unfortunately, there are no available data on different schizophrenia subtypes or at-risk mental state for schizophrenia, and further studies are needed to explore theseareas.

Table 1. Correlation between EEG sleep measures and clinical variables*

Clinical Variable	SL	TST	SE	SWS %/min	REM %/min	REM latency	REM density
Severity of Ilness		Neg	Neg		Pos/Neg	Neg	Neg
Outcome				Pos		Pos	
Positive Symptoms	Pos		Neg			Neg	Neg
Negative Symptoms				Neg		Neg	Neg
Cognitive Impairment			Neg	Neg			

Pos = positive correlation; Neg = negative correlation; SL = sleep latency;
TST = total sleep time; SE = sleep efficiency;
SWS %/min = minutes or percentage of slow wave sleep;
REM %/min = minutes or percentage of REM sleep
*= modified from Chors et al [41]

Associations between Sleep and Clinical Parameters

A number of relationships have been described between sleep variables and clinical variables, including severity of illness, positive symptoms, negative symptoms, neurocognitive impairment and outcome (Table 1). However, it should be considered that the limited number of methodologically rigorous studies limits the strength of these associations.

Several studies found significant associations between EEG sleep measures and severity of illness in patients with schizophrenia, usually assessing severity with eitherthe Positive and Negative Symptoms Scale (PANSS) or Brief Psychiatric Rating Scale (BPRS). Negative correlations have been described between TST and SE and the severity of psychosis in patients washed-out from haloperidol treatment [33]. Furthermore, REM latency inversely correlates with BPRS total score [21, 34, 35], and REM density shows negative associations with both BPRS and PANSS total scores [27, 30]. Eventually, REM duration has been associated both positively and negatively to BPRS total score [30, 36].

SWS and REM latency have been positively associated with outcomes from 4 weeks to 2 years after the baseline polysomnographic recording [37]. Another study replicated the association between shorter REM latency and poorer outcome, but did not confirm the role of SWS as a predictor of outcome [38].

The severity of positive symptoms has been negatively correlated with REM density in both medicated [39] and drug-free patients [30]. Moreover, REM latency showed a negative correlation with the degree of positive symptoms in both drug-naïvepatients and in patients withdrawn from medication for 2 [21] or 4 weeks[34]. Interestingly, the BRPS sub-factor "thinking disturbance", the analogue of positive symptoms for the PANSS, showed a positive relationship with sleep latency [40].

A decrease in SWS has been consistently associated with an increase in negative symptoms in a number of studies [41-43],and this association remained significant evenafter correction for age and depression [41]. Moreover,REM latency [21, 35] and REM density [42] inversely correlate with the severity of negative symptoms, and this seems to be independent of depression status [21]. Numerous sleep parameters have been associated with different neurocognitive tests. The PANSS cognitive symptom subscore has been negatively correlated with SWS in drug-free patients [30]. Another group reported an association between memory function and sleep in schizophrenia patients [43]: performancesin the recall of Rey-Osterrieth complex figure and a test for spatial memory were significantly impaired the morning after polysomnographic recording. These impairments were negatively correlated in SWS and SE. Overall, studies of correlates of sleep abnormalities in schizophrenia suggest that insomnia and REM variables are associated with psychotic state and positive symptoms, while SWS deficits seem to be related to negative symptoms and cognitive dysfunction.

Effect of Antipsychotics on Sleep

Notwithstanding the high prevalence of sleep disturbance in patients with schizophrenia and its correlation to many clinical features of the disorder, few studies have adequately studied the influence of antipsychotics on sleep either in healthy subjects or in patients with schizophrenic.Rigorous studies on the effects of antipsychotics on sleep areof additional interest since these drugs are very often used 'off-label' as sedatives and hypnotics in daily practice.Antipsychotics are usually classified as classical or first-generation drugs (which are often further divided into high-potency and low-potency antipsychotics) and second-generation antipsychotics. Although a precisedefinition for second-generation antipsychotics does not exist, their most important qualities are a considerably lower risk of extrapyramidal adverse effects and a better effect on cognitive deficits and negative symptomatology.Table 2 depicts the effects of different classes of antipsychotics on EEG sleep measures.

Table 2. The effects of administration of antipsychotics on sleep in patients

	TST		SE		SWS %/min		REM %/min		REM latency		REM density	
	Ctr	Sch	Ctr	Sch	Ctr	Sch	Ctr	Sch	Ctr	Sch	Ctr	Sch
Low potency 1st generation antipsychotics	↑	↑	↑	↑	↑	↑	(↑↓)	↓	(↑↓)	↓	n.s.	n.s.
High potency 1st generation antipsychotics	n.s.	↑	n.s.	↑	n.s.	n.s.	n.s.	n.s.	n.s.	↑	n.s.	n.s.
2nd generation antipsychotics	↑	↑	↑	↑	(↑↓)	(↑↓)	(↑↓)	(↑↓)	(↑↓)	(↑↓)	n.a.	↑

Ctr = healthy subjects; Sch = schizophrenic patients; TST = total sleep time; SE = sleep efficiency;
SWS %/min = minutes or percentage of slow wave sleep; REM %/min = minutes or percentage of REM sleep;
n.s. = not significant; n.a. = not available; ↑ indicates increase; ↓ indicates decrease;
(↑↓) indicates that some compounds determine an increase, while others a decreaseor no effect (see text for more information);

Given the small number of studies and their methodological limitations, it is difficult to define a specific profile for low-potency versus high-potency first-generation antipsychotic drugs.

The majority of the studies investigating low-potency antipsychotics, such as chlorpromazine, levomepromazine, mesoridazine and sulpirideshowed an increase in TST or SE in both healthy individuals and schizophrenia patients [44-50]. Interestingly, high-potency antipsychotics such ashaloperidol, thiothixene, fluphenazine and pimozide demonstrated a similar effect on TST and SE in schizophrenia patients[35, 51-54], while in healthy controls they seem to have negligible effects on the same measures [55-57]. The lower dose and acute administration in healthy individuals compared to the higher dose and chronic schedule in schizophrenic patients could partly account for this difference. Administration of some low-potency antipsychotics, like chlorpromazine, levomepromazine and promethazineshowed an increase in SWS sleep in healthy subjects andpatients with schizophrenia [44, 49, 58]. Conversely, high-potency antipsychoticsconsistently displayed no effect on SWS in the same populations [35, 51-57].

Concerning REM measures, the effects of first generation antipsychotics varies from one compound to another. The acute administration of two low potency antipsychotics, namely chlorpromazine and promethazine, in healthy subjects determined a decrease in REM sleep in some but not all studies [58-59]. Conversely, levomepromazine and mesoridazine increased REM sleep in healthy individuals [44, 60]. REM latency is increased by acute administration oflevomepromazine and promethazine in healthy subjects [44, 58], but a decrease was reported after the acute administration of chlorpromazinein healthy controls [61-63]. Moreover, chronic administration of chlorpromazine in schizophrenia patients may increase REM density [49]. Eventually, mostlow potency first generation antipsychotics showed no effects on REM density [58, 59, 63]. It has been consistently shown that high-potencydrugs mainly leave REM sleep unaffected in both healthy subjects and patients with schizophrenia [51-57]. Some drugs of this class were associated withan increase in REM latency [35, 52, 53], althoughpimozide andtrifluoperazine did not [56, 57].REM density showed to be uninfluenced by most high potency first-generation antipsychotics.

Most of the second-generation antipsychotics studied show an increase in TST and SE in both healthy subjects and schizophrenia patients [64-74]. Risperidone is the only memberof this group of drugs that leave these variables unaffected [57, 71]. On the contrary, the effects of second-generation drugs on REM and NREM parameters are extremely variable, and often each drughas its own profile.

Olanzapine and ziprasidone were associated with an increase in SWS in healthy individuals and schizophrenia patients [57, 67, 68], while clozapine displayed a decrease in the same populations [57, 64-66];risperidone, paliperidone and quietiapine seemed to have no effects on thismeasure [69, 70, 72, 74].Studies on olanzapine have generated conflicting data on its relationship with REM sleep duration: both an increase and decrease were observed in healthy individuals and schizophreniapatients[57, 65]. Two studies with clozapine found an increase in REM sleep durationin patients with schizophrenia[],whilemost studies on healthy controls and patients found no effect [64, 69-71, 77]. Risperidonecauses a decrease in REM sleep durationin healthy individuals [78], but no significant change in schizophrenia [71]. Concerning REM latency, the results are similar. Olanzapine caused an increase in REM latency in some, but not all studies, in healthy controls and schizophrenia patients [65, 66, 73]. Clozapine increases REM latency in schizophrenia patients [71], but not in healthy individuals [64, 77].Clozapine and olanzapine increase REM density in schizophrenia patients [71, 73].

Clinical Presentation and Treatment

As mentioned earlier, clinicians often overlook sleep disturbance in schizophrenia patients. Nevertheless, the implementation of a specific therapy to address this problem is of fundamental importance since sleep disturbance is one of the most important causes of antipsychotic drug discontinuation in schizophrenia patients [79]. Although schizophrenia has an extreme clinical variability, patients withsleep disturbance can be divided into two different categories.

The first is represented by psychotic episodes, characterized by hallucinations, delusions and cognitive and behavioural disorganization. During these episodes patients typically report intense emotional experiences.

Fear, anger and hostility together with motor and psychic hyperactivity maybe present during psychotic episodes and have an effect in sleep continuity measures and subjective quality, particularly if experienced during the evening. In this context, the emotional hyper-arousal is a determining factor. Therapy is aetiopathogenetic and based on the administration of antipsychotics.

Indeed, the improvement of psychotic symptoms determines an improvement in sleep disturbance. For this purpose, molecules with important sedating action (drugs acting on multiple receptor systems with high affinity for H1 receptors) are employed together with dose boost in the evening. Some drugs (e.g. clozapine) are effective in improving total sleep time without causing daily somnolence; others (e.g.selective D2 antagonists), when employed at sedating doses,cancause drug-induced sleep disturbance due to their extrapyramidal effects. Add-on therapy with phenothiazine derivatives in the evening hours produces symptomatic sleep improvement in some patients. In the acute psychotic episode, the use of hypnotics acting on GABA receptors such as benzodiazepines, zolpidem and zopiclone are of modest efficacy unless administered at sedating doses. More recently, the administration of melatonin appearedto be effective in improving residual insomnia, while bearing virtually no risk to induce sedation or daytime sleepiness in schizophrenia patients [80].

The second group of patients is characterized by schizophrenia phases when apathy, aboulia, alogia, adynamia and loss of programming ability are predominant symptoms. In this condition hyperarousal is not present, and the most frequent sleep disturbance is circadian rhythm alteration with a partial or total inversion of the waking-sleep cycle. Moreover, these patients typically spend more time in bed (up to 12 hours) than healthy individuals, but they have marked impairment in sleep efficiency usually resulting in normal total sleep time. Interestingly, antipsychotic drugs, even when administered at low doses as maintenance therapy, are associated with this wake-sleep phase delay as observed for the lack of stimuli and the abuse of legal and illegal psychostimulant drugs. Wake-sleep phase alteration in schizophrenia patients is difficult to manage. Indeed, both evening dose boosting of antipsychotics and GABAergic drugs have limited efficacy. Positive results have been obtained with non-pharmacological intervention that increment the patient's stimulation and progressively reduce morning sleep. Melatonin administration maybe beneficial in these patients given that they do not have the physiological circadian secretion of this wake-sleep phase regulating hormone [81].

Conclusion

Sleep-onset,the maintenance of insomnia and impaired sleep quality are characteristic hallmarks in schizophrenia patients regardless of either the phase of the disorder or themedication status. Moreover, most studies reported a decrease in SWS and REM latency, but no changes in REM sleep duration and density.Available therapies show some improvement in patients, but much remains to be done to improve efficacy and tolerability. Sleep disturbance in schizophrenia should be specifically targeted, given that the available data suggests thatthisis likely tohave a positive impact on the quality of life. In the future, studies overcoming current methodological shortcomings, together with advancements in our understating of the pathophysiology of sleep disturbance in schizophrenia, should provide more definitiveevidence for the management of this difficult clinical issue.

References

[1] McGrath J., Saha S., Chant D., Welham J. Schizophrenia: a concise overview of incidence, prevalence, and mortality. *Epidemiol. Rev.*, 2008; 30: 67–76.

[2] Castle D., Wessely S., Der G., et al. The incidence of operationally defined schizophrenia in Camberwell, 1965–84. *Br. J. Psychiatry.*, 1991;159:790–4.

[3] Wykes T., Reeder C., Landau S., et al. Cognitive remediation therapy in schizophrenia: randomised controlled trial. *Br. J. Psychiatry.* 2007 May; 190: 421-7.

[4] Lewis D. A., Levitt P. Schizophrenia as a disorder of neurodevelopment. *Ann. Rev. Neurosci.*, 2002; 25: 409-432.

[5] Siris S. G. Suicide and schizophrenia. *J. Psychopharmacol.*, 2001; 15(2): 127-135.

[6] Doi Y., Minowa M., Uchiyama M., et al. Psychometric assess- ment of subjective sleep quality using the Japanese version of the Pittsburgh Sleep Quality Index (PSQI-J) in psychiatric disordered and control subjects. *Psychiatry Res.*, 2000 Dec 27; 97 (2-3): 165-72.

[7] Ritsner M., Kurs R., Ponizovsky A., et al. Perceived quality of life in schizophrenia: relationships to sleep quality. *Qual. Life Res. May*, 2004; 13 (4): 783-91.

[8] Donlon P. T., Blacker K. H. Clinical recognition of early schizo- phrenic decompensation. *Dis. Nerv. Syst. Jun.*, 1975; 36 (6): 323- 7.

[9] Kumar S., Thara R., Rajkumar S. Coping with symptoms of relapse in schizophrenia. *Eur. Arch. Psychiatry Neurol. Sci.*, 1989; 239 (3): 213-5.

[10] Jorgensen P. Schizophrenic delusions: the detection of warning signals. *Schizophr. Res.*, 1998 Jun 22; 32 (1): 17-22.

[11] Hofstetter J. R., Mayeda A. R., Happel C. G., et al. Sleep and daily activity preferences in schizophrenia: associations with neurocognition and symptoms. *J. Nerv. Ment. Dis.*, 2003; 191:408-410.

[12] Mattai A. A., Tossell J., Greenstein D. K., et al. Sleep disturbances in childhood-onset schizophrenia. *Schizopr. Res.,* 2006; 86:123-129.

[13] Lee Y. J., Cho S. J., Cho I. H., et al. The relationship between psychotic-like experiences and sleep disturbances in adolescents. *Sleep med.,* 2012; 13: 1021-1027.

[14] Detre T. On the psychodynamics and the ego psychology of the depressive illnesses: sleep disorder and psychosis. *Can. Psychiatr. Assoc. J.,* 1966; 11 Spec Suppl.: S169-77.

[15] Haffmans P. M., Hoencamp E., Knegtering H. J., et al. Sleep disturbance in schizophrenia. *Br. J. Psychiatry.,* 1994 Nov; 165 (5): 697-8.

[16] Serretti A., Mandelli L., Lattuada E., et al. Depressive syndrome in major psychoses: a study on 1351 subjects. *Psychiatry Res.,* 2004 Jun 30; 127 (1-2): 85-99.

[17] Royuela A., Macias J. A., Gil-Verona J. A., et al. Sleep in schizo- phrenia: a preliminary study using the Pittsburgh Sleep Quality Index. *Neurobiol. Sleep Wakefulness Cycle,* 2002; 2 (2): 37-9.

[18] Chouinard S., Poulin J., Stip E., et al. Sleep in untreated patients with schizophrenia: a meta-analysis. *Schizophr. Bull.,* 2004; 30 (4): 957-67.

[19] Jus K., Bouchard M., Jus A. K., et al. Sleep EEG studies in untreated, long-term schizophrenic patients. *Arch. Gen. Psychiatry,* 1973; 29: 386–390.

[20] Ganguli R., Reynolds C. F., Kupfer D. J. Electroencephalographic sleep in young, never-medicated schizophrenics. *Arch. Gen. Psychiatry,* 1987; 44: 36–44.

[21] Tandon R., Shipley J. E., Taylor S., et al. Electroencephalographic sleep abnormalities in schizophrenia. *Arch. Gen. Psychiatry,* 1992; 49: 185–194.

[22] Lauer C. J., Schreiber W., Pollmächer T., et al. Sleep in schizophrenia: A polysomnographic study of drug-naive patients. *Neuropsychopharmacology,* 1997: 16; 51–60.

[23] Lauer C. J., Krieg J. C. Slow-wave sleep and ventricular size: A comparative study in schizophrenia and major depression. *Biol. Psychiatry,* 1998; 44: 121–128.

[24] Benson K. L., Faull K. F., Zarcone V. P. Evidence for the role of serotonin in the regulation of slow wave sleep in schizophrenia. *Sleep,* 1991: 14; 133–139.

[25] Benson K. L., Zarcone V. P. Rapid eye movement sleep eye movements in schizophrenia and depression. *Arch. Gen. Psychiatry,* 1993; 5: 474–482.

[26] Hiatt J. F., Floyd T. C., Katz P. H., et al. Further evidence of abnormal non-rapid-eye-movements sleep in schizophrenia. *Arch. Gen. Psychiatry,* 1987; 42: 797–802.

[27] Poulin J., Daoust A. M., Forest G., et al. Sleep architecture and its clinical correlates in first episode and neuroleptic-naive pa- tients with schizophrenia. *Schizophr. Res.,* 2003 Jul 1; 62 (1-2): 147-53.

[28] Benson K. L., Sullivan E. V., Lim K. O., et al. Slow wave sleep and computed tomographic measures of brain morphology in schizophrenia. *Psychiatry Res.,* 1996; 60: 125–134.

[29] Hoffmann R., Hendricks E. W., Rush A. J., et al. Slow-wave activity during non-REM sleep in men with schizophrenia and major depressive disorders. *Psychiatry Res.,* 2000; 95: 215–225.

[30] Yang C., Winkelman J. W. Clinical significance of sleep EEG abnormalities in chronic schizophrenia. *Schizophr. Res.,* 2006 Feb 28; 82 (2-3): 251-60.

[31] Sarkar S, Katshu M. Z. U. H., Nizamie S. H., et al. Slow wave sleep deficits as a trait marker in patients with schizophrenia. *Schizopr. Res.,* 2010; 124:127-133.

[32] Ferrarelli F., Peterson M. J., Sarasso S., et al. Thalamic Dysfunction in Schizophrenia Suggested by Whole-Night Deficits in Slow and Fast Spindles. *Am. J. Psychiatry*, 2010; 167: 1339-1348.

[33] Neylan T. C., van Kammen D. P., Kelley M. E., et al. Sleep in schizophrenic patients on and off haloperidol therapy: clinically stable vs relapsed patients. *Arch. Gen. Psychiatry*, Aug 1992; 49 (8): 643-9.

[34] Thaker G. K., Wagman A. M., Tamminga C. A. Sleep polygraphy in schizophrenia: methodological issues. *Biol. Psychiatry*, 1990 Aug 1; 28 (3): 240-6.

[35] Taylor S. F., Tandon R., Shipley J. E., et al. Effect of neuroleptic treatment on polysomnographic measures in schizophrenia. *Biol. Psychiatry*, 1991 Nov 1; 30 (9): 904-12.

[36] Keshavan M. S., Reynolds III C. F., Ganguli R, et al. Electroen- cephalographic sleep and cerebral morphology in functional psychoses: a preliminary study with computed tomography. *Psychiatry Res.*, 1991 Dec; 39 (3): 293-301.

[37] Strauss J. S., Carpenter W. T. The prediction of outcome in schizo- phrenia: I. Characteristics of outcome. *Arch. Gen. Psychiatry*, 1972 Dec; 27 (6): 739-46.

[38] Goldman M., Tandon R., DeQuardo J. R., et al. Biological predictors of 1-year outcome in schizophrenia in males and females. *Schizophr. Res.*, 1996 Aug 23; 21 (2): 65-73.

[39] Rotenberg V. S., Hadjez J., Indursky P., et al. Eye movements density in positive and negative schizophrenia. *Homeostasis*, 1997; 38: 97-102.

[40] Zarcone V. P., Benson K. L. BPRS symptom factors and sleep variables in schizophrenia. *Psychiatry Res.*, 1997 Feb 7; 66 (2- 3): 111-20.

[41] Chors S. Sleep disturbances in patients with schizophrenia: impact and effect of antipsychotics. *CNS Drugs*, 2008;22(11):939-62. Review.

[42] Riemann D., Hohagen F., Krieger S., et al. Cholinergic REM induction test: muscarinic supersensitivity underlies polysomnographic findings in both depression and schizo- phrenia. *J. Psychiatr. Res.*, 1994 May-Jun; 28 (3): 195-210.

[43] Goder R., Boigs M., Braun S., et al. Impairment of visuospatial memory is associated with decreased slow wave sleep in schizophrenia. *J. Psychiatr. Res.*, 2004 Nov-Dec; 38 (6): 591-9.

[44] Kanno O., Watanabe H., Kazamatsuri H. Effects of zopiclone, flunitrazepam, triazolam and levomepromazine on the tran- sient change in sleep-wake schedule: polygraphic study, and the evaluation of sleep and daytime condition. *Prog. Neuropsychopharmacol Biol. Psychiatry*, 1993 Mar; 17 (2): 229-39.

[45] Lewis S. A., Evans J. I. Dose effects of chlorpromazine on human sleep. *Psychopharmacologia*, 1969; 14 (4): 342-8.

[46] Hartmann E., Cravens J. The effects of long term administration of psychotrophic drugs on human sleep: IV. The effects of chlorpromazine. *Psychopharmacologia*, 1973; 33 (3): 203-18.

[47] Gaillard J. M., Moneme A. Modification of dream content after preferential blockade of mesolimbic and mesocortical dopa- minergic systems. *J. Psychiatr. Res.*, 1977; 13 (4): 247-56.

[48] Kupfer D. J., Wyatt R. J., Synder F., et al. Chlorpromazine and sleep in psychiatric patients. *Arch. Gen. Psychiatry*, 1971 Feb; 24 (2): 185-9.

[49] Kaplan J., Dawson S., Vaughan T., et al. Effect of prolonged chlorpromazine administration on the sleep of chronic schizophrenics. *Arch. Gen. Psychiatry*, 1974; 31 (1): 62-681.

[50] Brannen J. O., Jewett R. E. Effects of selected phenothiazines on REM sleep in schizophrenics. *Arch. Gen. Psychiatry*, 1969 Sep; 21 (3): 284-90.

[51] Gillin J. C., van Kammen D. P., Post R., et al. Effects of prolonged administration of pimozide on sleep-EEG patterns in psychiat- ric patients. *Commun. Psychopharmacol.*, 1977; 1 (3): 225-32.

[52] Keshavan M. S., Reynolds C. F., Miewald J. M., et al. A longitudinal study of EEG sleep in schizophrenia. *Psychiatry Res.*, 1996; 59 (3): 203-11.

[53] Maixner S., Tandon R., Eiser A., et al. Effects of antipsychotic treatment on polysomnographic measures in schizophrenia: a replication and extension. *Am. J. Psychiatry*, 1998; 155 (11): 1600-2.

[54] Wetter T. C., Lauer C. J., Gillich G., et al. The electroencepha- lographic sleep pattern in schizophrenic patients treated with clozapine or classical antipsychotic drugs. *J. Psychiatr. Res.*, Nov-Dec 1996; 30 (6): 411-9.

[55] Clarenbach P., Prunkl R., Riegler M., et al. Effects of haloperidol on afternoon sleep and on the secretion of growth hormone in man. *Neuroscience*, 1978; 3 (3): 345-8.

[56] Puca F. M., Dammacco F., Rigillo N., et al. Increzione somato- tropinica ed EEG durante il sonno notturno dell' adulto normale dopo pimozide. *Boll. Soc. Ital. Biol. Sper.*, 1978 Mar 15; 54 (5): 460-5.

[57] Gimenez S., Clos S., Romero S., et al. Effects of olanzapine, risperidone and haloperidol on sleep after a single oral morn- ing dose in healthy volunteers. *Psychopharmacology*, (Berl) Mar 2007; 190 (4): 507-16.

[58] Risberg A. M , Risberg J., Ingvar D. H. Effects of promethazine on nocturnal sleep in normal man. *Psychopharmacologia*, 1975 Sep 17; 43 (3): 279-84.

[59] Feinberg I., Wender P. H., Koresko R. L., et al. Differential effects of chlorpromazine and phenobarbital on EEG sleep patterns. *J. Psychiatr. Res.*, 1969 Dec; 7 (2): 101-9.

[60] Adam K., Allen S., Carruthers Jones I., et al. Mesoridazine and human sleep. *Br. J. Clin. Pharmacol.*, Feb 1976; 3 (1): 157-63.

[61] Lester B. K., Guerrero Figueroa R. Effects of some drugs on electroencephalographic fast activity and dream time. *Psycho- physiology*, Jan 1966; 2 (3): 224-36.

[62] Sagales T., Erill S., Domino E. F. Differential effects of scopolam- ine and chlorpromazine on REM and NREM sleep in nor- mal male subjects. *Clin. Pharmacol. Ther.*, 1969 Jul-Aug; 10 (4): 522-9.

[63] Lester B. K., Coulter J. D., Cowden L. C., et al. Chlorpromazine and human sleep. *Psychopharmacologia*, 1971; 20 (3): 280-7.

[64] Touyz S. W., Beumont P. J., Saayman G. S., et al. A psychophysio- logical investigation of the short-term effects of clozapine upon sleep parameters of normal young adults. *Biol. Psychiatry*, 1977 Dec; 12 (6): 801-22.

[65] Sharpley A. L., Vassallo C. M., Cowen P. J. Olanzapine increases slow-wave sleep: evidence for blockade of central 5- HT(2C) receptors in vivo. *Biol. Psychiatry*, 2000 Mar 1; 47 (5): 468-70.

[66] Sharpley A. L., Vassallo C. M., Pooley E. C., et al. Allelic variation in the 5-HT2C receptor (HT2RC) and the increase in slow wave sleep produced by olanzapine. *Psychopharmacol.*, (Berl) 2001 Jan 1; 153 (2): 271-2.

[67]   Cohrs S., Rodenbeck A., Guan Z., et al. Sleep-promoting proper- ties of quetiapine in healthy subjects. *Psychopharmacol.*, (Berl) 2004; 174 (3): 421-9.

[68]   Cohrs S., Meier A., Neumann A. C., et al. Improved sleep continui- ty and increased slow wave sleep and REM latency during ziprasidone treatment: a randomized, controlled, crossover trial of 12 healthy male subjects. *J. Clin. Psychiatry*, 2005 Aug; 66 (8): 989-96.

[69]   Hinze-Selch D., Mullington J., Orth A., et al. Effects of clozapine on sleep: a longitudinal study. *Biol. Psychiatry*, 1997; 42 (4): 260-6.

[70]   Lee J. H., Woo J. I., Meltzer H. Y. Effects of clozapine on sleep measures and sleep-associated changes in growth hormone and cortisol in patients with schizophrenia. *Psychiatry Res.*, 2001 Sep 20; 103 (2-3): 157-66.

[71]   Tandon R. Effects of atypical antipsychotics on polysomno- graphic measures in schizophrenia. In: Judd LL, Saletu B, Filip V, editors. *Basic and clinical science of mental and addictive disorders.* Vol. 167. Basel: Karger, 1997: 219-22.

[72]   Salin Pascual R. J., Herrera Estrella M., Galicia Polo L., et al. Olanzapine acute administration in schizophrenic patients in- creases delta sleep and sleep efficiency. *Biol. Psychiatry*, 1999 Jul 1; 46 (1): 141-3.

[73]   Muller M. J., Rossbach W., Mann K., et al. Subchronic effects of olanzapine on sleep EEG in schizophrenic patients with pre- dominantly negative symptoms. *Pharmacopsychiatry,* Jul 2004; 37 (4): 157-62.

[74]   Luthringer R., Staner L., Noel N., et al. A double-blind, placebo- controlled, randomized study evaluating the effect of paliper- idone extended-release tablets on sleep architecture in patients with schizophrenia. *Int. Clin. Psychopharmacol.*, 2007 Sep; 22 (5): 299-308.

[75]   Rüther E., Davis L., Papousek M., et al. Pharmakologische Beein- flussung zentraler serotonerger Mechanismen am Menschen und Auswirkungen auf den Schlaf. *Arzneimittelforschung,* 1976; 26 (6): 1071-3.

[76]   Blum A., Girke W. Marked increase in REM sleep produced by a new antipsychotic compund. *Clin. Electoencephalogr.*, 1973; 4 (2): 80-4.

[77]   Touyz S. W., Saayman G. S., Zabow T. A psychophysiological investigation of the long-term effects of clozapine upon sleep patterns of normal young adults. *Psychopharmacology,* (Berl) 1978 Jan 31; 56 (1): 69-73.

[78]   Sharpley A. L., Bhagwagar Z., Hafizi S., et al. Risperidone aug- mentation decreases rapid eye movement sleep and decreases wake in treatment-resistant depressed patients. *J. Clin. Psychiatry,* Feb 2003; 64 (2): 192-6.

[79]   Benson K. L. Sleep in schizophrenia: impairments, correlates, and treatment. *Psychiatr. Clin. North Am.,* 2006 Dec;29(4):1033-45.

[80]   Shamir E., Laudon M., Barak Y., et al. Melatonin improves sleep quality of patients with chronic schizophrenia. *J. Clin. Psychiatry*, 2000;61:373-7.

[81]   Bromundt V., Köster M., Georgiev-Kill A., et al. Sleep–wake cycles and cognitive functioning in schizophrenia. *Br. J. Psychiatry*, 2011; 198:269-76.

In: Sleep Medicine
Editors: A. Del Casale, R. Brugnoli and P. Girardi

ISBN: 978-1-62808-515-0
© 2013 Nova Science Publishers, Inc.

Chapter XII

Substance-Related Sleep Disorders

Alessandro E. Vento[1,] and Paolo Girardi[1]*
[1]Sapienza University, NESMOS (Neuroscience, Mental Health and Sensory Organs)
Department, School of Medicine and Psychology, Rome, Italy

Abstract

The consumption of a wide variety of substances determines, through different mechanisms, the onset of sleep disturbances, which has a considerable impact on the neurobiology of sleep-wake circadian rhythm. Many substances are widely used and easy to find, such as alcohol, nicotine and caffeine and are frequently the cause of degradation in quality and quantity of sleep. Furthermore, substance abuse is often associated with poor sleep hygiene. In this case, the regularity of sleep-wake cycle is affected not only by the direct effect of the substances, but also by the presence of correlated disturbing factors in the sleep environment that do not support the synchronization of circadian cycle [1]. Even illicit substances, both psychostimulants and inhibitors of central nervous system - such as heroin, cocaine and ecstasy - have mechanisms of action that lead to a high potential for dysregulation of sleep. The current literature describes sleep abnormalities related to the use/abuse of many other substances sold on the street market or on the internet: cannabis, hallucinogens, methamphetamine, novel psychoactive drugs, etc. In a considerable number of cases, sleep disturbances are caused by prescribed substances - such as corticosteroids, beta-blockers, benzodiazepines and hypnotics, antidepressants, chemotherapy, etc. - which can adversely affect sleep through several different mechanisms. In particular, a significant impact on the above phenomenon is represented by the long-term use of sedative-hypnotics compounds, mainly benzodiazepines, that may generate a dysregulation of sleep through the onset of dependence patterns [2]. From 3-7% of all sleep disorders are caused by use/abuse of psychotropic substances, and 12-16% do have not an apparent cause. It is possible to hypothesize that a variable percentage of these cases could be drug-related cases, underestimated for various reasons. Furthermore, sleep disturbances and substance use correlate with an increased prevalence of psychiatric disorders. It has been reported that 51% of patients with psychiatric disorders become addicted to at least one substance, and

---

* E-mail: ventoalessandro@hotmail.com.

41-66% of individuals with substance dependence/addiction have a psychiatric disorder. Mental disorders are the main cause of sleep disturbances (e.g. psychiatric illness represents about 30-40% of all cases of insomnia). This fact emphasizes the strong correlation between psychopathology, use/abuse of substances and sleep disorders [3, 4, 5]. The discussion of the molecular and neurobiological mechanisms that bring into connection the use/abuse of substances with qualitative and quantitative alterations of sleep is the central focus of this chapter.

Introduction

Sleep disorders frequently occur while using psychotropic substances as result of both acute *intoxication* - due to the pharmacodynamic effect - and *withdrawal* syndrome - such a consequence of drug-related neurobiological long-term changes. In fact, the conditions of drug dependence and addictionare a key elementin the pathogenesis of substance-related sleep disorders. In particular, drug addiction is a chronically relapsing disorder that is characterized by compulsion to seek and take the drug, loss of control in limiting intake, and emergence of a negative emotional state (e.g. dysphoria,anxiety, irritability that frequently results in insomnia or hypersomnia). This condition reflects a motivational withdrawal syndrome when access to the drug is prevented (defined as Substance Dependence by the DSM-IV-TR) [6]. According to Koob and Volkow, "the occasional but limited use of an abusable drug is clinically distinct from escalated drug use, loss of control over limiting drug intake, and the emergence of chronic critical nature of the distinction between drug use, abuse and dependence has been demonstrated by data showing that approximately 15% of the adult population will engage in non-medical or illicit drug use at some time in their lives, with approximately 3% going on to substance dependence on illicit drugs". The focus of current studies on drug addiction is shifting to chronic administration and the acute and long-term neuroadaptive changes in the brain that result in relapse and onset of many symptoms (among which insomnia, hypersomnia and parasomnias) [7].

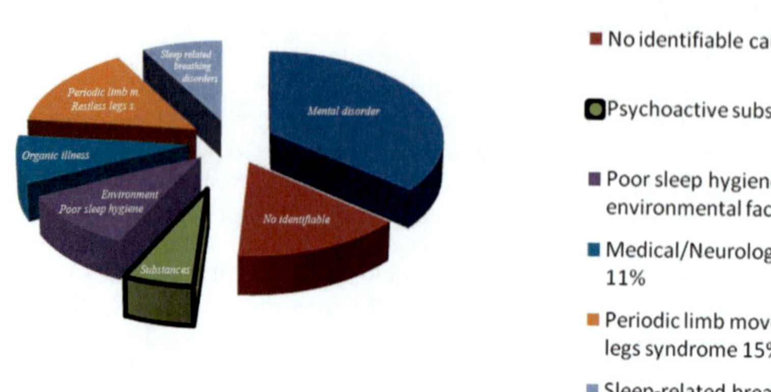

Source: NIH – U.S.A. 2010.

Figure 1. Causes of Sleep Disorders.

Furthermore, sleep disorders can play an important role in the outcome of addiction, sometimes acting as a balance or as a trigger for the relapse. Regarding this, a relevant mechanism is the increase of cortisol and corticosterone resulting in activation of the hypothalamic-pituitary-adrenal axis due to the long-term abuse of substances. These hormones increase brain arousal and frequently cause insomnia [8].

Matching the neurobiological mechanisms of sleep regulation, described in the previous chapters, with the pharmacodynamic knowledge on the effects of drugs and the changes that occur due to the chronic exposure to a substance, we can argue that several neurotransmitter systems are involved in substance-related sleep disorders as a common target. In this context, many studies have reported the role of serotonin in the regulation of sleep (e.g. as a precursor of melatonin - N-acetyl-serotonin - and through the involvement of neurons in the raphe area). As previously shown, even noradrenergic neurons are involved in the regulation of the sleep-wake cycle and N-methyl-D-aspartate (NMDA) transmission. Neurons that release acetylcholine in the pontine reticular formation and in other regions of the basal forebrain (REM-ON neurons), also involved in depression-related insomnia, are involved in substance-related sleep disorders. The GABAergic system, strongly influenced by alcohol and benzodiazepines, is the main inhibitory system of the brain and, therefore, plays a delicate role in regulating the sleep-wake cycle. We must also include the meso-limbic dopamine system, as it is the main target in the onset of addiction, in addition to the meso-cortical and tuber-infundibular dopamine system, which are both involved in the regulation of arousal levels and the circadian cycle. The secretion of melatonin by the pineal gland, usually inhibited by the light of day, would seem to be influenced by the use of several substances. Thus, the suprachiasmatic nucleus of the hypothalamus, usually with circadian pacemaker function for the melatonin secretion and on the entire 24 hour sleep-wake cycle, may be desynchronized by the use of psychotropic substances [2, 8, 9].

On the other hand,from a clinical perspective,when a physician encounters a case of sleep disorder the possibility of use/abuse or the existence of dependence/addiction to psychoactive substances should be investigated. Nonetheless, when there is evidence that the sleep disturbance is directly due to exposure to medications, alcohol or other drugs, it is appropriate to make a diagnosis of substance-induced sleep disorder [6].

In the DSM-IV-TR, this diagnostic category requires fulfillment of the following criteria:

A. a prominent disturbance in sleep that is sufficiently severe to warrant independent clinical attention.

B. there is evidence from history, physical examination, or laboratory findings of either 1 or 2:

1. the symptoms in criterion A developed during, or within a month of, substance intoxication or withdrawal;

2. medication use is aetiologically related to the sleep disturbance;

C. the disturbance is not better accounted for by a sleep disorder that is not substance induced. Evidence that the symptoms are better accounted for by a sleep disorder that is not substance induced might include the following: the symptoms precede the onset of the substance use (or medication use); the symptoms persist for a substantial period of time (e.g. about a month) after cessation of acute withdrawal or severe intoxication, or are substantially in excess of what would be expected given the type or amount of the substance used or the duration of use; or there is other evidence that suggests the existence of an independent non-substance-induced sleep disorder (e.g. a history of recurrent non-substance-related episodes);

D.　the disturbance does not occur exclusively during the course of a delirium;

E.　the sleep disturbance causes clinically significant distress or impairment in social, occupational or other important areas of functioning.

This diagnosis should be made when the sleep symptoms are in excess of those usually associated with the intoxication or withdrawal syndrome and when symptoms are sufficiently severe to warrant independent clinical attention. Sleep disorders can be induced by many substances, including alcohol, amphetamine, caffeine, cocaine, opiates, sedative-hypnotic and/or other substances. It is required to specify the predominant type of sleep disorder, such as *insomnia, hypersomnia, parasomnia* or mixed type and, as mentioned above, if with onset during intoxication or during withdrawal.

In the following section, we will try to describe the mechanisms that can trigger the sleep alterations for each single substance category.

Alcohol and Benzodiazepines

Alcohol and benzodiazepines (BDZs) mainly act on γ-aminobutyric acid receptor type A (GABA-A-R). Alcohol also activates nicotinic receptors for acetylcholine, serotonin type 3 receptors (5-HT-3-R) and inhibits glutamate and calcium channel voltage-dependent receptors. Therefore, both alcohol and BDZs produce similar sedative-hypnotic effects and can influence the sleep cycle in terms of hypersomnia or parasomnia - during acute administration - and insomnia or parasomnia after discontinuation of intake or as a consequence of habituation [10]. Alcohol is one of the cultural habits of our society and, unfortunately, is widely used from a young age. BDZs are the most widely prescribed class of psychoactive drugs worldwide. Both can produce addiction. Therefore, screening for current or previous alcohol use/abuse or BZD use is essential in evaluating sleep disorder.

The acute effect of alcohol intake is dose-related and frequently causes drowsiness. As for all the substances described below, the effect varies from individual to individual, and in cases of strong intoxication can lead to coma and death. Therefore, when an individual starts drinking alcohol, and after a long time as well, he/she can develop alcohol-induced hypersomnia.

Even if alcohol intake in the evening is generally associated with an increased ease of falling asleep (i.e. a decreased latency to induction of sleep), alcohol has negative effects on the architecture of sleep. In particular, the use of alcohol is associated with the decrease in the duration of the cycles of REM sleep and deep sleep (stage 4) and therefore is related to increased fragmentation of sleep, as well as longer and more numerous awakening episodes. Considering this, it can be argued that alcohol consumption causes insomnia in the central and late phases of sleep [2]. According to the literature, chronic alcohol assumption (with subsequent habituation and withdrawal when access is prevented) can produce long-lasting changes in neurotransmission, and particularly upon the inhibitory function - involving the γ-aminobutyric acid type A receptors (GABA-A-R) – that are directly related to the onset of sleep disturbances.

The propensity for dependence on alcohol involves both brain reward mechanisms and withdrawal syndrome, leading to increased consumption. Clinical studies have shown that poor objective sleep during the first two weeks of abstinence predicts relapse to alcohol five months after treatment.

Moreover, withdrawal syndrome frequently includes sleep disorders and tolerance to the sedative actions of alcohol and sleep aids. In a rat model of alcohol dependence, involving chronic intermittent ethanol administration, with multiple episodes of intoxication and withdrawal, it is been possible to deduce that multiple withdrawals produce a kindling-like phenomenon. It is also been demonstrated that behavioral changes are induced by a single dose of alcohol and result from changes in subunit composition, subcellular location, pharmacology and function of GABA receptors. In fact, ethanol-sensitive extrasynaptic $\alpha4/\delta$-containing GABA-R-mediated tonic inhibitory currents are rapidly down-regulated, followed by a slower down-regulation of benzodiazepine-sensitive $\alpha1/\gamma2$-mediated inhibitory synaptic currents and increased compensatory $\alpha4/\gamma2$ synaptic GABA-R currents in parallel with increased sensitivity to low mM concentrations of ethanol. While these changes are transient and normalize in a few days, chronic intermittent ethanol exposure (>30 doses) makes remodeling of GABA receptors persistent. In consequence of that, it is possible to affirm that GABA receptor plasticity is essential to the development of alcohol dependence, and at the same time provide a model for sleep disorders in chronic ethanol consumers or ex-consumers [11]. From a clinical point of view, the above fact leads to the appearance of strong/progressive chronic insomnia in long-time alcohol consumers.

Many studies have described secondary forms of REM sleep behavior disorder (a sleep parasomnia characterized by enactment of dream content during REM-sleep associated with loss of muscle atonia) or with narcolepsy, which are associated with neurodegenerative diseases belonging to the model of glutamate-related neurotoxicity or to α-synucleinopathies. However, RBD (REM behavior disorders) may occur in subjects witha history of alcohol abuse or withdrawal [12]. Furthermore, alcohol use is also related to the onset of sleep-disordered breathing, as consequence of obstructive sleep apnea syndrome or internal disorders such as gastro-esophageal reflux [13].

A similar pharmacodynamic and clinical profile may be observed with the acute or chronic use of BDZs. In fact, this category of drugs and alcohol often results in cross-tolerance and cross-dependence. BZDs early users often show sleepiness or hypersomnia and then progress over time toward a state of altered mixed sleep patterns (insomnia alternating with hypersomnia).

The chronic use of BDZs is strictly related to the high prevalence of sleep disorders. BDZs initially result in a reduction of nocturnal awakenings and a prolongation of the total hours of sleep by changing the architecture of sleep, with a strengthening of high frequency electroencephalogram waves and a reduction of slow wave sleep. This is the main reason why these molecules are commonly used in the treatment of insomnia.

However, the subsequent occurrence of tolerance – mainly due to changes in GABA inhibitory neurotransmission - and/or the discontinuation of BDZs intake, with the consequence of rebound phenomenon, may be the cause of sleep disorders, particularly the insomnia type [14].

Nicotine and Caffeine

Nicotine and caffeine are the most consumed psychostimulant drugs worldwide, and at the same time are easy to find in Western countries. The World Health Organization estimated that the prevalence of smoking in Europe is 28.6% (with a large gender difference: 40% among men and 18.2% among women), and that the prevalence of caffeine users is higher than nicotine [15]. According to their wide diffusion, both substances have a high potential for inducing addiction and sleep disorders. At high doses, they are highly toxic and frequently induce insomnia.

Usually, nicotine is taken through cigarette smoke, but is also present in a wide variety of products used for smoking cessation (trans-dermal patches, chewing gum, inhaler and others) and insecticides. The average content of nicotine in a cigarette is 10-20 mg/g of tobacco and by smoking one cigarette the user absorbs about 1-3 mg of nicotine, depending on the mode of "suction" of the smoke and the absorption capacity. For each "shot" in a matter of seconds (about 7 seconds), the substance is absorbed through the lungs and to a lesser extent by the pharyngeal and gastrointestinal mucosa. Its half-life in plasma is approximately 1.5-3 hours, while the half-life of its principal metabolite, cotinine, is around 12-20 hours [16]. Plasma cotinine levels correlate negatively with slow wave sleep in smokers, and subjective quality of sleep is impaired in smokers compared with non-smokers [17]. Nicotine and cotinine work in the CNS by binding to nicotinic acetylcholine receptor (nAChR) expressed in the meso-limbic system and determine a dopamine spike in the nucleus accumbens shell.

High doses of nicotine can produce different symptoms, including agitation and insomnia. The current literature describes the occurrence of some cases of nicotine poisoning [16]. Nicotine activates, on a massive scale, the mesolimbic reward pathway, resulting in an increase of dopaminergic transmission in these areas - through activation of cholinergic receptors (pre-synaptic nicotinic receptors) on dopaminergic neurons, projecting to the nucleus accumbens - producing a sense of gratification and temporary alleviation of negative moods.

We premised that the nicotine reaches the central nervous system in few seconds, determining its pharmacological effect. Thus, each single aspiration constitutes a positive reinforcement. With 10 aspirations per cigarette, a smoker of a pack/day reinforces the habit of smoking 200 times a day. Nicotine quickly generates tolerance and withdrawal [10]. This is the main reason for the onset of sleep disorders in nicotine addicted individuals, and sleep disturbances are also a known risk factor for early relapse after initial tobacco abstinence.

Heavy smokers (>20 cigarettes/day), in order to fight withdrawal because of the short half-life of nicotine, wake up during the night to smoke and restore normal levels of nicotine in the blood, giving rise to a form of secondary insomnia based on withdrawal syndrome. Furthermore, nicotine induces potent inhibition of monoamine oxidase B (MAO-B) and therefore, insomnia in heavy smokers is also supported by a reduced degradation of catecholamines in the brain.

In a polysomnography (PSG) sleep characteristics study, smokers showed a shorter sleep period time, longer sleep latency, higher rapid eye movement sleep density, more sleep apneas and leg movements in sleep than non-smokers (insomnia-like sleep impairments) [17].

Another relevant factor to consider when evaluating sleep problems is the occurrence of mental disorders. As previously mentioned, this factor correlates with both the trend to use/abuse cigarettes and insomnia, making it difficult to distinguish between primary and secondary forms of sleep disorders in this population.

Another link between use of cigarettes and sleep disorders (both parasomnia and insomnia type associated with daytime sleepiness) is the occurrence of chronic obstructive pulmonary disease, frequently present in heavy smokers. Airway obstruction generates the phenomena of obstructive apnea during sleep, often associated with the occurrence of both dyssomnias and parasomnias [18].

All these findings suggest that it is important for sleep researchers to always control smoking status in their analyses.

Caffeine (1,3,7-trimethylxanthine) is a mild psychostimulant contained in plants of coffee, cocoa, tea, cola, guarana, mate, etc., and inside beverages made from them, as well as in many analgesic compounds. This natural alkaloid, due the widespread use of beverages in which it is contained, is largely the most used psychoactive substance. Caffeine blocks, through competitive antagonism, adenosine receptors on membranes thereby increasing the secretion of norepinephrine in several brain areas. The dose of caffeine contained in consumer beverages depends on the concentration of the infusion and quality of the product. On average, a cup of coffee contains 90-100 mg of caffeine, a cup of tea about 50 mg, a can of cola 35 mg; some energy drinks contain 80 mg of caffeine per can. The pharmacological effects of caffeine include the appearance of anxiety, tachycardia, tremor, agitation, and insomnia. There are death reports regarding caffeine in subjects taking about 10 grams (the equivalent of 100 cups of coffee or 50 tablets of 200 mg). Regular consumers of caffeine develop tolerance that results in weakening of the stimulating effect, and simultaneously in a heightened sensitivity to adenosine. Subsequent symptoms include anxiety, irritability, and insomnia. However, the most frequent means through which caffeine generates insomnia is the appearance of its acute effects after consumption. Caffeine has a slow absorption in the digestive tract and a half-life of 5 hours. Therefore, the ingestion of coffee, energy drinks (such as Red Bull, Planet Energy, Coca-Cola) or other beverages containing caffeine later than the early afternoon can cause, because of its stimulating effect, marked insomnia and other sleep disorders. In rare cases, abuse of caffeine meets criteria for addiction, including the unsuccessful attempt to reduce the dose, loss of control in use or prolonged use despite the presence of harmful effects on the user [10, 19]. Furthermore, sleepiness associated with the discontinuation of caffeine assumption is a very frequent occurrence in users of this substance.

Cocaine and Other Psychostimulants (MDMA, Methamphetamine)

Considering that the use of psychostimulants causes sleep disturbance primarily through the acute effect, during the intoxication, we will try to review all the neurobiological mechanisms that can affect sleep in stimulant abusers. In fact, stimulant-related sleep disturbances are very common in clinical practice. The most frequent cases of this condition are linked to the abuse of crack and hydrochloride cocaine, MDMA (ecstasy), other ecstasy-like compounds, methamphetamine (crystal ice or shaboo) and kathinons. Due to their considerable acute stimulating effect on dopaminergic and noradrenergic neurotransmission, these substances generate, among other symptoms, increase of arousal, euphoria and a decreased need for sleep.

Chronic cocaine abusers may feel they are sleeping better during early abstinence, but objective measures show that the opposite happens. A team of NIDA-funded addiction and sleep researchers at the Yale and Harvard Schools of Medicine found evidence of insomnia on days of taking the drug and after 2-3 weeks of abstinence. The researchers believe that cocaine may impair the brain's ability to gauge its own need for sleep, and patients' ability to benefit from early treatment may suffer as a result. After 14 to 17 days of abstinence, the study group exhibited sleep deficits on several measures, relative to healthy, age-matched peers who participated in prior studies. For example, they had less total sleep time (336 versus 421-464 minutes) and took longer to fall asleep (19 versus 6-16 minutes). The time participants took to fall asleep and their total time asleep transiently improved during the first week of abstinence, but then reverted to the patterns recorded on days of cocaine taking. On abstinence days 14-17, participants took an average of 20 minutes to fall asleep (from a low of 11) and slept 40 minutes less than their minimum. Slow-wave sleep rose during a binge and on abstinence days 10-17. Unlike most people with chronic insomnia, cocaine abusers do not perceive sleep problems and may not ask clinicians for treatment to improve sleep. Furthermore, the insidious nature of cocaine-related insomnia may directly trigger relapse in addicted individuals, who may take cocaine to improve sleep-related cognitive functioning deficits. Some medications – such as tiagabine and modafinil - can improve cognitive performance and restore sleep in cocaine abusers. In fact, sleep deprivation constitutes an unmet public health problem in the general population. These findings highlight this important problem in cocaine abusers [20, 21].

MDMA-ecstasy works by binding to the type 2 serotonin receptor (5-HT-2). Ecstasy users report a variety of disorders after taking the drug, including sleep disorders. However, mechanisms that link ecstasy use to sleep disorders - such as sleep domains involved or factors that might predict that ecstasy users may have poor sleep quality and / or excessive daytime sleepiness – are not entirely known [22]. In a study on 395 recreational ecstasy users, about 70% reported sleep disturbance.

Although the frequency of ecstasy use did not affect the degree of reported sleep disturbance, participants who used larger amounts of ecstasy had poorer sleep. In addition, participants who perceived harmful consequences arising from their ecstasy use or had experienced remorse following ecstasy use had poorer sleep. Clinically relevant levels of sleep disturbance were still evident after controlling for polydrug use. Risk factors for poor sleep quality were younger age, injury following ecstasy use and having been told to cut down on ecstasy use.

According to a recent study by Di Iorio et al. [23], sleep disturbance are related to the status of serotonin receptors in the cerebral cortex of a group of MDMA young women consumers. The use of this substance causes a chronic reduction of serotonergic transmission by increasing the number of 5-HT-2A receptors in the occipito-temporo-parietal, frontal, fronto-parietal and fronto-limbic areas even in cases of occasional or recreational ecstasy intake. The degree of functional impairment correlated proportionally with both the increase in number of 5-HT-2A receptors and early age of intake of the substance. In addition, the phenomenon does not seem to decrease with abstinence. This is considered an important neurobiological base for sleep disorders in MDMA consumers.

There is evidence of methamphetamine-induced sleep disturbances in both adolescents and adults. Cloak and co-workers have shown, in a magnetic resonance spectroscopy study, that teenage users of methamphetamine have reduced levels of choline compounds at the level of the anterior cingulate cortex. This finding would seem to interfere with the inhibitory functions of the Stroop Test and with a regular alternation in the sleep-wake cycle, as well as a disturbance in the normal brain maturation [24]. At any rate, various methamphetamine and derivatives induced brain damage have been extensively described and, from a clinical point of view, were all related to the presence of sleep disorders. Using both structural and functional neuroimaging, it has been amply demonstrated that the strong use of methamphetamine is related to long-term alterations of the serotoninergic and dopaminergic systems [25, 26].

The main areas affected are those involved in selective attention (striatum, prefrontal cortex and amygdala) and memory processes (hippocampus). A picture of general hypertrophy of the white matter with decreased gray matter related to sleep disturbance has also been clearly shown.

Cannabis

Cannabis use is widespread in Europe and the rest of the world. The rate of lifetime prevalence in individuals between 15 and 64 years is more than 30% in countries such as Italy and the United Kingdom [27]. A proportion of cannabis users start smoking as an attempt to self-medicate states of hyper-arousal or insomnia in individuals with hyperthymic, cyclothimic or irritable type temperament [28]. Other individuals start smoking for reasons that relate to social interaction with a peer group. However, subsequent cases of sleep disturbance arising from use of cannabis have been described, and the above premise should not be viewed as a master key for the use of this substance treating sleep disorders. Cannabis acts by binding to specific receptors for endogenous cannabinoids (anandamide, 2-arachidonoylglycerol and subsequently 2-arachidonyl glyceryl ether, virodamine, N-arachidonyldopamine, palmithoilethanolamine) located in several regions around the brain. Many studies have shown metabolic changes of CNS resulting from the use of cannabis. In a study by 4 Tesla proton magnetic resonance spectroscopy (H1-MRS) in two-dimensional sequences (2D) it was possible to quantify cannabis metabolites at the level of the basal ganglia, thalamus, cortex and white matter in individuals with cannabis addiction. It was possible to highlight an imbalance in the relationship between inositol and creatine compared to the control group of cannabis non-smokers. Furthermore, this imbalance would have been associated with the onset of behavioral and affective disorders (including sleep disorders), often referred by cannabis users, especially if young males [29]. In another study by Vaidya et al., the difficulty in falling asleep (initial insomnia) of young people cannabis addicts abstained from the assumption of cannabis for at least 24 hours is highlighted. In this study, the great difficulties of these individuals to make decisions are also described, due to an alteration in the ventral medial prefrontal cortex (vmPFC). From the results of positron emission tomography (PET) it can be noticed that these individuals likely use larger areas of the brain, with greater cognitive effort, to make decisions and choices [30]. Therefore, the onset of insomnia during periods of abstinence constitutes a reinforcement to the onset of cannabis addiction.

Opiates

As described for other substances with a sedative effect, heroin and other opiates (such as codeine, methadone/buprenorphine) may induce hypersomnia - as a result of acute intoxication - and insomnia when access to the substance is prevented – during withdrawal – or as a consequence of habituation. Cases of parasomnias associated with the use of opiates have also been described. Opiates dependency is the strongest and most relevant withdrawal syndrome in clinical practice and frequently causes sleep disorders. Heroin and other opiates act by binding different types of opioid receptors (μ-type, k-type and δ-type) in the CNS. The onset of insomnia and parasomnias in chronic opiates users is due to the emergence of alterations that go beyond the up / down regulation of opioid, dopaminergic and GABAergic receptors. According to Nestler et al., it would seem that there are modifications in gene expression that cause qualitative and quantitative changes in addicted neurons. The cascade of signal transduction via cAMP appears compromised, as well as that of phospholipase A2. A regulatory protein of gene transcription at the neuronal level, CREB (cAMP-related element binding), is the main marker of biological processes induced neuronal adaptation after taking long-time heroin. CREB determines an imbalance by activating a massive transcription of genes that encode for dynorphin (endogenous ligand of the k opioid receptors). This imbalance induces, becoming stable over time, insomnia and dysphoria in individuals with heroin addiction [31]. Based on the above information, also considering the addiction as a chronic relapsing disorder, it can be assumed that sleep disorders (particularly insomnia and parasomnia) are to be expected in individuals with past or current use of opiates, whenever they do not receive adequate treatment with substitution compounds (methadone, buprenorphine). This clinical element affects the rate of relapse and often leads to a switch to other drugs, such as alcohol, cocaine, cannabis, etc. Because of the frequent comorbidity with sleep disorders, it is necessary to prescribe pharmacotherapy for opiate dependence. It is worth remembering that it is necessary to set up a program for long-term treatment (called maintenance) with opioid receptor agonists. The gold standard drugs are methadone and buprenorphine, the latter in single formulation or in combination with naloxone in a proportion of 4:1. The following four therapeutic phases are indicated: induction, stabilization, maintenance, and interruption (optional) under medical monitoring.

Other Prescribed Compounds

Many studies have reported on sleep disturbances caused by prescribed substances other than benzodiazepines. The most frequent cases in clinical practice involve *corticosteroids, beta-blockers, antidepressants* and *chemotherapy*, which can adversely affect sleep through several different mechanisms. Therefore, in the anamnesis regarding individuals with insomnia, hypersomnia and parasomnias it is necessary to screen for these compounds and, when present, to determine any correlation with the sleep disorder [1, 10, 32, 33]. To avoid a discussion beyond the scope of this chapter, we have only listed these categories of prescription medications, referring to specific publications that can clarify the mechanisms through which they induce sleep disorders.

Novel Psychoactive Drugs

A new trend has to be considered in the evaluation of sleep disorders that affects mostly teenagers and young adults. According to the European Monitoring Centre for Drugs and Drug Addiction (EMCDDA), the widespread use of new psychoactive substances is today a phenomenon of considerable epidemiological importance [34]. Approximately 600 new compounds - new molecules or new psychoactive compositions – are circulating on the web and street market [35]. For many of these compounds, still poorly studied, an association with sleep disorders is been highlighted. A good example of a novel psychoactive drug, which can be used as a paradigm, is mephedrone. This is a synthetic form of the active substance present in the plant Khat (Catha Edulis Forsk). The plant, of varying sizes (which vaguely resembles an asparagus that can grow up to several meters), is widely chewed in East Africa and Yemen for its stimulant effects. These effects are due to the presence of an alkaloid that is pharmacologically similar to amphetamine, called cathinone. In addition to its stimulating properties, cathinone is strongly anorectic and induces insomnia. Khat is widely distributed within communities from these countries, after having been introduced to different parts of Europe. Mephedrone (4-methyl-meth-cathinone or 4-MMC, street/internet name "meow meow") appeared around 2007 and its effects have been largely associated with those of cocaine, amphetamines and ecstasy. The molecule is sold at a low price on the web in the form of crystalline powder or capsules (5 euro for a 250 mg capsule) formally used as fertilizer or as bath salts, always with the words "not for human consumption" (forbidden consumption). The request for mephedrone on the web has increased exponentially over the past years, making it necessary in some countries to ban sales as a plant fertilizer or a salt bath (in the UK it has been illegal since April 2010). On the web, however, there are also instructions for use as a recreational drug. Several deaths related to the misuse of mephedrone in Europe have been reported. It is usually taken on an empty stomach if swallowed or inhaled, but there have been reports in which it was smoked or taken intravenously. The mean dose indicated by consumers is between 100 and 500 mg, but assumptions with doses greater than 4 grams have been recorded. The desired effect, which occurs within 10-20 minutes and reaches a peak after about an hour, and then ceases after a further two hours, consists of an elevation of mood, with euphoria, increased empathy and self-esteem, fatigue reduction and enhancement of sensory experience, up to illusions or hallucinations. Adverse symptoms are frequent after taking mephedrone, and include strong insomnia and other sleep disturbances.

Another example of novel psychoactive drugs related to the onset of sleep disorders are the "spice drugs". These are composed of a similar texture to dried plants, formally sold on the web as air fresheners, inside envelopes of varying colors. These compounds contain doses of synthetic cannabinoids and produce a boosted cannabis-like effect.

GBL-GHB (liquid ecstasy) is to be counted, along with flunitrazepam and ketamine, among the "date-rape drugs". GHB abuse can lead to hypersomnia, during acute intoxication, and insomnia in consequence of abstinence.

Table 1. Synopsis of the effect of substances on sleep

	INSOMNIA	HYPERSOMNIA	PARASOMNIA
Alcohol and Benzodiazepines	*Chronic Use* *Withdrawal*	*Intoxication* *Chronic Use*	*Intoxication* *Chronic Use* *Withdrawal*
Nicotine	*Withdrawal*	-	*Intoxication* *Withdrawal*
Caffeine	*Intoxication*	*Withdrawal*	*Intoxication* *Withdrawal*
Cocaine	*Intoxication* *Chronic Use* *Withdrawal*	*Withdrawal*	*Intoxication* *Chronic Use* *Withdrawal*
MDMA and Amphetamines	*Intoxication* *Chronic Use* *Withdrawal*	*Withdrawal*	*Intoxication* *Chronic Use* *Withdrawal*
Cannabis	*Withdrawal*	*Intoxication*	*Intoxication* *Chronic Use* *Withdrawal*
Opiates	*Withdrawal* *Chronic Use*	*Intoxication* *Chronic Use*	*Intoxication* *Chronic Use* *Withdrawal*

Sleep disorders (insomnia and parasomnia) are related to the use of other substances, such as piperazine, Hawaiian woodrose seeds, ecstasy-like drugs (MDA, MDEA, etc.) or dimethyltryptamine.

Other substances that have been anecdotally related to sleep disorders are: Phalaris Arundinacea (a plant of the grass family containing dimethyltryptamine). There is evidence of recreational use of this plant. The extract is inhaled or injected and produces a state of psychic alteration within about 10 minutes characterized by intense hallucinations and other psychedelic phenomena; Heimia salicifolia is a plant native to Mexico once used by shamans during their rituals. The infusion of this plant or the smoke arising from it produce intense euphoria associated with auditory hallucinations and reduced need for sleep; Poppy Straw is derived from a plant of the family Papaveraceae (Papaver somniferum) and it is widely used in medicine for its analgesic properties (opium, morphine, which is extracted). Recently, it has been inhaled or swallowed for its relaxing and euphoric effects, which also antagonize the effect of stimulants. It can induce hypersomnia type disorder; Kava-Kava, Yage, Ayahuasca, Salvia divinorum, MDPV (MethyleneDioxyPyroValerone), Ibogaine and Ivory Wave are other examples of plant-derived substances related to the onset of sleep disturbances [36].

Conclusion

As described in this chapter, the central issue is that sleep disorders are frequently associated with the use of psychotropic substances, both legal and illegal, possibly in combination with poor sleep hygiene. On this background, we can argue that stimulants most frequently generate insomnia during the acute effect and hypersomnia during withdrawal; vice versa, "downers" (sedative substances) most frequently cause hypersomnia as an acute effect, and insomnia during chronic use or withdrawal syndrome. Both categories increase the extent of qualitative sleep disorders, such as several parasomnias. Frequently, the use of these substances is underrated by clinicians and this fact complicates the treatment of symptomatic syndromes and exposes the patient to an increased risk of adverse effects. A screening for recent or past use / abuse of substances (including alcohol, nicotine, caffeine and prescribed drugs) is essential when investigating the history of patients who present with a sleep disorder. This is very complicated, however, because the interviewee is often reluctant to talk about an illegal phenomenon (for illicit drugs), or does not want to be subject to moral criticism from society, with the possible presence of a feeling of shame. Nonetheless, when this disturbance is identified the physician will need a specific program for treatment and relapse prevention that targets not only the treatment of sleep disorder *in se*, but also the detoxification and addiction treatment. The description of specific treatments for the use / abuse of various substances mentioned above, is beyond the central purpose of this chapter and would require discussion that is oversized for the present work. Therefore, we refer to the literature in the field of integrated therapy of substance addiction, keeping in mind that the acquisition of tools for the recognition of sleep disorders related to substance use is an essential goal for the clinician.

References

[1] Riemann D., Nissen C. 2011. Substance-induced sleep disorders and abuse of hypnotics. *British Journal on Health Research,* 54(12):1325-31.

[2] Kaplan H. I., Sadock B. J., Grebb J. A. 1997. Synopsis of psychiatry: behavioural sciences, clinical psychiatry – seventh edition. Williams and Wilkins- Baltimore, Maryland, USA.

[3] Ohayon M. M. 2009. Observation of the natural evolution of insomnia in the american general population cohort. *Sleep Med. Clin.,* 4(1): 87–92.

[4] Kessler R. C., McCongale K. A., Zhao S., Nelson C. B., Hughes M. et al. 2001. Lifetime and 12-month prevalence of DSM-III psychiatric disorders in the United States. Results from the National Comorbidity Survey. *Archives of General Psychiatry,* 51(1), 8-19.

[5] Ohayon M. M., Roth T. J. 2001. What are the contributing factors for insomnia in the general population? *Psychosom. Res.,* 51(6):745-55.

[6] American Psychiatric Association. 2000. Diagnostic and Statistical Manual of Mental Disorders – Fourth Edition - Text Revision. Washington DC: American Psychiatric Association.

[7] Koob G. F., Volkow N. G. 2010. Neurocircuitry of addiction. *Neuropsychopharmacology,* 35, 217–238.

[8] Nestler E. J. 2002. From neurobiology to treatment: progress against addiction. *Nat. Neurosci.,* 5 suppl. 1076-1079.

[9] Leu-Semenescu S., Arnulf I. et al. 2010. Sleep and Rhythm Consequences of a Genetically Induced Loss of Serotonin. *Sleep,* 2010 March 1;33(3):307-314.

[10] Goodman A. G., Hardman J. G., Limbird L. E. 2003. The pharmacological basis of therapeutics. 10' ed. – McGraw-Hill.

[11] Olsen R. W. and Spigelman I. 2012. GABAA Receptor Plasticity in Alcohol Withdrawal. In: Jasper's Basic Mechanisms of the Epilepsies [Internet]. 4th edition. Noebels J. L., Avoli M. et al. editors. Bethesda (MD): National Center for Biotechnology Information, USA.

[12] Zanigni S., Calandra-Buonaura G., Grimaldi D., Cortelli P. 2011. REM behavior disorder and neurodegenerative diseases. *Sleep Med.*, 12 Suppl 2:S54-8.

[13] Sakurai S., Cui R., Tanigawa T., Yamagishi K., Iso H. 2007. Alcohol consumption before sleep is associated with severity of sleep-disordered breathing among professional Japanese truck drivers. *Alcohol Clin. Exp. Res.*, 31(12):2053-8.

[14] Hirase M., Ishida T., Kamei C. 2008.Rebound insomnia induced by abrupt withdrawal of hypnotics in sleep-disturbed rats.*Eur. J. Pharmacol.*, 597(1-3):46-50.

[15] World Health Organization – Regional Office for Europe. 2012. Available at: http://www.euro.who.int/en/what-we-do/health-topics/disease-prevention/tobacco/facts-and-figures.

[16] Corkery J. M., Button J., Vento A. E., Schifano F. 2010. Two UK suicides using nicotine extracted from tobacco employing instructions available on the Internet. *Forensic. Sci. Int.*, 199(1-3):e9-13.

[17] Jaehne A., Unbehaun T., Feige B., Lutz U. C., Batra A., Riemann D. 2012. How smoking affects sleep: A polysomnographical analysis. *Sleep Med.*,13(10):1286-92.

[18] Kim K. S., Kim J. H., Park S. Y., Won H. R., Lee H. J., Yang H. S., Kim H. J. 2012. Smoking induces oropharyngeal narrowing and increases the severity of obstructive sleep apnea syndrome. *J. Clin. Sleep Med.*, 8(4):367-74.

[19] Bergin J. E., Kendler K. S. 2012. Common psychiatric disorders and caffeine use, tolerance, and withdrawal: an examination of shared genetic and environmental effects. *Twin Res. Hum. Genet.*, 15(4):473-82.

[20] Morgan P. T. et al. 2006. Sleep, sleep-dependent procedural learning and vigilance in chronic cocaine users: Evidence for occult insomnia. *Drug and Alcohol Dependence*, 82(3):238-249.

[21] Whitten L. 2008. National Institute of Health, National Institute On Drug Abuse (NIDA). Chronic cocaine abusers have occult insomnia in early abstinence. Available at: .http://www.drugabuse.gov/news-events/nida-notes/2008/03/chronic-cocaine-abusers- have-occult-insomnia-in-early-abstinence

[22] Ogeil R. P., Rajaratnam S. M., Phillips J. G., Redman J. R., Broadbear J. H. 2011. Ecstasy use and self-reported disturbances in sleep.*Hum. Psychopharmacol.*, 26(7): 508-16.

[23] Di Iorio C. R., Watkins T. J., Dietrich M. S., Cao A., Blackford J. U., Rogers B., Ansari M. S., Baldwin R. M., Li R., Kessler R. M., Salomon R. M., Benningfield M., Cowan R. L. 2012. Evidence for chronically altered serotonin function in the cerebral cortex of female 3,4-methylenedioxymethamphetamine polydrug users. *Arch. Gen. Psychiatry.*, 69(4):399-409.

[24] Cloak C., Alicata D., Chang L. et al. 2011. Age and sex effects levels of choline compounds in the anterior cingulated cortex of adolescent methamphetamine users. *Drug and alcohol dependence*, 207-215.

[25] Zhou F. C. and Bledsoe S. 1996. Methamphetamine causes rapid varicosis, perforation and definitive degeneration of serotonin fibers: an immunocytochemical study of serotonin transporter. *Neuroscience-Net*, 1-17.

[26] Ricaurte G. A., Seiden L. S., Schuster C. R. 1984. Further evidence that amphetamines produce longlasting dopamine neurochemical deficits by destroying dopamine nerve fibers. *Brain Res.*, 303: 359-364.

[27] European Monitoring Centre for Drugs and Drug Addiction (EMCDDA). 2012. Lifetime prevalence of drug use among all adults (aged 15 to 64 years) in nationwide surveys among the general population.

[28] Unseld M., Dworschak G., Tran U. S., Plener P. L., Erfurth A., Walter H., Lesch O. M., Kapusta N. D. 2012. The concept of temperament in psychoactive substance use among college students. *J. Affect Disord.*, 141(2-3):324-30.

[29] Gruber S. A., Silveri M. M., Dahlgren M. K., Yurgelun-Todd D. 2011. Why so impulsive? White matter alterations are associated with impulsivity in chronic marijuana smokers. *Exp. Clin. Psychopharmacol.,* 19(3):231-42.

[30] Vaidya J. G., Block R. I., O'Leary D. S., Ponto L. B., Ghoneim M. M., Bechara A. 2012. Effects of chronic marijuana use on brain activity during monetary decision-making. *Neuropsychopharmacology,* 37(3): 618-29.

[31] Nestler E. J. 2001. Molecular basis of long-term plasticity underlying addiction. *Nature Rev. Neurosci.*, 2: 119-128.

[32] Turner R., Elson E. 1993. Sleep disorders. Steroids cause sleep disturbance. *BMJ.*306(6890):1477-8.

[33] Ryan P. W. 1987. Beta blocker side-effects.*Can. Fam. Physician*, 33:831.

[34] European Monitoring Centre for Drugs and Drug Addiction. 2012. Annual report on the state of the drugs problem in Europe (launched 15.11.2012).

[35] Deluca P., Davey Z., Corazza O., Di Furia L., Farre M., Flesland L. H., Mannonen M., Majava A., Peltoniemi T., Pasinetti M., Pezzolesi C., Scherbaum N., Siemann H., Skutle A., Torrens M., van der Kreeft P., Iversen E., Schifano F. 2012. Identifying emerging trends in recreational drug use; outcomes from the Psychonaut Web Mapping Project. *Prog. Neuropsychopharmacol. Biol. Psychiatry,* 39(2):221-6.

[36] Vento A. and Di Tommaso A. 2013. Indagini su sostanze stupefacenti - chapter 4 in "Il Sopralluogo nel processo penale"; Graphisoft edition, Rome.

Part III.
Diagnostic Techniques

In: Sleep Medicine
Editors: A. Del Casale, R. Brugnoli and P. Girardi

ISBN: 978-1-62808-515-0
© 2013 Nova Science Publishers, Inc.

Chapter XIII

EEG and Polysomnography in Sleep Disorders

Carla Buttinelli, Michela Ferraldeschi, Miriam Tasillo
and Manuela Giuliani*
Sapienza University, NESMOS Department, Rome Italy

Abstract

In the International Classification of Sleep Disorders (ICSD-2)[1] eight major categories of sleep disorders are listed: 1) insomnia; 2) sleep-related breathing disorder (SRBD); 3) hypersomnia not due to a sleep-related breathing disorder; 4) circadian rhythm sleep disorder; 5) parasomnia; 6) sleep-related movement disorder 7) isolated symptoms, apparently normal variants, and unresolved issues; and 8) other sleep disorders. In this chapter will be summarize the procedures for monitoring and evaluating the main sleep disorders.

Keywords: Sleep disorders, polysomnography, multiple sleep latency test, actigraphy

Introduction

The assessment of human sleep stages using polysomnography (PSG) requires the acquisition of three core measures: electroencephalogram (EEG), electro-oculogram (EOG), and electro-myogram (EMG); sleep is divided into two states with independent functions and controls: NREM and REM sleep (called macrostructure of sleep). In an ideal situation, NREM and REM alternate in a cyclic manner, each cycle lasting on average from 90 to 110 min. During a normal sleep period in adults, 4-6 cycles are noted. NREM sleep accounts for 75-80% of sleep time in an adult human. [2]

---

* Corresponding author: Carla Buttinelli, Sapienza University, Rome, email: carla.buttinelli@uniroma1.it

According to the current American Academy of Sleep Medicine (AASM) [3] scoring manual, the terminology of sleep stages include the following: stage wakefulness (W), stage NREM (N 1), stage NREM 2 (N 2), stage N3 [NREM 3(N3)] and stage REM (R). Stage W (Figure 1) represents the waking state, ranging from full alertness through early stages of drowsiness. The dominant rhythm during this study consists of alpha rhythm (8-13 Hz), noted predominantly in the posterior region, intermixed with a small amount of beta rhythm (>13 Hz) seen mainly in the anterior head regions. [3] The EOG during wakefulness may demonstrate rapid eye blinks at a frequency of about 0.5-2 Hz. As drowsiness develops, the frequency of blinking slows, and eye blinks maybe replaced by slow eye movements, even in the presence of continued alpha rhythm. The chin EMG during this stage is of variable amplitude. [3] NREM sleep is divided into three stages: N1, N2, and N3, primarily on the basis of EEG criteria. [3]

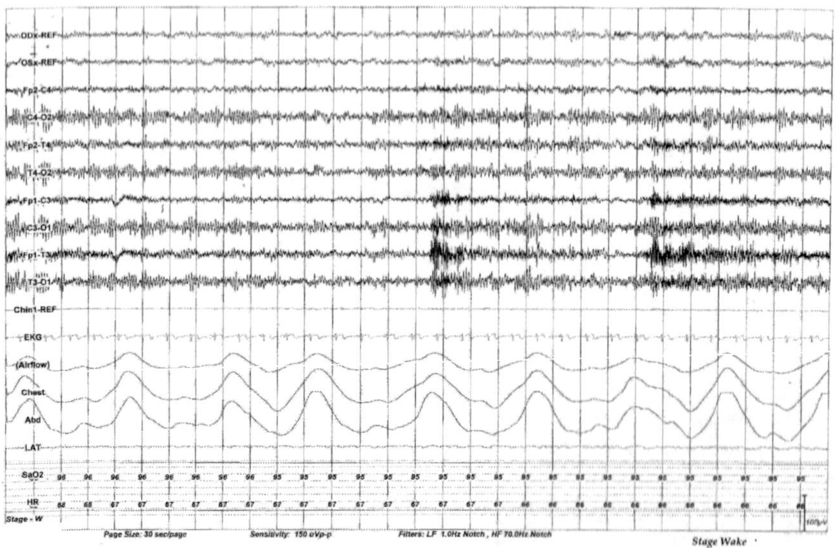

Figure 1. Stage Wake.

In NREM sleep, N1 occupies 3-8% of total sleep time; N2 comprises 45-55% and N3 makes up 15-20% of total sleep time. [3]

In N1 (Figure 2), the alpha rhythm diminishes to less than 50% in an epoch (a 30-sec segment of the polysomnographic tracing with the monitor screen speed of 10 mm/sec) intermixed with slower theta rhythms (4-7 Hz) and beta waves. Sharply contoured waves with duration < 0.5 sec over the central region (vertex sharp waves) may be present. The EOG shows slow eye movement, but these are not required for scoring. During this stage, the chin EMG amplitude is variable, but often lower than in stage W. [3].

Stage N2 (Figure 3) begins after approximately 10-12 min of stage N1. Sleep spindles (11-16 Hz) and K complex (negative sharp wave followed by a positive component) intermixed with vertex sharp waves herald the onset of stage N2 sleep. After about 30-60 min of N2, N3 begins and delta waves comprise 20% or more of an epoch. (Figure 4) In this stage, eye movements are not typically seen and the chin EMG is of variable amplitude. [3]

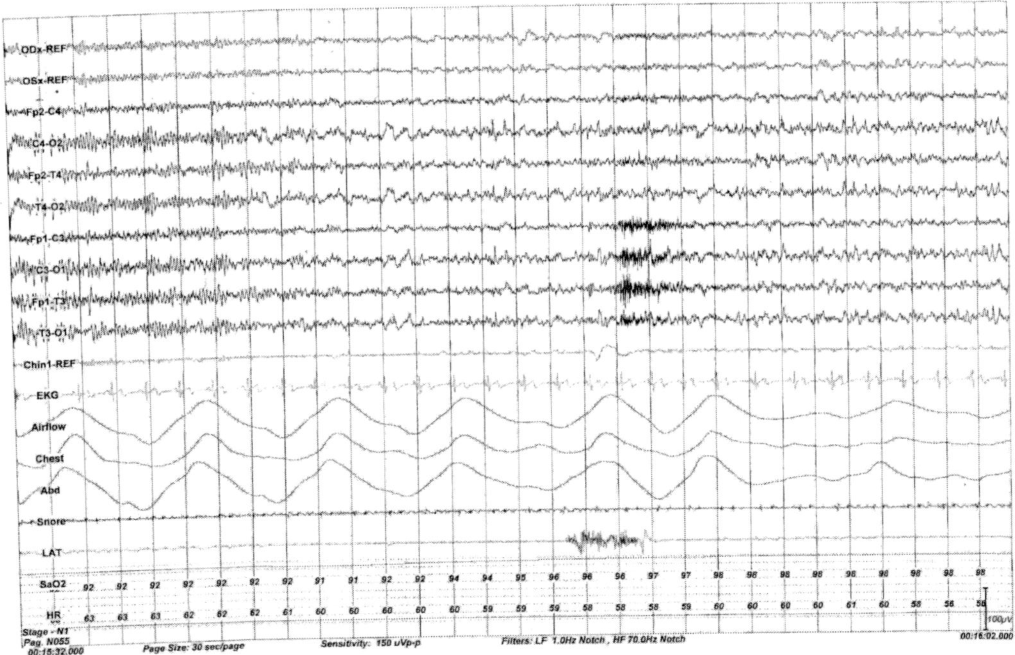

Figure 2. Stage N1.

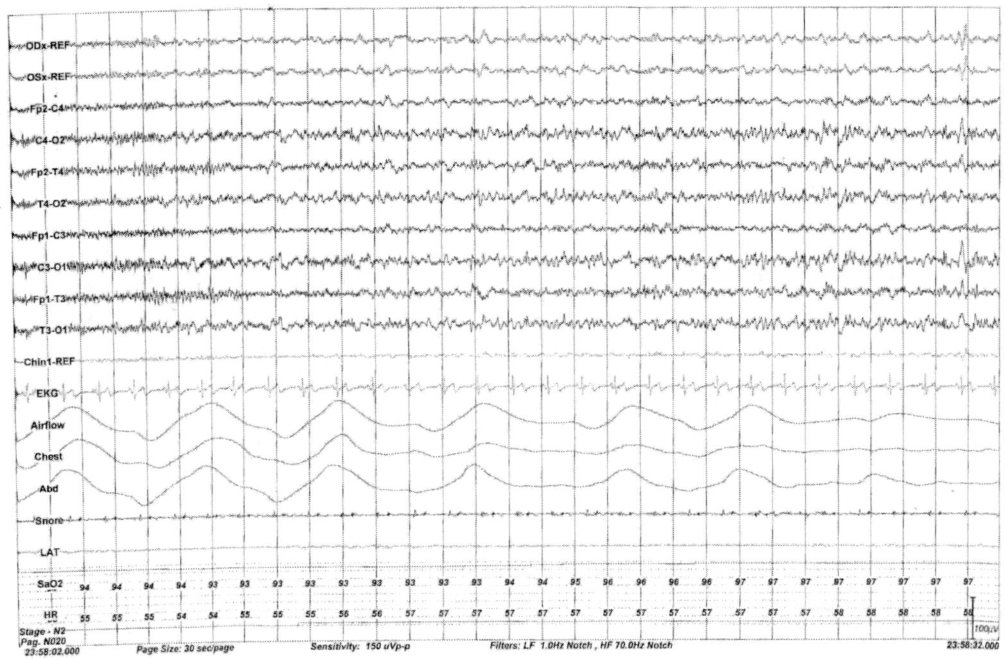

Figure 3. Stage N2.

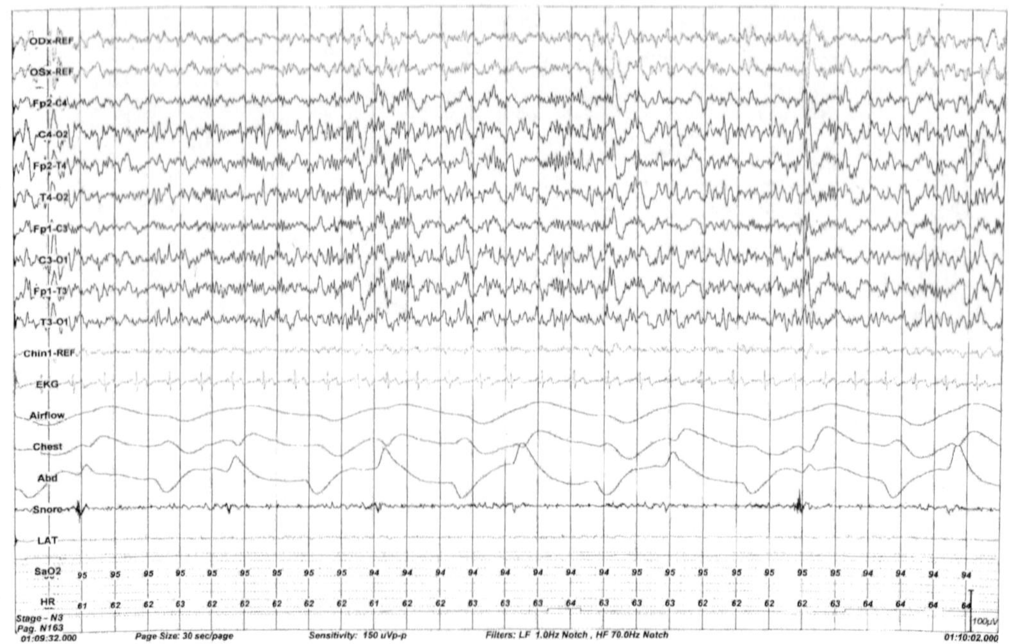

Figure 4. Stage N3.

REM sleep (Figure 5) accounts for 20-25% of total sleep time. EEG during REM sleep consists of a low amplitude, fast pattern in the beta frequency range mixed with a small amount of theta rhythms. Trains of sharply contoured or triangular 2-6 Hz waves (sawtooth waves) are maximal in amplitude over the central regions and often preceding a burst of rapid eye movements. EMG activity in the chin derivation is no higher than in any other sleep stage, and it is usually at the lowest level of the entire recording.

The cycling alternating pattern (CAP) [4-5] represents the so-called microstructure of sleep and indicates sleep instability. A CAP sequence is composed of a succession of CAP cycles. A CAP cycle is composed of a phase A and the following phase B.

The phase A of CAP is the EEG marker of cerebral activation, including cortical arousal, and for this reason it is a potential trigger of somatomotor activities. Arousals are transient phenomena resulting in fragmented sleep without behavioral awakenings. An arousal is characterized by an abrupt shift in EEG frequency lasting from 3-14 sec and including alpha, beta or theta activities, but not spindles or delta waves. Phase B is an EEG indicator of rebound deactivation which induces somatomotor inhibition and becomes a potential limiting factor for the duration of any body movement during the NREM sleep period.

All CAP sequences begin with a phase A and end with a phase B. Each phase of CAP has a duration of is 2-60 sec. This cut-off relies on the consideration that the great majority (about 90%) of A phases occurring during sleep are separated by an interval <60 sec. The absence of CAP for >60 sec is scored as non-CAP. CAP sequences have no upper limits on overall duration or the number of CAP cycles.

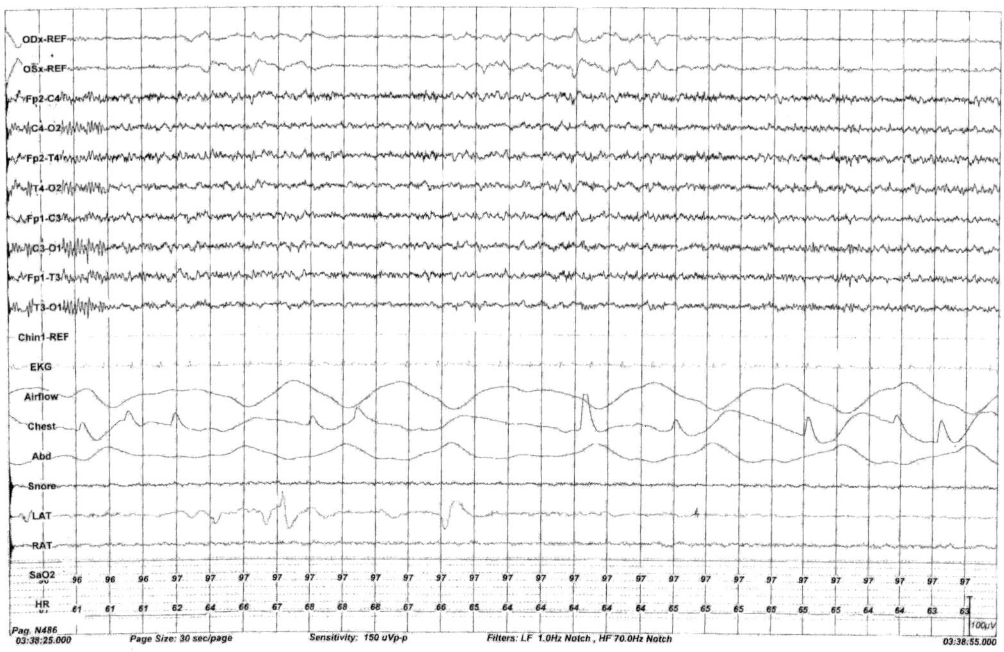

Figure 5. REM.

In this chapter, the procedures for monitoring and evaluating the main sleep disorder will be summarized. Sleep disorders will be described according to the International Classification of Sleep Disorders (ICSD-2) [1], which lists eight major categories of sleep disorders:

1) insomnia;
2) sleep-related breathing disorder;
3) hypersomnia not due to a sleep-related breathing disorder (SRBD);
4) circadian rhythm sleep disorder;
5) parasomnia;
6) sleep-related movement disorder
7) isolated symptoms, apparently normal variants, and unresolved issues; and
8) other sleep disorders.

Measurement Techniques in Sleep Disorders

Polysomnographic Technique

Polysomnography is the most important laboratory test used in diagnoses of sleep disorders and includes recording, analysis, and interpretation of several parameters during sleep, which include the following: 1) electroencephalogram (EEG), 2) electro-oculogram (EOG), 3) electro-myogram (EMG); 4) electrocardiogram (ECG), 5) oximetry; 6) pH meter and change in pressure in positive airway pressure treatment. 7) snoring; 8) nasal/oral airflow 9) thoracic and abdominal effort 10) body position.

The examination is made by a technician using a polygraph, an instrument which contains a series of amplifiers (some channels of alternating and direct current), and the data from the amplifiers is stored by a computer for analysis. Alternating current amplifiers are used to record EEG, EOG, EMG, and ECG. Direct current amplifiers are used to record oximeters, pH, and change in pressure in positive airway pressure. The quality of the examination depends on the quality of the electrode application according to the International 10-20 System. [6]

According to the AASM Manual for the Scoring of Sleep and Associated Events [3], for monitoring EEG activity during sleep the recommended derivations are: F4-M1, C4-M1, and O2-M1. Other alternative acceptable derivations are F2-C2, C2-O2, and C4-M1. EEG electrode position is determined by International 10-20 System [2] and a minimum of three EEG derivations are required for monitoring frontal, central, and occipital activity. M1 and M2 refer to the left and right mastoid processes.

The EOG records movement of corneo-retinal potential difference in the eye. Two derivations are recommended [3]: E1-M2 (E1 is placed 1 cm below the left outer canthus) and E2-M2 (E2 is placed 1 cm above the right outer canthus).

EMG activity is recorded by three electrodes: one in the midline 1 cm above the inferior edge of the mandible, one 2 cm below the inferior edge of the mandible and 2 cm to the right of the midline, and last 2 cm below the inferior edge of the mandible and 2 cm to the left of the midline. [3] Electrodes placed in this area record mylohyoid and the anterior belly of the digastric muscles which are innervated by the fifth cranial nerve. These also record activities from the genioglossus and hypoglossus muscle to identify the degree of muscle tone for sleep stage scoring. Another electrode can be added over the masseter muscle in patients with history of bruxism.

In patients with suspected sleep related breathing disorder it is important to record respiratory muscle activities: the intercostals and the diaphragmatic muscles, the upper airway muscles, and facial muscles. Electrodes are placed to the right or left of the umbilicus or over the anterior costal margin. ECG electrodes to record ECG activity are applied on the skin from the right clavicle and on the left side at the level of the seventh rib.

According to the guidelines of AASM [4], the indications to perform a PSG study are: 1) diagnosis of sleep-related breathing disorders; 2) positive airway pressure titration in patients with SRBD; 3) evaluate the presence of obstructive sleep apnea (OSA) before upper airway surgery and for follow-up after surgical treatment; 4) neuromuscular disorders with sleep-related symptoms; 5) narcolepsy; 6) parasomnia and seizures disorders; 7) restless leg syndrome and periodic limb movement; 8) circadian rhythm sleep disorders.

The use of polysomnography for evaluating sleep-related breathing disorders requires a minimum of the following recordings: EEG, EOG, chin EMG, airflow, arterial oxygen saturation, respiratory effort, and ECG or heart rate. Anterior tibialis EMG is useful to assist in detecting movement arousals and may have the added benefit of assessing periodic limb movements, which coexist with sleep-related breathing disorders in many patients. [3] Due to the high costs of PSG, cardiorespiratory monitoring (CRM) is increasingly used to detect breathing disorders.

According to the parameters indicated by AASM [3], the minimum channels required for the diagnosis of narcolepsy include EEG, EOG, chin EMG, and ECG.

The minimum channels required for the diagnosis of parasomnia or sleep-related seizure disorder include sleep-scoring channels (EEG, EOG, chin EMG); EEG using an expanded bilateral montage; and EMG for body movements (anterior tibialis or extensor digitorum). Audiovisual recording and documented technologist observations during the period of study are also essential. [3]

PSG is not required for common, uncomplicated, non-injurious parasomnias (such as typical disorders of arousal, nightmares, enuresis, sleep talking, and bruxism,) because diagnosis is based on clinical features. Moreover, PSG, with additional EEG derivations and video recording, is indicated in evaluating sleep-related behaviors that are violent or otherwise potentially injurious to the patient or others. PSG is indicated when evaluating patients with sleep behaviors suggestive of parasomnias that are unusual or atypical because of the patient's age at onset, the time, duration, or frequency of occurrence of the behavior or the specifics of the particular motor patterns in question (e.g. stereotypical, repetitive, or focal). Polysomnography may be indicated in situations with forensic considerations, (e.g. if onset follows trauma or if the events themselves have been associated with personal injury), and is also indicated in patients in which an epileptic seizure is suspected. PSG is not routinely indicated for patients with a seizure disorder who have no specific complaints consistent with a sleep disorder. [3]

PSG is further indicated when a diagnosis of periodic limb movement disorder is considered because of complaints by the patient or an observer of repetitive limb movements during sleep and frequent awakenings, fragmented sleep, difficulty maintaining sleep, or excessive daytime sleepiness. PSG is not routinely indicated to diagnose or treat restless legs syndrome, except where uncertainty exists in diagnosis. The minimum channels required for the evaluation of periodic limb movements and related arousals include EEG, EOG, chin EMG, and left and right anterior tibialis surface EMG. [3]

Usually, PSG is not required to diagnose circadian rhythm sleep disorders since diagnosis is based on clinical features; it may be useful when the causes are uncertain or when pharmacologic treatment is unsuccessful.

Multiple Sleep Latency Test

Multiple Sleep Latency Test (MSLT) is an important test used for diagnosis of excessive daytime sleepiness (EDS), which is defined as sleepiness that occurs in a situation when an individual would usually be expected to be awake. [7] The first publication about MSLT was in 1992 by the AASM [8], and after 13 years, in 2005, the Standards of Practice Committee and the Board of Directors of AASM recommended practice parameters for the clinical use of MSLT and Maintenance of Wakefulness Test (MWT), another laboratory test to measure sleepiness/wakefulness. [7]

The MSLT is a validated objective measure of the ability or tendency to fall asleep, and is intended to measure physiological sleep tendency under standardized conditions in the absence of external alerting factors. The test is based on the premise that the degree of sleepiness is reflected by sleep latency.

The MWT is a validated objective measure of the ability to stay awake for a defined time and measures the ability to stay awake for a defined period of time. The clinical relevance of the MWT is based on the premise that the volitional ability to remain awake provides important information regarding the ability to stay awake and response to intervention for a disorder associated with excessive sleepiness. [7]

Specific indications for use of the MSLT, according to the AASM Report [7], are: 1) evaluation of patients with suspected narcolepsy to confirm the diagnosis; 2) evaluation of patients with suspected idiopathic hypersomnia to help differentiate diagnosis.

The test is not routinely indicated in the initial evaluation and diagnosis of OSA, SRBD, and circadian rhythm disorders, but when patients continue to have excessive sleepiness despite treatment they may require evaluation for possible narcolepsy with MSLT. [7]

MWT has specific indications to assess an individual's ability to remain awake when his/her inability to remain awake constitutes a public or personal safety issue, and is also indicated in patients with excessive sleepiness to assess response to treatment. The MSLT protocol, according to the recommendations of AASM [7], consists of five nap opportunities performed at two hour intervals. The initial nap opportunity begins 1.5 to 3 hours after termination of the nocturnal recording. A shorter four-nap test may be performed, but this test is not reliable for the diagnosis of narcolepsy unless at least two sleep onset REM periods have occurred.

The MSLT must be performed immediately following PSG recorded during the individual's major sleep period. The test should not be performed after a split night sleep study. Sleep logs may be obtained for 1 week prior to the MSLT to assess sleep-wake schedules. Standardization of test conditions is critical for obtaining valid results. Sleep rooms should be dark and quiet during testing. Room temperature should be set based on the patient's comfort level. Stimulants, stimulant-like medications, and REM suppressing medications should ideally be stopped 2 weeks before MSLT. [7] The conventional recording montage for the MSLT includes central EEG (C3-A2, C4-A1) and occipital (O1-A2, O2-A1) derivations, left and right eye EOGs, mental/submental EMG, and ECG. [7]

Sleep onset for the clinical MSLT is determined by the time from lights out to the first epoch of any stage of sleep, including stage 1 sleep. Sleep onset is defined as the first epoch of greater than 15 sec of cumulative sleep in a 30-sec epoch. The absence of sleep on a nap opportunity is recorded as a sleep latency of 20 min. This latency is included in the calculation of mean sleep latency (MSL). In order to assess for the occurrence of REM sleep, in the clinical MSLT the test continues for 15 min from after the first epoch of sleep. A nap session is terminated after 20 min if sleep does not occur. [7]

The MWT consists of four trials performed at two hour intervals, with the first trial beginning about 1.5 to 3 hours after the patient's usual wake-up time. Performance of a PSG prior to MWT should be decided by the clinician based on clinical circumstances. The conventional recording montage for the MWT includes central EEG (C3-A2, C4-A1) and occipital (O1-A2, O2-A1) derivations, left and right eye electrooculograms (EOGs), mental/submental electromyogram (EMG), and electrocardiogram (EKG). Sleep onset is defined as the first epoch of greater than 15 sec of cumulative sleep in a 30-sec epoch. [7]

Actigraphy

Actigraphy is a method used to study sleep-wake patterns and circadian rhythms by assessing movement, most commonly of the wrist. [9] Actigraphy is based on the principle that there is reduced movement during sleep and increased movement during wake.

Actigraphy utilizes a portable device (actigraph) that records movement over extended periods of time and is worn most commonly on the wrist. Sleepwake patterns are estimated from periods of activity and inactivity based on this movement. [9] A modern actigraph uses accelerometers to detect wrist (alternatively ankle and trunk) movement, which is sampled several times a second. These data are stored within the actigraph for up to several weeks. The length of time the actigraph is able to record data is typically dependent on the actigraph epoch length (i.e. the period of time that the actigraphy data is averaged), which is usually 30 sec or 1 min.

The individual is advised to wear the actigraph continuously for a given period of time (usually a minimum of 1 week). In addition, a sleep diary is frequently given to the individual to complete during the monitoring period. This latter information is often used to establish the lights off and lights on time for each 24-hour period. At the end of this period, the actigraph is returned to the clinician's office for analysis. [9]

Thus, the estimated sleep-wake parameters such as sleep latency, total sleep time, number and frequency of awakenings, sleep efficiency can be derived. Circadian rhythm parameters, such as amplitude actigraphy, are reliable and valid for detecting sleep in normal, healthy adult individuals. [10-11] Two studies found no difference between data collected from actigraphs placed on different locations (e.g. dominant wrist, non dominant wrist, ankle, or trunk). [12-13]

Actigraphy is not indicated for routine diagnosis, assessment of severity, or management of sleep disorders. However, it may be a useful adjunct to a detailed history, examination, and subjective sleep diary in situations where a more standard technique, such as the MSLT, is not practical and above all for the assessment of specific aspects of some disorders such as insomnia (assessment of sleep variability, measurement of treatment effects, and detection of sleep phase alterations in insomnia secondary to circadian rhythm disturbance), restless legs syndrome/periodic limb movement disorder. [10-11]

Evidence has suggested that actigraphy might have some value in the assessment of sleep disorders. For insomnia, actigraphy may be most valuable in assessing treatment effects or night-to-night variations in sleep. It has been demonstrated that actigraphy has the ability to detect sleep phase alterations associated with circadian rhythm disturbances. Additionally, actigraphy is capable of distinguishing moderate to severe sleep apnea from normal control subjects, due to its greater sensitivity, compared to sleep logs, in detecting brief arousals from sleep; it is also useful for detecting periodic limb movements. [14]

It is important to remember that actigraphy may not be 100% accurate when compared to PSG. In fact, actigraphy is one-dimensional, whereas polysomnography comprises at least 3 distinct types of data (EEG, EOG, EMG), which jointly determine whether a person is asleep or awake. It is therefore doubtful whether actigraphic data will ever be informationally equivalent to PSG, although progress on hardware and data processing software is being made. [15]

However, actigraphy makes home recordings more accessible, permitting the evaluation of patients in their natural sleep environment, thereby minimizing laboratory effects that may alter a patient's typical sleep patterns. [15] It may also provide an opportunity for subjects to adhere more closely to their scheduled bedtime and wakeup time than a PSG recording, thus providing a more accurate estimate of typical sleep duration than does PSG. [15]

The actigraph's limitations, however, continue to restrict its value as a stand-alone diagnostic device. [14-15]

Clinical Applications

1. Insomnia

Insomnia is the most prevalent sleep disorder and affects large proportions of the population. It is often under-recognized and untreated because of barriers in assessment and management. Insomnia is characterized by a complaint of difficulty initiating sleep, maintaining sleep, and/or non-restorative sleep that causes clinically significant distress or impairment in social, occupational or other important areas of functioning. [16]

Overnight PSG is a standard tool in sleep medicine for evaluating sleep-related pathophysiology, sleep architecture, and sleep integrity. Measures such as latency to sleep onset, total sleep time, number of arousals and awakenings, and sleep efficiency are routinely calculated to characterize a night of sleep. Disturbance in such measures provides objective verification of complaints in difficulty initiating and maintaining sleep. [16-17]

Polysomnographic evaluation of self-defined insomniacs can reveal more impairments of sleep continuity parameters (e.g. longer sleep latencies, more time awake after sleep onset, lower sleep efficiency) and reduced total sleep time compared to self-defined good sleepers.

Sleep architecture shows an increased amount of stage N1, reduced stages N3 and more frequent stage shifts throughout the night. The cortex is more active in people with insomnia than in good sleepers, both around sleep onset and during NREM sleep; this is consistent with the general state of hyperarousal in people with insomnia. [18]

Evidence of the microstructure of sleep reveals increased beta activity in primary insomniacs relative to healthy controls, both around the sleep onset period and during NREM.

The role of actigraphy in insomnia evaluation and treatment monitoring is not well established. In the research environment, actigraphy is useful for examining night-to-night variability and for identifying individuals with circadian rhythm disorders. Insomnia is primarily diagnosed by clinical evaluation through a careful, detailed medical, psychiatric and thorough sleep history (which includes assessment of sleep patterns and waking processes). PSG is not indicated for routine evaluation of transient or chronic insomnia, for routine evaluation of insomnia due to psychiatric disorders or in differentiating insomnia associated with dementia from other forms of insomnia, including insomnia associated with depression. [16]

PSG is, however, indicated when sleep-related breathing disorders or periodic limb movement disorder are suspected and when initial diagnosis is uncertain, treatment fails (behavioral or pharmacologic) or precipitous arousals occur with violent or injurious behavior. [16]

2. Sleep-Related Breathing Disorder (SRBD)

Individuals with OSA are rarely aware of their sleep disorder, even upon arousal. Apnea is usually recognized as a problem by family members who witness apneic episodes or by a primary care doctor because of the individual's risk factors and symptoms.

Most commonly, patients present with vague complaints. Clinical symptoms can include EDS that usually begins during quiet activities (e.g. reading, watching television), daytime fatigue, feeling tired despite a full night's sleep, morning headaches, personality and mood changes, dry or sore throat, gastroesophageal reflux, and sexual dysfunction. [19]

Diagnosis of OSA is based on the evaluation of clinical symptoms and risk factors, as well as a formal sleep study evaluation (polysomnography, or a portable home-based test. [19] In fact, confirmation of a diagnosis of OSA requires documentation of sleep-related breathing disturbances.

Snoring is a common finding in individuals with OSA. Although not everyone who snores is experiencing sleep apnea, snoring in combination with obesity has been found to be highly predictive of increased risk of OSA. [20]

The volume of the snoring is not indicative of the severity of obstruction. However, snoring with witnessed apneas has 94% specificity for OSA. The AASM defines an apnea as a cessation in airflow lasting at least 10 sec; apneic episodes can last anywhere from 10 sec to a few min, and may occur multiple times per hour. [21]

There are three types of apneas: obstructive, mixed, and central. The AASM defines an obstructive apnea (Figure 6) as a drop in peak thermal sensor excursion by ≥90% of baseline lasting at last 10 sec, with continued or increased inspiratory effort noted throughout the entire period of absent airflow. Central apnea (Figure 7) is defined as a drop in peak thermal sensor excursion by ≥90% of baseline lasting at last 10 sec with absent inspiratory effort noted throughout the entire period of absent airflow. [21] Mixed apnea (Figure 6) is defined as a drop in peak thermal sensor excursion by ≥90% of baseline lasting at least 10 sec, with absent inspiratory effort during the initial portion of the respiratory event, followed by resumption of inspiratory effort during the latter part of the event. [21] Hypopnea (Figure 8) is defined as a recognizable transient reduction (but not complete cessation) of breathing for at least 10 sec.

This differs from apnea in that there remains some flow of air. In the context of sleep disorders, a hypopnea event is only considered to be clinically significant if there is a 30% or more reduction in flow with or without an associated 4% or greater desaturation in O2 level, lasting for 10 sec or longer. An alternative definition is also provided, characterized by a drop of ≥50% of the nasal pressure signal at last 10 sec accompanied by a ≥3% oxygen desaturation or associated with an arousal. [21].

Apneas and hypopnea are both considered when assessing the severity of a person's sleep disorder. [22]

The apnea-hypopnea index (AHI) is used to assess the severity of sleep apnea based on the total number of apneas and hypopneas occurring per hour of sleep. In general, an individual is considered to have an OSA syndrome if they demonstrate an AHI of at least 5 with the presence of daytime symptoms or AHI of 15 or more independently of symptoms. The AHI can also be used to stratify severity of the disease; an AHI of 5-15 is classified as mild, 15-30 is considered moderate and >30 is considered severe. Obstructive apneas and hypopnea are typically distinguished from central events by the detection of respiratory efforts during the event. [23]

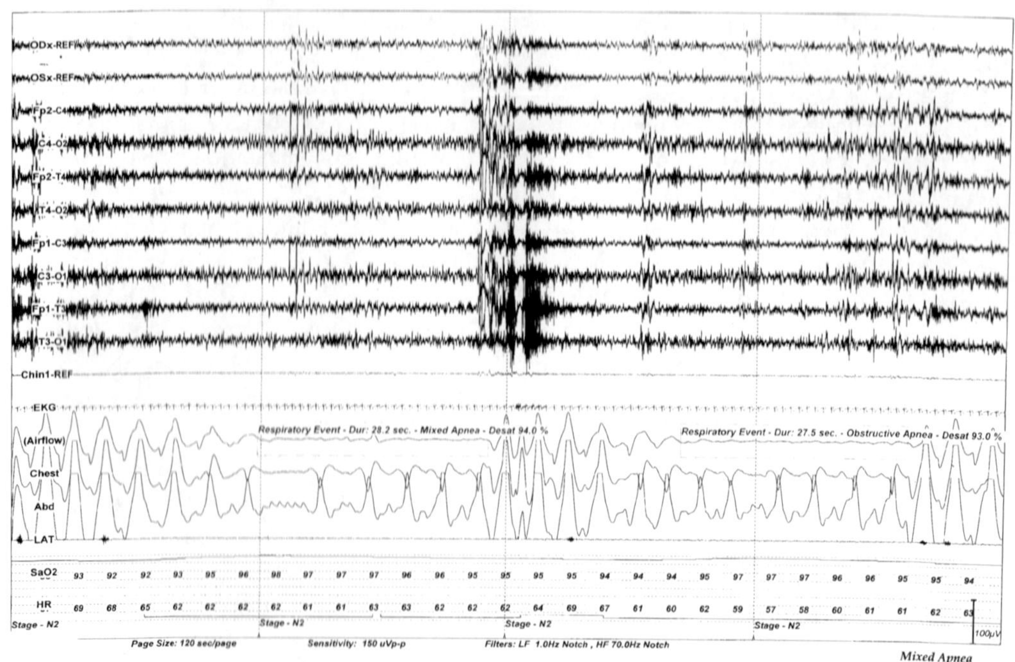

Figure 6. Obstructive and mixed apnea.

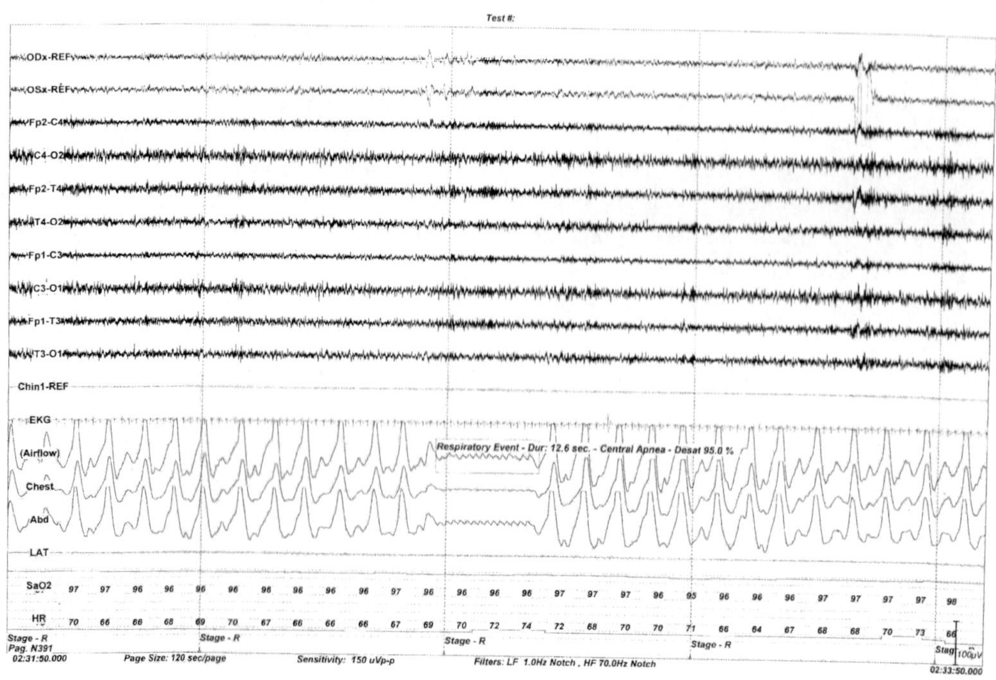

Figure 7. Central apnea.

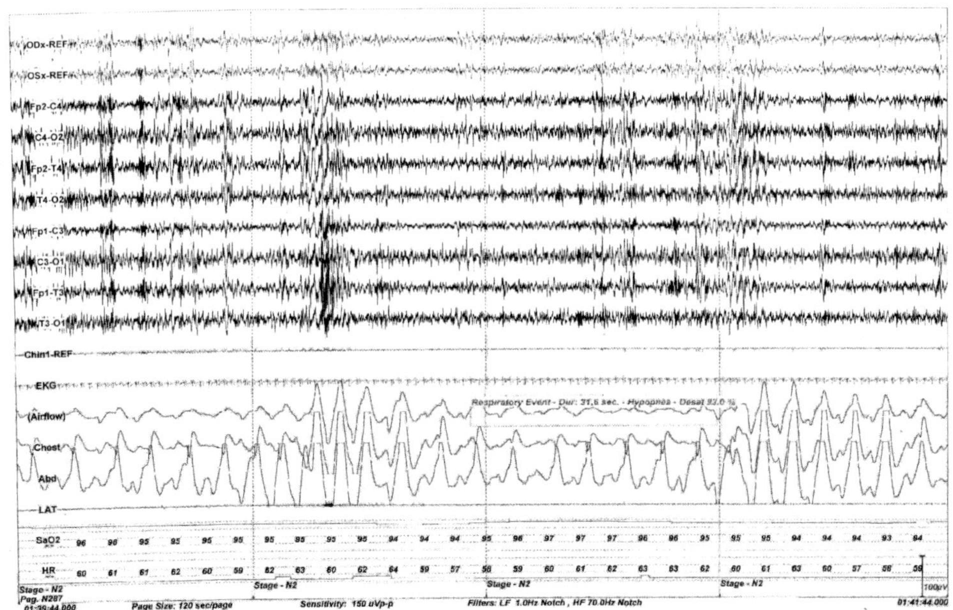

Figure 8. Hypopnea.

A respiratory effort-related arousal (RERA) is an event characterized by increasing respiratory effort for ≥10 sec leading to an arousal from sleep, but which does not fulfill criteria for hypopnea or apnea. [25] The respiratory disturbance index (RDI) is defined as the number of obstructive apneas, hypopneas, and RERAs/hour averaged over the course of at last 2 hours of sleep as determined by PSG [25]

An overnight PSG is recorded during the normal sleeping hours of a patient. Patients sleep 6-8 hours before either awakening spontaneously or being awakened. PSG includes simultaneously recording and analysis of EEG, EOG, EMG, oronasal airflow, chest wall effort, body position, snore microphone, ECG, and oxyhemoglobin saturation. Nasal airflow is best measured with a nasal cannula, and thoraco-abdominal movement with a respiratory inductive plethysmography. [26] Audio-visual recordings are included in most studies and PSG is supervised by a technician. Analysis requires manual scoring. With the inclusion of an EEG, sleep disruption caused by apneas and hypopneas and even more subtle respiratory effort related arousals are registered. Periodic limb movements are also routinely recorded with electromyogram electrodes to the fibular muscles. Limb movements may provoke repeated arousals which are easily recognized on EEG and may also cause daytime sleepiness. [27]

With the custom addition of video-surveillance, even more information is taken from in laboratory sleep studies, e.g. the occurrence of parasomnias, epilepsy or sleep-choking. The duration of a diagnostic PSG is typically at least 6 hours. A 6 hour minimum duration of a diagnostic nocturnal polysomnogram is preferred, which allows for the assessment of variability related to sleep stage and position compared to the frequency of obstructive respiratory events and the occurrence of other types of nocturnal events, such as periodic limb movements. [24]

The goal of the PSG is to quantify the amount of time spent in various stages of sleep during the night and to document clinically-relevant events such as cardiopulmonary abnormalities and/or changes in sleep stages. [22]

A portable home-based sleep study has recently emerged as an alternative to the PSG. Cardiorespiratory monitoring (CRM) incorporates a minimum of four channels, including signals of airflow (at last two channels of respiratory movement, or respiratory movement and airflow) heart rate or ECG, and oxygen saturation. Some CRM devices also register snoring sounds, body position, and leg movements. CRM may be performed attended or unattended in a hospital room or as an outpatient study in the patient's home with potential advantages in terms of improved sleep quality in their hospital environment. [28]

The main limitation of the portable home sleep study is that it does not have the EEG component; it is therefore not able to assess an individual's sleep architecture and will not be able to assess arousals based on changes in sleep stages. As a consequence, it can underestimate the prevalence of OSA. However, due to the high costs of PSG, CRM is increasingly used to detect breathing disorders.

3. Hypersomnia Not Due to a Sleep-Related Breathing Disorder

The ICDS-2 [1] classifies narcolepsy into three categories: narcolepsy with cataplexy, narcolepsy without cataplexy, and secondary narcolepsy. Cataplexy is a muscle weakness, typically provoked by strong emotion. The loss of tone can be total, leading to a fall, and/or partial, affecting only some muscles (facial, shoulders, knees, etc.). The attack has a rapid onset, short duration, bilateral involvement with consciousness fully preserved. Narcolepsy can also be accompanied by other REM sleep phenomena, such as sleep paralysis and hypnagogic or hypnopompic hallucinations.

The diagnosis of narcolepsy should be confirmed by nocturnal PSG followed by a MSLT. Moreover, continuous 24 or 36 hour PSG monitoring provides information about the actual, number duration, time, and type of daytime sleep episodes and confirms disrupted nighttime sleep.

PSG should reveal sufficiently long nocturnal sleep (at least 6 hours). Nocturnal sleep is fragmented not only by frequent awakenings, but also by symptoms that reflect abnormal motor control during sleep, such as periodic limb movements, restless legs syndrome (RLS) and REM sleep behavior disorder [29,30], and/or by sleep related breathing disorders [31].

Nevsimalova et al. [32] enrolled 148 narcoleptic patients in order to identify the association of narcolepsy with other sleep disorders in different age groups. They showed an increasing age-related proportion of associated sleep disorders with obstructive sleep apnea, periodic leg movements, and restless leg syndrome (p < 0.001). Patients affected by narcolepsy without cataplexy showed sleep comorbidities less frequently than those with narcolepsy cataplexy. A close connection with narcolepsy cataplexy was found particularly in REM behavior disorder (RBD) (p < 0.05). RBD affected a third of the patients in the youngest as well as in the oldest groups. However, association with other sleep disorders had no significant effect on nocturnal sleep (with the exception of obstructive sleep apnea), and the sleep comorbidities under investigation had no noticeable effect on daytime sleepiness.

With MSLT the latency between lights-out time and sleep onset is calculated for each nap, and the number of sleep onset REM periods (SOREMPs) is noted. SOREMPs are defined as REM sleep that occurs within 15 min of sleep onset. In normal population, MSLT scores vary with age among pediatric, adolescent, and adult populations, with young adults having the shortest latencies and the pre-pubescent children having the longest latencies. In adults, mean sleep latencies scores under 8 min are generally considered to be in the pathological range, while those over 10 min are considered normal. The ICSD-2 criteria [1] for narcolepsy utilize a mean sleep latency of ≤ 8 min. Within the context of objective marked sleepiness, the occurrence of 2 or more SOREMPs during MSLT are suggestive of narcolepsy.

The MWT measures the ability to remain awake under soporific conditions for a defined period of time. It is primarily used to follow the treatment of hypersomnia with stimulant medications to objectively document the ability to stay awake. The latest AASM Standards of Practice Committee considered mean sleep latency <8 min on the 40 min MWT protocol as abnormal, whereas values between 8 and 40 min were considered to be of uncertain significance.

ICSD-2 diagnostic criteria [1] of narcolepsy with cataplexy are as follows: 1) The patient has a complaint of excessive daytime sleepiness occurring almost daily for at least three months. 2) A denoted history of cataplexy, defined as sudden and transient episodes of loss of motor tone triggered by emotions is present. 3) The diagnosis of narcolepsy with cataplexy should, whenever possible, be confirmed by nocturnal polysomnography followed by a MSLT; the mean sleep latency on MSLT is ≤ 8 min and two or more SOREMPs are observed following sufficient nocturnal sleep (minimum 6 hours) during the night prior to the test. Alternatively to the PSG criteria, hypocretin-1 levels in the CSF are ≤ 110 pg/ml or one-third of mean normal values. 4) The hypersomnia is not better explained by another sleep disorder or neurological disorder, mental disorder, medication use, or substance use disorder. The diagnostic criteria of narcolepsy without cataplexy echoed those of narcolepsy with cataplexy, the main differences being the absence of typical cataplexy and the necessity to confirm the clinical diagnosis by nocturnal PSG followed by an MSLT showing two or more SOREMPs to avoid the risk of over-diagnosis in the absence of cataplexy. [1]

Patients with idiopathic hypersomnia have a complaint of EDS occurring almost daily for at least three months. The PSG studies of such patients have excluded other causes of daytime sleepiness. In the ICSD-2 [1], idiopathic hypersomnia has been separated in two entities: idiopathic hypersomnia with long sleep time and a form with short sleep time.

According to ICSD-2 criteria [1] in idiopathic hypersomnia with long sleep time, patients have prolonged nocturnal sleep time (>10 h) documented by interview, actigraphy or sleep logs; wake up in the morning or at the end of naps is almost always laborious; the PSG demonstrates a short sleep latency and a major sleep period that is prolonged to more than 10 hours in duration. If an MSLT is performed following overnight PSG, a mean sleep latency of less than 8 min is found and fewer than two SOREMPs are recorded. Mean sleep latency in idiopathic hypersomnia with long sleep time has been shown to be 6.2 ±3.0 min. In idiopathic hypersomnia without long sleep time, patients have normal nocturnal sleep that is greater than 6 hours but less than 10 hours. [1]

4. Circadian Rhythm Sleep Disorder

In the ICSD-2 [1], six distinct circadian rhythm sleep disorders (CRSDs) are described: 1) delayed sleep phase type, 2) advanced sleep phase type, 3) irregular sleep-wake phase type, 4) free-running type, 5) jet lag type, and 6) shift work type. The ICSD-2 also recognizes CRSDs secondary to medical conditions and drug or substance abuse, as well as a general category, CRSD Not Otherwise Specified (NOS). According to the ICSD-2 [1], "The essential feature of CRSDs is a persistent or recurrent pattern of sleep disturbance due primarily to alterations in the circadian timekeeping system or a misalignment between the endogenous circadian rhythm and exogenous factors that affect the timing or duration of sleep." The diagnosis also requires that the disorder is not "better explained" by another primary sleep disorder. The scientific literature on the clinical evaluation and treatment of CRSDs was reviewed by an AASM Task Force of experts in 2007 [33-34], and practice parameters were later developed based on the two accompanying comprehensive reviews.[33-34] The recommendations included were divided in three levels of strength: standard, guideline, and optional based on evidence from published studies. The main diagnostic tools considered include sleep logs, actigraphy, the morningness-eveningness questionnaire (MEQ), circadian phase markers, and polysomnography.

Sleep-wake diaries (sleep logs) are consistently recommended to evaluate sleep schedules in CRSD patients; however, there are no widely accepted, standardized sleep logs, and investigators and clinicians often construct their own. Sleep logs have apparent validity and can provide data on qualitative as well as quantitative aspects of sleep. [33]

Among general recommendations, the committee [35] concluded that: actigraphy is indicated to assist in evaluation of patients suspected of CRSDs, including irregular sleep-wake disorder (ISWR), free-running disorder (FRD) (with or without blindness) (optional), and in advanced sleep phase disorder (ASPD), delayed sleep phase disorder (DSPD), and shift work disorder (SWD) (guideline). Actigraphy is useful as an outcome measure in evaluating the response to treatment for CRSDs (guideline). PSG is indicated to rule out another primary sleep disorder in patients with symptoms suggestive of both a CRSD and another primary sleep disorder, but is not routinely indicated for diagnosis of CRSDs (standard).

ICSD-2 [1] diagnostic criteria for most CRSDs require that abnormalities in the timing of the habitual sleep pattern be documented with either sleep logs or actigraphy for seven days or more.

Parasomnia

REM sleep behavior disorder (RBD) is a parasomnia manifested by vivid, often frightening dreams associated with simple or complex motor behavior during REM sleep. Patients appear to "act out their dreams," in which the exhibited behaviors mirror the content of the dreams, and the dream content often involves a chasing or attacking theme. The PSG features of RBD include increased EMG tone +/- dream enactment behavior during REM sleep, so-called REM sleep without atonia RSWA [36]

Frauscher et al. framed the current state of affairs in assessing EMG tone during REM sleep very well [37]. The ICSD-2[1] defined REM sleep without atonia (RSWA) as the 'electromyographic (EMG) finding of excessive amounts of sustained or intermittent elevation of submental EMG tone or excessive phasic submental or (upper or lower) limb EMG twitching.' This definition has several limitations. First, a precise definition of 'excessive amounts of tonic and phasic EMG activity' was not provided, since normal values of these measures are unknown. Second, it is not stated how the tonic and phasic EMG activity should be measured. Third, it is unclear which muscle or combination of muscles of the body (either axial or extremity muscles, lower or upper extremity muscles, or proximal or distal extremity muscles) provides the highest rates of abnormal REM sleep EMG activity in RBD. Thus, some authors have developed scoring systems to not only qualify the EMG tone as normal or abnormal, but also to quantify the degree to which EMG tone is abnormal. [37-38-39]

The ICSD-2 [1] requires the following for a clinical diagnosis of RBD [1]: A. Presence of RSWA on PSG; B. At least one of the following: 1. sleep-related, injurious, potentially injurious, or disruptive behaviors by history (i.e. dream enactment behavior), and/or 2. abnormal REM sleep behavior documented during PSG monitoring; C. Absence of EEG epileptiform activity during REM sleep unless RBD can be clearly distinguished from any concurrent REM sleep related seizure disorder [3]; D. The sleep disorder is not better explained by another sleep disorder, medical or neurological disorder, mental disorder, medication use, or substance use disorder.

The AASM [3] has critically evaluated the scoring methods of PSGs, and the formal diagnosis of RBD has changed slightly. The differential diagnosis of recurrent RBD includes non-REM parasomnias (somnambulism, night terrors, confusional arousals), nocturnal panic attacks, nocturnal seizures, nightmares, nocturnal wandering associated with dementia, and OSA. The history usually allows differentiation of these disorders from RBD. When diagnostic clarification is necessary, particularly when the risk for injury is high, the behaviors occur at any time of the night, other features suggesting an evolving neurodegenerative are present, or loud snoring and observed apnea suggestive of OSA is present, PSG with simultaneous video monitoring is warranted [36]

The new AASM Manual for the Scoring of Sleep and Related Events [3] has maintained many of the criteria and definitions for REM sleep (stage R), primarily low amplitude mixed frequency EEG background, rapid eye movements, and low chin EMG tone. RSWA can be applied when there is: 1) sustained muscle activity in REM sleep with 50% of the epoch having increased chin EMG amplitude, and/or; 2) excessive transient muscle activity, defined by the presence of 5 or more mini-epochs (a 30 second epoch is divided into ten 3-sec mini-epochs) in an epoch having transient muscle activity lasting at least 0.5 sec. There was no minimum number of epochs showing abnormal muscle activity required for the RSWA designation – this was purposefully not stated as there is little good normative data. [3]

Simultaneous video/PSG recording is essential for evaluating patients with suspected RBD so that vocalizations and limb movements can be captured and viewed concurrently with PSG data. When vocalizations and/or limb movements emerge during REM sleep, without associated epileptiform activity on EEG derivations, a diagnosis of RBD is established [36]. It is relatively uncommon during single night PSG to record violent and complex dream enactment behavior; rather, increased EMG tone during REM sleep and sparse limb jerks are the norm.

PSG is essential to establish a diagnosis of RBD, but the procedure does require appropriate monitoring equipment, including time synchronized video recordings, specially trained technologists, bed availability in a sleep laboratory, and clinicians who can interpret the data.

Fantini et al. [40] performed quantitative analyses of waking and REM sleep EEG in 15 patients with idiopathic RBD (iRBD) and in 15 matched controls. EEG slowing was demonstrated in the RBD group, suggesting impaired cortical activity during both wakefulness and REM sleep. The authors interpreted these findings as possibly reflecting a very early sign of central nervous system dysfunction.

In a study by Massicotte-Marque et al. [41], 14 patients with iRBD and 14 healthy control subjects underwent waking EEG recordings. Compared to controls, patients with iRBD showed EEG slowing (higher delta and theta power) during wakefulness in all brain areas compared to controls. The authors concluded that waking EEG slowing in patients with iRBD is similar to that observed in early stages of some synucleinopathies.

About 70% of patients with iRBD have periodic limb movement (PLMS) (see below for the scoring criteria) index (number of PLMS per hour of sleep) greater than 10, which, in the past, has been usually been considered to be pathologic. [42]

Manconi et al. confirmed the high prevalence of PLMS in RBD [43] and the significant differences in PLMS time structure that are present between patients with RBD and those with RLS. Firstly, PLMS were clearly associated with NREM sleep in RLS and with REM sleep in RBD, at least in terms of number per hour. Moreover, PLMS were shorter, less often bilateral, and had with a higher intermovement interval in patients with RBD compared to those with RLS [43]. This might have important prognostic implications in distinguishing between different RBD subtypes.

Sleep Related Movement Disorder

The sleep-related movement disorders (SRMD) comprise five different disorders: restless legs syndrome (RLS), periodic limb movement disorder (PLMD), sleep-related leg cramps, sleep-related bruxism, and sleep-related rhythmic movement disorder (RMD).

The four essential criteria for diagnosis of RLS and the additional supportive clinical features are listed in the report of the International Restless Legs Syndrome Study Group (IRLSSG) and are as follows: an urge to move the legs usually accompanied or caused by uncomfortable or unpleasant sensations in the legs that begin or worsen during periods of rest or inactivity; symptoms are worse in the evening/night than during the day or only occur in the evening or night, and are partially or totally relieved by movement. [44]

Supportive features useful for diagnosing of RLS [44] in uncertain clinical cases are follows: response to dopaminergic therapy, positive family history, and presence of periodic limb movements during sleep (PLMS; see below for PLMS scoring criteria).

Although diagnosis of RLS is based on clinical features, some instrumental examinations, such as PSG and actigraphy (ACT), can be performed. PSG and ACT may help to confirm the diagnosis or exclude other underlying primary sleep disorders, such as sleep apnea, or assess efficacy of drug treatment. A PSG may also be helpful in patients with RLS in whom conventional therapy does not yield positive results.

In patients with RLS, PSG and ACT may identify the presence of PLMS (see below). A PSG performed with surface EMG of the tibialis anterior muscles is the gold standard for PMLS diagnosis. Due to the high costs of PSG, ACT is increasingly used to detect PLMS in RLS patients.

The symptoms due to RLS cause difficulties in falling asleep by interfering with sleep onset or through frequent and prolonged awakenings with difficulty in going back to sleep. As a consequence, a large proportion of RLS patients refers poor sleep quality, insomnia and EDS.

PLMD is characterized by periodic episodes of repetitive and stereotyped limb movements occurring during sleep and by clinical sleep disturbance that cannot be explained by another primary sleep disorder. PLMS is similar to the Babinski response and is characterized by dorsiflexion of the ankle, toes, partial flexion of the knee, and sometimes the hip. [1]

In the ICSD-2 [1], the four criteria for PLMD are described as follows: (1) PSG demonstrates repetitive, highly stereotyped, limb movements that satisfy the criteria for PLMS (see below); (2) the PLMS index, i.e. the number of PLMS divided the number of hours of sleep with limb movement recording, exceeds 5 per hour in children and 15 per hour in adults; (3) presence of clinical sleep disturbance or daytime fatigue; (4) the PLMS are not better explained by another sleep disorder, medical or neurological disorder, mental disorder, medication use, or substance use disorder. Although the ICSD-2 reports that many individuals affected by PLMD suffer from insomnia and EDS [1], there are controversies over the clinical significance of PLMS. [45, 46]

It is known that periodic leg movements are frequently accompanied by full awakenings or by signs of EEG arousals on PSG studies with a consequent sleep fragmentation. Recent studies report that EEG and autonomic arousals may herald PLMS [45]. The time relationship of these EEG arousals with leg movements seems to vary from patient to patient. They may precede or follow leg movements or occur simultaneously. It is not clear whether these arousals trigger leg movements or, alternatively, whether both EEG arousals and leg movements are separate expressions of a common pathophysiological mechanism.

PLMS can be detected by PSG or ACT. Scoring criteria for PLMS were first proposed by Coleman in 1982. [47] In 1993, the American Sleep Disorders Association (ASDA) committee developed scoring rules for PLMS. [48] In 2006, a task force of PLM Scoring of the IRLSSG revised the previous criteria in order to adapt detection of PLMS to the new requirements of computerized sleep recordings and to the developing understanding of the different pathologies associated with PLMS. [49] These new guidelines apply to adults and are expected to be valid for children, but are recommended for cautious use with children until there are further pediatric evaluations of PLM. [49]

For correct electromyographic recording during PGS studies, surface electrodes should be placed at 2-3 cm apart or one-third of the length of the anterior tibialis muscle, whichever is shorter. Electrodes should be placed longitudinally on the muscles, symmetrically around the middle. Two channels, one for each leg, are strongly recommended for all studies and required for research.

The electromyographic activation of leg muscles (in particular the anterior tibialis muscle), defines a leg movement (LM) event. A LM event starts when the EMG voltage increases to ≥ 8 μV above resting baseline, while the event ends when the EMG voltage decreases to < 2 µV above resting level and remains below that value for 0.5 sec. The duration of a LM event must be at least 0.5 sec and no longer than 10 sec.

The period length (from limb-movement onset to limb-movement onset) for two consecutive events to be considered as PLM must be at least 5 and no longer than 90 sec. The number of consecutive candidate events meeting the period criteria must be ≥4.

An arousal event and movement event are considered associated with each other when there is less than 0.5 sec between the end of one event end the onset of the other event, regardless of which is first. A critical breath event (apnea/hypopnea) and an LM are assumed to be associated with each other if they overlap or if the end of one event and the beginning of the other event are within 0.5 sec or less of each other, regardless of which event is first [49]

Activity monitoring of leg or foot movements by a motion detector system provides another measure of leg movements in sleep. These devices provide the possibility of multiple nights of recording in a home environment, reducing somewhat the vexing problems caused by the relatively large night-to-night within-subject variation reported to occur for PLM [50, 51].

The presence of PLMS is very common in a variety of sleep disorders such as RLS, RBD (see above), narcolepsy, insomnia, and obstructive sleep apnea syndrome (OSAS). Patients affected by sleep-related leg cramps report painful sensations due to sudden and intense involuntary contractions of single muscles or muscle groups affecting lower limbs, usually the calf or the feet. According to ICSD-2 criteria [1], PSG is not routinely recommended for identifying isolated nocturnal leg cramps. Sleep studies reveal non-periodic bursts of leg EMG activity.

In patients affected by sleep-related leg cramps nocturnal sleep may be impaired with difficulty in falling asleep and/or frequent awakenings at night. Moreover, persisting discomfort after the cramps often delays subsequent return to sleep. Accordingly, the major complications include insomnia and sleepiness due to interruptions in sleep.

Sleep-related bruxism is characterized by grinding or clenching of the teeth during sleep; although diagnosis of sleep-related bruxism is clinically assessed, an audio-video PSG can be performed in dubious cases. If EMG artifacts on EEG derivations referenced to ear electrodes occur in routine PSG, sleep bruxism can be hypothesized. [52] To confirm a diagnosis of sleep bruxism, the EMG from at least one masseter muscle with audio recording to associate muscular activity with grinding sound production should be included in the PSG. Patients with sleep bruxism show three different patterns of EMG activity in masseter or temporalis muscles: 1) tonic, isolated sustained contractions lasting more than 2 s; 2) phasic, rhythmic masticatory muscle activities (RMMA) lasting from 0.25 to 2 sec; 3) mixed, both tonic and phasic types. [52]

PSG diagnosis of sleep bruxism is based on (1) more than four bruxism episodes per hour; (2) more than six bruxism bursts per episode and/or 25 bruxism bursts per hour of sleep; and (3) at least two episodes with grinding sounds.

Rhythmic movement (RMs) during sleep can involve any part of the body. There are several subtypes of RMD. The most frequent forms of RMD are body rocking, body rolling, head banging, and head rolling, while leg rolling and leg banging are less common. The frequency of RMs can vary, but it is generally between 0.5 and 2 per second, lasting less than 15 min. [1] Usually patients with RMD show only one form of RMs and rarely two forms in the same night [53,54]. Sleep-related rhythmic movement disorder can be diagnosed based on clinical features, and PSG is often reserved when the differential diagnosis includes epilepsy.

These movements occurs during all sleep stages, most commonly during NREM sleep (N1, N2), less frequently during N3, and only rarely during REM sleep. A sleep study with expanded EEG montage may be necessary to differentiate the behavior from that of epilepsy. EEG studies have shown normal activity between episodes of rhythmic behavior.

Differential Diagnosis of Paroxysmal Events during Sleep

The widespread use of EEG recordings under audiovisual monitoring has revealed several pathological conditions characterized by paroxysmal motor events during sleep. Two broad nosological categories with episodes of motor activity during NREM sleep stages have been identified, namely parasomnias such as sleep terror and sleep-walking, which are thought to represent disorders of arousal during sleep, and epileptic seizures arising during sleep (nocturnal or morpheic epilepsy). [55]

The differential diagnosis of paroxysmal events during sleep includes [56]: parasomnias; NREM arousal disorders (confusional arousals, sleep walking, sleep terrors); parasomnias associated with REM sleep (RBD); sleep-related movement disorders; psychogenic non-epileptic seizures; sleep-related dissociative disorder.

Differentiating between nocturnal seizures and NREM parasomnias can be challenging, especially in nocturnal frontal lobe epilepsy (NLFE) because of the typically unusual, bizarre presentation of NLFE seizures, along with its common association with a normal EEG. [56]

NFLE has been delineated as a distinct syndrome in the heterogeneous group of paroxysmal sleep-related disturbances. The variable duration and intensity of the seizures distinguish three non-rapid eye movement-related subtypes: paroxysmal arousals, characterized by brief and sudden recurrent motor paroxysmal behavior; nocturnal paroxysmal dystonia, motor attacks with complex dystonic–dyskinetic features; and episodic nocturnal wanderings, stereotyped, agitated somnambulism. [55]

The features supporting an epileptic etiology of paroxysmal events are: (1) stereotyped nature of spells; (2) high frequency and tendency to cluster [57]; (3) timing of the events (NREM parasomnias usually emerge from slow wave sleep, which typically occurs within 2 h of sleep onset, whereas frontal lobe seizures may occur during any sleep stage, but are common shortly after falling asleep) [58]; (4) semiology of events (although frontal lobe seizures may have variable manifestations, the occurrence of prominent unilateral tonic stiffening favors an epileptic origin rather than a parasomnia); (5) duration of events (parasomnias are usually relatively prolonged events, whereas epileptic seizures, especially frontal lobe seizures, tend to be very brief, lasting <2 min on average) [58]; and (6) presenting age (NREM parasomnias are often limited to childhood, but can occur in adulthood, whereas NFLE often persists into adulthood).

Although many seizures are easily distinguished from non-epileptic events on the basis of patient history, this can be difficult in the case of NFLE. However, it is important to note that in NFLE the EEG can frequently be normal even during the ictal episodes, for multiple reasons, including deep generators, few electrodes, and poor field coverage with the international 10-20 system. [56] Therefore, differentiating an epileptic from a parasomnia attack using an EEG recording alone is not straightforward when the epileptic focus is located in the deep or mesial frontal regions and the attacks are restricted to NREM sleep. [55] In addition, the EEG can be frequently obscured by muscle artifacts.

Moreover, even when epileptiform activity is recorded, it may difficult to correctly lateralize the onset, especially from a parasagital focus in which the near-midline ictal focus can create an electrical dipole directed toward the contralateral electrodes. There are several semiological features that can be seen in both NFLE and psychogenic non-epileptic seizures: eye closure, hypermotor activity, and partial recall during the events. [56]

Nocturnal video-polysomnography is the gold standard for diagnosing and differentiating parasomnias from other arousals with atypical motor behaviors such as NFLE. [58] In fact, with more prolonged monitoring of patients, it is possible to confirm the stereotypical nature of the events on video and to record several seizures. [56] On occasion, patients show no difference from classical sleep parameters, while microstructure analysis shows sleep instability and arousal fluctuations in parasomnias and NFLE. [58]

References

[1]   American Academy of Sleep Medicine. The international classification of sleep disorders. Sateia M, editor. Diagnostic and coding manual. 2nd edition. Westchester (IL): *American Academy of Sleep Medicine*; 2005. pp. 1-297.

[2]   Mecarelli O. Manuale teorico pratico di elettroencefalografia. 2007

[3]   Iber C, Ancoli-Israel S, Chessonn A, Quan SF. In The AASM Manual for the scoring of sleep and associated events: rules, terminology and technical specifications. 1st ed. Westchester, IL: *American Academy of Sleep Medicine*; 2007.

[4]   Terzano MG, Mancia D, Salati MR, Costani G, Decembrino A, Parrino L.The cyclic alternating pattern as a physiologic component of normal NREM sleep. *Sleep*. 1985;8(2):137-45.

[5]   Parrino L, Ferri R, Bruni O, Terzano MG. Cyclic alternating pattern (CAP): the marker of sleep instability. *Sleep Med Rev*. 2012 Feb;16(1):27-45.

[6]   Klem GH, Lüders HO, Jasper HH, Elger C. The ten-twenty electrode system of the International Federation. The International Federation of Clinical Neurophysiology. *Electroencephalogr Clin Neurophysiol Suppl*. 1999;52:3-6.

[7]   Michael R. Littner MD1; Clete Kushida MD, PhD2; Merrill Wise MD3et al. Practice Parameters for Clinical Use of the Multiple Sleep Latency Test and the Maintenance of Wakefulness Test. *Sleep*, Vol. 28, No. 1, 2005

[8]   Thorpy MJ, Westbrook P, Ferber R, Fredrickson P, Mahowald M, Perez-Guerra, Reite M, Smith P. An American Sleep Disorders Association Report: The clinical use of the multiple sleep latency test. *Sleep* 1992; 15:268-276.

[9]   Michael Littner MD et al. Practice Parameters for the Role of Actigraphy in the Study of Sleep and Circadian Rhythms: An Update for *2002SLEEP*, Vol. 26, No. 3, 2003 337

[10]   Standards of Practice Committee of the American Sleep Disorders Association. Practice parameters for the use of actigraphy in the clinical assessment of sleep disorders. *Sleep* 1995;18(4):285-287.

[11]   Sackett D. Rules of evidence and clinical recommendation. Can J Cardiol 1993;9:487-489.

[12] Jean-Louis G, von Gizycki H, Zizi F, Spielman A, Hauri P, Taub H. The actigraph data analysis software: I. A novel approach to scoring and interpreting sleep-wake activity. *Percept Mot Skills* 1997; 85(1):207-216.

[13] Sadeh A, Sharkey KM, Carskadon MA. Activity-based sleep-wake identification: An empirical test of methodological issues. *Sleep* 1994; 17:201-207.

[14] Chambers MJ. Actigraphy and insomnia: A closer look Part I. Sleep 1994; 17(5):405-408.

[15] Sonia Ancoli-Israel PhD et al. The Role of Actigraphy in the Study of Sleep and Circadian Rhythms. *SLEEP*, Vol. 26, No. 3, 2003

[16] Practice parameters for using polysomnography to evaluate insomnia: an update. Littner M, Hirshkowitz M, Kramer M, Kapen S, Anderson WM, Bailey D, Berry RB, Davila D, Johnson S, Kushida C, Loube DI, Wise M, Woodson BT; American Academy of Sleep Medicine; Standards of Practice Committe. *Sleep.* 2003 Sep;26(6):754-60

[17] Chronic insomnia. Morin CM, Benca R. Lancet. 2012 Mar 24;379(9821):1129-41.

[18] Perlis ML, Smith MT, Andrews PJ, Orff H, Giles DE. Beta/Gamma EEG activity in patients with primary and secondary insomnia and good sleeper controls. *Sleep* 2001; 24: 110–17.

[20] Morris L, Kleinberger A, Lee K, et al. Rapid risk stratification for obstructive sleep apnea, based on snoring severity and body mass index. *Otolaryngology-Head and Neck Surgery* 2008;139:615-8.

[21] Sleep Apnea: What Is Sleep Apnea?. NHLBI: Health Information for the Public. U.S. Department of Health and Human Services. 2009-05.

[22] American Academy of Sleep Medicine.International Classification of Sleep Disorders. In: Diagnostic and Coding Manual. Second Edition. Westchester, Ill: *American Academy of Sleep Medicine*;2005.

[23] Sleep –related breathing disorders in adults:recommendations for syndrome definition and measurement technoques in clinical research. *Sleep* 1999; 22:667-689.

[24] Mosko SS, Dickel MJ,Ashurst J. Night to night variability in sleep apnea and sleep related periodic leg movement in the elderly. *Sleep* 1988; 11:340-348.

[25] Loube DI, Andrada TF. Upper airway resistance syndrome:detection with respiratory indictutive plethysmography. *Chest* 1999; 115:1333-1337.

[26] Thurnheer R, Xie X, Bloch KE. Accuracy of nasal cannula pressure recordings for assessment of ventilation during sleep. *Am J Resp Crit Care Med* 2001; 164:1914-9.

[27] Chervin RD.Periodic leg movements and sleepiness in patients evaluated for sleep-dosordered breathing. *Am J Resp Crit Care Med* 2001;164:1454-8.

[28] Kingshott RN, Douglas NJ. The effect of in-laboratory polysomnography on sleep and objective daytime sleepiness. *Sleep* 2000; 23:1109-13.

[29] Plazzi G, Pizza F, Palaia V et al (2011) Complex movement disorders at disease onset in childhood narcolepsy with cataplexy. *Brain* 134:3480–3492

[30] Nevsimalova S, Prihodova I, Kemlink D et al (2007) REM behavior disorder (RBD) can be one of the first symptoms of childhood narcolepsy. *Sleep Med* 8:784–786

[31] Pataka AD, Frangulyan RR, Mackay TW, Douglas NJ, Riha RL (2012) Narcolepsy and sleep-disordered breathing. *Eur J Neurol* 19:696–702

[32] Nevsimalova S, Pisko J, Buskova J, Kemlink D, Prihodova I, Sonka K, Skibova J. Narcolepsy: clinical differences and association with other sleep disorders in different age groups. *J Neurol.* 2012 Oct 16.

[33] Circadian rhythm sleep disorders: part I, basic principles, shift work and jet lag disorders. An American Academy of Sleep Medicine review. Sack RL, Auckley D, Auger RR, Carskadon MA, Wright KP Jr, Vitiello MV, Zhdanova IV; American Academy of Sleep Medicine. *Sleep*. 2007 Nov;30(11):1460-83.

[34] Circadian rhythm sleep disorders: part II, advanced sleep phase disorder, delayed sleep phase disorder, free-running disorder, and irregular sleep-wake rhythm. An American Academy of Sleep Medicine review. Robert L Sack, MD1; Dennis Auckley, MD2; R. Robert Auger, MD3; Mary A. Carskadon, PhD4; Kenneth P. Wright Jr, PhD5; Michael V. Vitiello, PhD6; Irina V. Zhdanova, MD7

[35] Practice parameters for the clinical evaluation and treatment of circadian rhythm sleep disorders. An American Academy of Sleep Medicine report. Morgenthaler TI, Lee-Chiong T, Alessi C, Friedman L, Aurora RN, Boehlecke B, Brown T, Chesson AL Jr, Kapur V, Maganti R, Owens J, Pancer J, Swick TJ, Zak R; Standards of Practice Committee of the American Academy of Sleep Medicine. *Sleep*. 2007 Nov;30(11):1445-59.

[36] Bradley F. Boeve, M.D. Ann N Y Acad Sci. Author manuscript; available in PMC 2011 January 1.

[37] Frauscher B, Iranzo A, Högl B, et al. Quantification of electromyographic activity during REM sleep in multiple muscles in REM sleep behavior disorder. *Sleep* 2008;31:724–731.

[38] Lapierre O, Montplaisir J. Polysomnographic features of REM sleep behavior disorder: development of a scoring method. *Neurology* 1992;42:1371–1374.

[39] Bliwise D, Rye D. Elevated PEM (phasic electromyographic metric) rates identify rapid eye movement behavior disorder patients on nights without behavioral abnormalities. *Sleep* 2008;31:853–857.

[40] Fantini ML, Gagnon JF, Petit D, et al. Slowing of electroencephalogram in rapid eye movement sleep behavior disorder. *Ann Neurol* 2003;53:774–780.

[41] Massicotte-Marquez J, Carrier J, Decary A, et al. Slow-wave sleep and delta power in rapid eye movement sleep behavior disorder. *Ann Neurol* 2005;57:277–282.

[42] Fantini ML, Michaud M, Gosselin N, Lavigne G, Montplaisir J. Periodic leg movements in REM sleep behavior disorder and related autonomic and EEG activation. *Neurology* 2002;59:1889-94.

[43] Manconi M; Ferri R; Zucconi M; Fantini ML; Plazzi G; Ferini-Strambi L. Time structure analysis of leg movements during sleep in REM sleep behavior disorder. *SLEEP* 2007;30(12):1779-1785.

[44] Allen RP, Picchietti D, Hening WA, Trenkwalder C, Walters AS, Montplaisir J; Restless Legs Syndrome Diagnosis and Epidemiology workshop at the National Institutes of Health in collaboration with members of the International Restless Legs Syndrome Study Group (2003) Restless Legs Syndrome: diagnostic criteria, special considerations, and epidemiology. A report from the restless legs syndrome diagnosis and epidemi- ology workshop at the *National Institutes of Health. Sleep Med* 4:101–119

[45] Hogl B (2007) Periodic limb movements are associated with disturbed sleep. Pro J Clin Sleep Med 3:12–14 124.

[46] Mahowald MW (2007) Periodic limb movements are NOT associated with disturbed sleep. *Con J Clin Sleep Med* 3:15–17

[47] Coleman RM (1982) Periodic movements in sleep (nocturnal myoclonus) and restless legs syndrome. In: Guilleminault C (ed) Sleep and waking disorders: indications and techniques. Addison-Wesley, Menlo Park, pp 265–295

[48] The atlas task force (1993) Recording and scoring leg movements: the atlas task force. *Sleep* 16:748–759

[49] Zucconi M, Ferri R, Allen R, Baier PC, Bruni O, Chokroverty S, Ferini-Strambi L, Fulda S, Garcia-Borreguero D, Hening WA, Hirshkowitz M, Ho ¨gl B, Hornyak M, King M, Montagna P, Parrino L, Plazzi G, Terzano MG, International Restless Legs Syndrome Study Group (IRLSSG) (2006) The official World Association of Sleep Medicine (WASM) standards for recording and scoring periodic leg movements in sleep (PLMS) and wakefulness (PLMW) developed in collaboration with a task force from the International Restless Legs Syndrome Study Group (IRLSSG). *Sleep Med* 7:175–183

[50] Allen RP. The resurrection of periodic limb movements (PLM): leg activity monitoring and the restless legs syndrome (RLS). *Sleep Med* 2005;6:385–7.

[51] Hornyak M, Kopasz M, Feige B, et al. Variability of periodic limb leg movements in various sleep disorders: implications for clinical and pathophysiological studies. Sleep 2005;28:331–5.

[52] Merlino G, Gigli GL. Sleep-related movement disorders. *Neurol Sci.* 2012 Jun;33(3):491-513.

[53] Kohyama J, Matsukura F, Kimura K, Tachibana N (2002) Rhythmic movement disorder: polysomnographic study and summary of reported cases. *Brain Dev* 24:33–38

[54] Mayer G, Wilde-Frenz J, Kurella B (2007) Sleep related rhythmic movement disorder revisited. *J Sleep Res* 16:110–116

[55] Federica Provini, Giuseppe Plazzi, Paolo Tinuper, Stefano Vandi, Elio Lugaresi and Pasquale Montagna. Nocturnal frontal lobe epilepsy. A clinical and polygraphic overview of 100 consecutive cases. *Brain* (1999), 122, 1017–1031

[56] Lana Jeradeh Boursoulian, M.D.,1 Carlos H. Schenck, M.D.,2,3 Mark W. Mahowald, M.D.,2,4 and Andre H. Lagrange, M.D., Ph.D. Differentiating Parasomnias from Nocturnal Seizures. *J Clin Sleep Med.* 2012 February 15; 8(1): 108–112.

[57] Provini F, Plazzi G, Lugaresi E. From nocturnal paroxysmal dystonia to nocturnal frontal lobe epilepsy. *Clin Neurophysiol.* 2000;111(Suppl 2):S2–8.

[58] Zucconi M, Ferini-Strambi L. NREM parasomnias: arousal disorders and differentiation from nocturnal frontal lobe epilepsy. *Clin Neurophysiol.* 2000;111(Suppl 2):S129–35.

[59] Schenck CH, Milner DM, Hurwitz TD, Bundlie SR, Mahowald MW. A polysomnographic and clinical report on sleep-related injury in 100 adult patients. *Am J Psychiatry.* 1989;146:1166–73.

In: Sleep Medicine
Editors: A. Del Casale, R. Brugnoli and P. Girardi

ISBN: 978-1-62808-515-0
© 2013 Nova Science Publishers, Inc.

Chapter XIV

Neuroimaging in Sleep Medicine

Antonio Del Casale, Valentina Corigliano, Chiara Rapinesi,
Daniele Serata, Anna Comparelli and Stefano Ferracuti*
[1]Sapienza University, Rome, NESMOS (Neuroscience, Mental Health and Sensory
Organs) Department, School of Medicine and Psychology

Abstract

Functional and structural neuroimaging provide a means to understand brain function in patients affected by sleep disorders. Herein, we describe neuroimaging findings of primary sleep disorders, including types of dyssomnia related to intrinsic sleep impairments (i.e., idiopathic insomnia, narcolepsy, and obstructive sleep apnea) and abnormal motor behaviors during sleep (i.e., periodic limb movement disorder, restless legs syndrome and rapid-eye-movement sleep behavior disorder). We also include functional neuroimaging studies in sleep complaints secondary to specific psychiatric disorders.

Functional neuroimaging may address different kinds of issues in sleep medicine. Functional and structural neural changes can have a causal role in the pathophysiology of sleep disorders. Other changes in brain structure or regional activity can be considered as secondary consequences of long-term sleep disruption.

Neuroimaging studies can help to better understand the cognitive and neural responses to various therapeutic approaches. In the future, neuroimaging studies will probably lead to modify the nosography of sleep disorders on the basis of their underlying and characteristic neural correlates.

Keywords: Sleep Disorders; Sleep Medicine; Neuroimaging; Computed Tomography; Magnetic Resonance Imaging; Functional Neuroimaging; Positron Emission Tomography; Single Photon Emission Computed Tomography; Proton Magnetic Resonance Spectroscopy; Functional Magnetic Resonance Imaging

[*] Corresponding author: Antonio Del Casale, M.D. "Sapienza" University of Rome. NESMOS (Neuroscience, Mental Health and Sensory Organs) Department, School of Medicine and Psychology. Email: antonio.delcasale@uniroma1.it.

Introduction: Human Physiological Sleep

Functional and structural brain imaging techniques provides clues for understanding the basic mechanisms and functional properties of human sleep. Several studies aimed to showing brain functional changes related to physiological sleep and its disturbances by using Positron Emission Tomography (PET), Single Photon Emission Computed Tomography (SPECT), Proton Magnetic Resonance Spectroscopy (^{1}H-MRS), and functional Magnetic Resonance Imaging (fMRI). Other studies with the aim of identifying brain morphometric changes correlated with sleep and its disorders/disturbances have used structural neuroimaging techniques, mainly Computed Tomography (CT), Magnetic Resonance Imaging (MRI) with Voxel Based Morphometry (VBM), and Diffusion Tensor Imaging (DTI).

Globally, several studies have shown a decrease in brain activity during non-rapid-eye-movement (NREM) sleep and a sustained level of brain function during the rapid-eye-movement (REM) sleep compared to wakefulness [1-8]. In addition, these studies have specifically characterized segregated patterns of regional neural activity for each sleep stage.

NREM sleep has been associated with relative reduction in activations of the brainstem, thalamus, and several cortical areas, mainly including the medial prefrontal cortex (mPFC) [9-11]. Deactivations in the thalamo-cortical circuits during NREM sleep reflect the homeostatic need for brain energy recovery, which appear to be crucial for several activities, including waking, conscious, and directed behavior [12, 13].

On the other hand, REM sleep has been associated with hyperactivation of the pons, thalamus, limbic areas, and temporo-occipital cortices, and with deactivation of prefrontal areas [5,8,14,15]. A meta-analysis by Maquet and colleagues [15] showed that during REM sleep quiescent regions are confined to the inferior and middle frontal cortex and to the inferior parietal lobule. In line with the theories of REM sleep generation and dreaming properties, these data suggest an important role of REM sleep in emotional behavior, given the involvement of limbic and paralimbic structures in the regulation of affects and in motivated behavior [16-19].

Idiopathic Insomnia

Idiopathic insomnia is the most common sleep disorder in the general population and consists of difficulty in initiating or maintaining sleep or in a non-restorative sleep, with daytime consequences [20]. Even if it can be related with various etiopathogenesis to different causes, both medical and neurological, including pain, dyspnea, agitation, delusions, increased alertness or forced positions [21], primary insomnia seems to depend on an abnormality of the neurological control of the sleep-wake system [20]. This can be due to an imbalance between arousal and sleep promoting system, which would cause a global cortical hyperactivity, so that hyperarousal is widely believed to be the final common pathway of the disorder [22].

Previous EEG studies have confirmed this hypothesis, reporting an increase in beta-gamma activity, which was proposed as an EEG marker of arousal during sleep, at sleep onset, and during NREM sleep in insomnia [23].

The hyperarousal theory has also been supported by a number of functional neuroimaging studies, which showed an increase of cortical functions in insomnia.

Using ^{18}F-fluorodeoxyglucose (^{18}F-FDG) PET in 7 patients affected by idiopathic insomnia compared to 20 healthy subjects, Nofzinger et al. [24] found a global increase of the cerebral metabolic rate of glucose consumption (CMRglu) during sleep and wakefulness in insomnia. Several brain areas, mainly including the ascending reticular activating system, thalamus, hypothalamus, and insular, anterior cingulate and mesial temporal cortices, did not show decreased metabolic rate from waking to sleep states in patients with insomnia (see Figure 1) [24].

From waking to NREM sleep states, insomniacs also showed a smaller CMRglu decline in the ascending reticular activating system, hypothalamus, thalamus, amygdala, hippocampus, and insular, anterior cingulate, and medial prefrontal cortices. These findings suggest a failure in the brain activity system that normally provides a progressive, controlled, and gradual decline in the functions of the brainstem, thalamus and prefrontal cortices during the transition from waking to sleep [8]. The CMRglu changes observed in the thalamus might reflect a persistent sensory processing that results in shallower sleep. In contrast, during wakefulness patients showed relative CMRglu reductions in the bilateral prefrontal, left superior temporal, parietal and occipital cortices, and in the thalamus, hypothalamus and brainstem reticular formation. The observed wakefulness-related CMRglu reduction in the thalamus and parietofrontal cortices is in agreement with a chronic state of sleep deprivation in insomniac patients, since previous studies showed in the same regions hypofunctioning subsequent sleep deprivation [25]. This hypofunctioning has been correlated with the greater fatigue and the impaired cognition resulting from inefficient nocturnal sleep [25, 26].

A PET study by Smith et al. [27] conducted on 5 insomniacs compared to 4 normal sleepers during NREM sleep showed a major decrease of regional cerebral blood flow (rCBF) of cortical regions, including the frontal medial, occipital, and parietal cortices. This study also showed an abnormal pattern of regional brain function measured by tomographs of rCBF during NREM sleep that particularly involves basal ganglia. Interestingly, after cognitive behavioral therapy 4 of the insomniac patients showed rCBF normalization, particularly in the basal ganglia [28]. These results, in addition to stimulating further investigations focused on the effects of psychotherapies on sleep disturbances, can suggest that the rCBF recovery reflects the normalization of the sleep homeostatic process.

Narcolepsy

Narcolepsy is characterized by excessive daytime sleepiness (EDS), cataplexy (sudden bilateral loss of muscle tone), and disturbed nocturnal sleep, including parasomnias, OSAS, and periodic leg movements [29,30]. Moreover, frequent occurrences of REM sleep onset periods during daytime and numerous awakenings during nocturnal sleep reflect a disruption of the sleep-wake cycle [30,31]. Narcolepsy with cataplexy is considered secondary to loss of hypothalamic hypocretin neurons in patients genetically predisposed by the human leukocyte antigen DQB1*0602 [32,33]. Hypocretin neurons produce dorsolateral hypothalamic neuropeptides that function in regulating sleep-wake cycles and have widespread excitatory projections throughout the brain stem, basal forebrain and spinal cord [34].

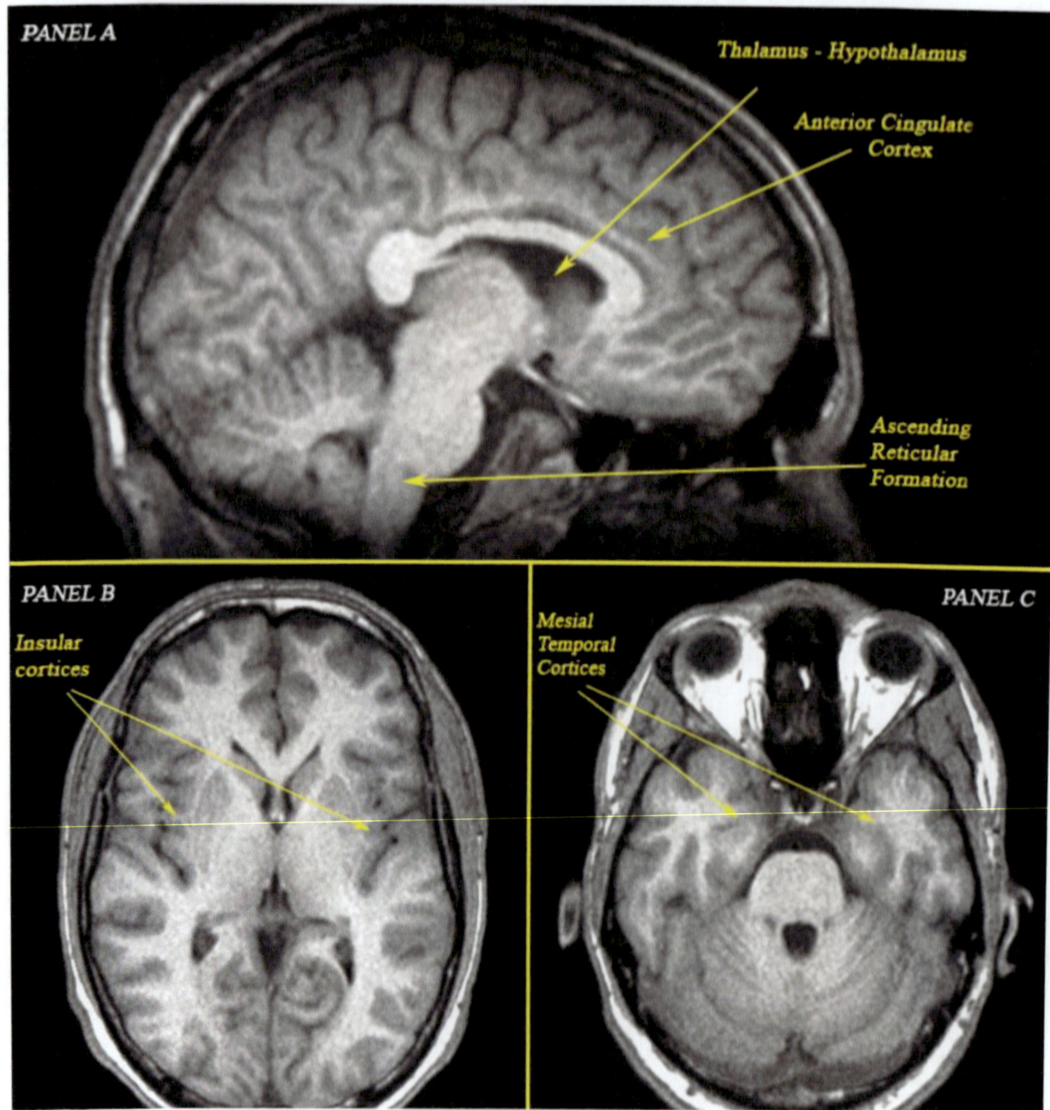

Figure 1. Brain regions that did not show decreased metabolic rate from waking to sleep states in patients with insomnia [24].

Hence, most neuroimaging studies focused on narcolepsy have had the aim of analyzing hypothalamic or pontine tegmentum abnormalities.

Structural Magnetic Resonance Imaging (MRI) studies found no pontine abnormalities in idiopathic narcolepsy [35,36], with the exception of a study by Plazzi et al. [37] who found pontine tegmentum abnormalities in three patients with narcolepsy, even if they were indistinguishable from ischemic changes, which probably reflected nonspecific age-related pontine vascular changes rather than a narcolepsy-related phenomenon.

However, some MRI studies conducted with the voxel-based morphometry (VBM) technique showed anatomical brain changes in narcoleptic patients, who showed cortical gray matter loss predominantly in frontal regions [38,39] and inferior temporal brain regions [39], as well as in the cerebellum (vermis), superior temporal gyrus right nucleus accumbens [40], and hypothalamus [40,41], although there were some exceptions [42]. This loss of gray matter could reflect disease-related atrophy due to the destruction of specific hypocretin projections.

Two studies used ^{1}H-MRS to verify if narcolepsy could be linked to neuronal loss or reduced activity of existing hypothalamic and pontine neurons, assessing the N-acetylaspartate (NAA) and creatinine-phosphocreatinine (Cr+PCr) content in narcoleptic patients.

Ellis et al. [43] reported decreased N-acetyl aspartate/creatine plus phosphocreatine (NAA/Cr+PCr) ratio in the ventral pontine areas of 12 narcoleptic patients compared to 10 control subjects, while Lodi et al. [44] reported the same decreased ratio in the hypothalamus of 23 narcoleptic patients compared with 10 unaffected controls, suggesting reduced neuronal function in these brain areas in narcolepsy.

Other functional neuroimaging studies conducted during wakefulness in narcoleptic patients showed lower waking baseline activity. Two subsequent ^{18}F-FDG PET studies [45,46] found reduced CMRglu in the bilateral precuneus, bilateral anterior and posterior hypothalamus, and mediodorsal thalamic nuclei.

Nonetheless, comparing regional brain activity during wakefulness and sleep states, functional neuroimaging studies have reported equivocal results in narcoleptic patients. A PET study by Meyer et al. [47] showed lower brainstem and cerebellar rCBF during wakefulness, as well as increased rCBF in all other areas, particularly in the temporo-parietal regions (i.e. cortical brain regions possibly related to visual dreaming and hypnagogic hallucinations) after sleep onset. In contrast, a study conducted on six narcoleptic patients subjected to a SPECT with technetium [99]m-hexamethylpropyleneamine-oxime ([99]mTC-HMPAO) reported no difference between the waking state and REM sleep, suggesting similar overall cortical activity across these two states [48].

Since cataplexy is a characteristic symptom of narcolepsy [30], some brain imaging studies have provided major insight into its neural correlates. Some emotional processing is often reported as a trigger of cataplexy [49,50], and different neuroimaging studies have shown changes in different limbic and striatal regions [16,18,19]. A SPECT study by Hong and colleagues [51] on 2 patients during a cataplexy episode showed increased blood flow in limbic areas, basal ganglia, thalami, premotor and sensorimotor cortices, and brainstem, as well as decreased perfusion in prefrontal cortex and occipital lobe, comparing the cataplectic state to REM sleep or baseline wakefulness. Another fMRI study by Schwartz et al. [52] showed enhanced amygdalar responses, as well as reduced hypothalamic responses, in narcoleptic patients compared to healthy controls while watching sequences of amusing pictures. An exception can be found in the study performed by Chabas et al. [53] using SPECT during an episode of cataplexy in a 68-year-old woman with hypocretin-deficient narcolepsy-cataplexy, who found no such hyperperfusion in limbic areas but showed increased activity in the cingulate and orbitofrontal cortices, and right putamen.

Acetylcholine plays an important role in the generation of REM sleep [54]; thus, some ligand neuroimaging studies have assessed the involvement of disorders within the cholinergic system in narcolepsy. However, the available PET data has shown no changes in muscarinic cholinergic receptors in narcoleptic patients [55].

Other theories argue that the dopaminergic system is also involved in narcolepsy, given that increased dopamine D2 binding was shown in post-mortem human narcoleptic brains [56,57]. In this regard, the results are still controversial. While one SPECT study found elevated D2-receptor binding correlated with the frequency of cataplectic and sleep attacks in narcolepsy [58], other PET or SPECT studies did not confirm these findings [59-62]. Interestingly, while some PET data did not show differences in striatal dopamine transporter availability in drug-free narcoleptic patients compared to healthy controls [63], Staedt et al. [62] reported a significant increase of the dopamine D2 receptor ligand uptake after drug treatment compared to pretreatment scans in 4 of 5 narcoleptic patients. It is possible that these discrepancies within ligand neuroimaging studies may relate to the drug treatments received, while reported post-mortem dopamine binding increases may correlate with long-term treatment effects rather than with dopamine system modifications.

Other functional neuroimaging studies have explored the effect of modafinil (a stimulant drug used in the treatment of narcolepsy) on cerebral function. An fMRI study by Ellis et al. [64], conducted with a multiplexed visual and auditory stimulation paradigm, showed no appreciable differences between mean pretreatment and post-treatment visual and auditory cortical activation levels, either in healthy subjects or in patients with narcoleptic syndrome given modafinil. Considering visual/auditory stimuli, another fMRI study by Howard et al. [65] reported a small reduction in the extent of the brain response to auditory and visual stimulation after amphetamine administration in controls, and an increase in the extent of induced activation within primary and association sensory cortex in narcoleptic patients, suggesting a possible enhancement of sensory processing mediated by amphetamine only in an arousal-deficit condition.

Obstructive Sleep Apnea Syndrome

Obstructive sleep apnea syndrome (OSAS) is characterized by repetitive complete (apnea) and partial (hypopnea) obstruction of the upper airway during sleep, and results in oxygen desaturation and arousals from sleep [20]. Such episodic events may in turn lead to systemic and pulmonary hypertension, increased incidence of cardiovascular or cerebrovascular disease, arrhythmias, and failure to thrive in children [66-68]. Common complications of OSAS include mood disorders [69], reduced quality of life [70], and cognitive problems [71,72], with the latter due to both excessive daytime sleepiness and nocturnal hypoxemia [73,74].

The precise neuropathophysiology of the cognitive and psychological complications associated with OSAS is still incompletely defined. The use of neuroimaging methodologies can however contribute to understanding the neuropathophysiology of OSAS. Macey et al. [75], using VBM on high resolution MRI scans, reported a gray matter loss in frontal, temporal and parietal regions, anterior cingulate cortex, hippocampus and cerebellum in OSAS patients, which are all involved in various cognitive functions and in motor regulation of the upper airway. Other structural MRI studies reported left hippocampal gray matter loss [76], as well as no difference in total gray matter volume [77].

Interestingly, Gale and Hopkins [78] reported hippocampal atrophy in both patients with OSAS and subjects with carbon monoxide poisoning. In the same study, the neuropathological features were compared with neuropsychological effects of hypoxia. Hippocampal volume positively correlated with performance on non-verbal tasks in both groups, and negatively correlated with performances on a subset of memory tests only in the patient group, suggesting a link between hippocampal damage and memory performance in patients affected by OSAS. In line with these results, a ^{1}H-MRS study by Bartlett et al. [79] reported a decrease of creatine (Cr)-containing compounds (an indicator of reduced neural function) in the left hippocampus, which correlated with the increase of the OSAS severity and worsening of neurocognitive performance. Later, Halbower et al. [80] showed also in a pediatric population a decrease of N-acetylaspartate/choline (NAA/Cho) ratio in the left hippocampus and right frontal cortex.

Several other studies have emphasized deterioration of executive functions associated with prefrontal-subcortical brain circuits [81] in OSAS patients [71,72,82]. A ^{1}H-MRS study by Alchanatis and colleagues [83] confirmed this hypothesis, showing that the N-acetyl aspartate/creatine (NAA/Cr) and the choline/creatine (Cho/Cr) ratios were significantly lower in the frontal white matter of OSAS patients compared to controls. Additionally, a previous ^{1}H-MRS by Kamba et al. [84] reported a lower brain white matter NAA/Cr ratio in patients with moderate to severe OSAS compared to patients with mild OSAS and healthy subjects, suggesting progressive cerebral damage likely caused by repeated apneic episodes.

Functional neuroimaging studies utilizing cognitive tasks have resulted either in reduced activation of the dorsolateral prefrontal cortex or in increased neural response in frontal lobe, cingulated, thalamus, cerebellum and temporoparietal junction depending on the cognitive task employed.

In particular, Thomas et al. [85] compared 16 untreated OSAS patients with 16 matched controls using fMRI during a 2-back verbal working memory task. They found a significant decreased dorsolateral prefrontal activity in the OSAS group. Eight of the OSAS patients were rescanned after successful treatment with continuous positive airway pressure (CPAP) and showed a significant increase in activation in posterior parietal areas. In addition, Castronovo et al. [86] found hypoactivation in the prefrontal and hippocampal areas together with an improvement in neuropsychological test performance in 17 OSAS patients after 3 months of treatment with CPAP.

Another fMRI study, conducted by Ayalon et al. [87] with a verbal learning task on 12 non-treated OSAS patients compared to matched controls, showed over-recruitment in several brain regions (bilateral inferior frontal and middle frontal gyri, cingulated gyrus, thalamus and cerebellum) in the OSAS population, despite no differences in performance between groups. The study by Castronovo et al. [86] also confirmed these results, showing over-recruitment of different brain regions, including prefrontal areas, hippocampus, cerebellum, and precuneus in OSAS patients compared with 15 normal controls, and a comparable level of working memory performances in an N-back test. Such over-activations can be attributed to adaptive compensatory mechanisms, supporting a relatively unimpaired level of performance.

Few studies have been conducted on the neural consequences of long-term treatment of OSAS patients. The first line of treatment is the application of CPAP via nasal mask [88], while surgery is used only in selected cases [89]. Ficker et al. [90] reported a completely reversion after CPAP therapy of a previous reduced perfusion in the left parietal site that was detected with [99]mTC-HMPAO SPECT on 14 OSAS patients during sleep. More recently, Tonon et al. [91] found NAA reduction in parietal-occipital cortices in 14 OSAS patients using ^{1}H-MRS, which persisted after CPAP therapy despite clinical, neurophysiological, and neuropsychological normalization.

Another fMRI study by Hashimoto et al. [92], performed during respiratory stress induced by resistive inspiratory loading on 12 healthy subjects, analyzed the effect of mandibular advancement, which is a frequent OSAS treatment, and showed hypoactivation of the left cingulate and bilateral prefrontal cortices.

Taken together, these studies demonstrate that efficient treatment of nocturnal apnea can alleviate some cerebral dysfunctions, despite the persistence of structural brain changes even after treatment.

Nasal CPAP has also been associated with improved vigilance and sustained attention [93]. However, some neurocognitive functions, including constructional abilities and psychomotor functioning, did not improve after treatment, suggesting an intrinsic neuronal dysfunction in OSAS patients.

Other series of studies aimed at elucidating the neural mechanisms of sleep respiratory control alterations in OSAS patients by using physiological challenges in fMRI probes. For instance, Harper et al. [94] used fMRI to examine neural responses to cold pressure challenge in 16 OSAS patients compared to 10 controls. They found that OSAS subjects have significant increases of signal in the anterior cingulate, posterior cingulate, cerebellar, and frontal cortices, and lower signals in the ventral thalamus, hippocampus, insula, and in medullary, midbrain areas, and cerebellar nuclei.

In another fMRI study by Henderson et al. [95], conducted during the Valsalva maneuver, OSAS patients showed attenuated signal changes in the left inferior parietal cortex, superior temporal gyrus, posterior insular cortex, cerebellar cortex, fastigial nucleus, and hippocampus, and enhanced signals emerged in the left lateral precentral gyrus, left anterior cingulate, and superior frontal cortices. Previously, gray matter loss was reported in the same regions in patients with OSAS [75]. The same Henderson and colleagues [95] pointed out that patients affected by OSAS showed altered neural responses to the Valsalva maneuver in regions involved in motor control of airway muscles, in cerebellar cortical and nuclear sites involved in blood pressure and breathing control, and in limbic areas involved in inspiratory onset and in blood pressure modulation. Macey et al. [96] evaluated the neural mechanisms underlying OSAS alterations in sleep respiratory control with fMRI procedures during baseline and expiratory loading conditions in 9 medication-free OSAS patients and 16 control subjects. They found reduced neural signals in the frontal and anterior cingulate cortices, cerebellar dentate nucleus, dorsal pons, anterior insula, and lentiform nuclei, while increases in signals were found in the dorsal midbrain, hippocampus, amygdala, quadrangular cerebellar lobule, ventral midbrain, ventral pons, and fastigial nuclei. A more recent fMRI study by the same group [97] evaluated brain activity changes during baseline and inspiratory loading in 7 drug-free OSAS patients and 11 control subjects. OSAS subjects showed altered signals in the thalamus, deep nuclei (basal ganglia), right hippocampus, and midbrain, as well as in the sensory, supplementary motor, cerebellar cortex, cingulate, medial temporal, and insular cortices. These brain regions are involved in sensory and autonomic processes, and motor timing, and play a major role in the neuropathophysiology of the OSAS.

Restless Legs Syndrome and Periodic Limb Movement Disorder In Sleep

Restless legs syndrome (RLS) and periodic limb movements in sleep (PLMS) are distinct disorders, although they can be considered superimposable for certain aspects. RLS is a sensorimotor neurological disorder characterized by an irresistible urge to move the legs, while PLMS consists of repetitive, highly stereotyped movements of the arms or legs occurring during sleep [20,98]. Treatments with dopaminergic agents are effective in both RLS and PLMS, suggesting a likely central dopaminergic dysfunction underlying the pathophysiology of these disorders [99].

Recently, an MRI with VBM technique study by Etgen et al. [100] showed structural abnormalities in idiopathic RLS, mainly including bilateral pulvinar gray matter increase. Changes in thalamic structure might be a primary neuropathophysiological intrinsic modification of this disorder, or they could be a consequence of dopaminergic therapy and/or of a chronic increase in afferent input due to sensory leg discomfort.

Different functional neuroimaging studies have attempted to identify brain areas involved in the induction of leg discomfort and periodic leg movements in RLS. Bucher et al. [101], in fMRI studies performed during wakefulness, showed bilateral activation of the cerebellum and contralateral activation of the thalamus in 19 RLS patients who experienced leg discomfort. When the same patients experienced periodic limb movements together with sensory leg discomfort, there was additional activation in red nuclei and brainstem reticular formation. Furthermore, during voluntary imitation of limb movements, patients showed additional activation in the globus pallidus and motor cortex, with no brainstem activation. These results exclude the involvement of cortical brain regions in the induction of periodic leg movements, suggesting a subcortical origin of the syndrome.

Given the evidence of RLS worsening after dopamine antagonist administration, as well as an improvement with dopaminergic drugs [99], some ligand neuroimaging studies have examined both presynaptic dopamine transporter and postsynaptic D2-receptor binding in the striatum of RLS/PLMS patients.

Staedt et al. [102-104] conducted a series of studies to test the hypothesis of decreased dopaminergic activity in patients with PLMS. In these studies, they measured central D2-receptor occupancy with ^{123}I-iodobenzamide (^{123}I-IBZM), reporting a reduction of the striatal ^{123}I-IBZM binding in PLMD patients [102-104] and a higher binding following dopaminergic therapy [103]. In agreement with these results, the ^{123}I-IBZM SPECT study by Michaud et al. [105] showed lower D2 receptor occupancy in 10 drug-naïve patients affected by both PLMS and RLS compared to 10 age-matched healthy controls. However, using ^{123}I-methyl-3-beta-(4-iodophenyl) tropane-2 beta-carboxylate (^{123}I-beta-CIT, a ligand of dopamine transporter), they found no difference in presynaptic dopamine transporter binding. The data indicated a decreased number of D2-receptors or decreased affinity of D2-receptors for the ^{123}I-IBZM, supporting the involvement of central striatal D2-receptor abnormality in the pathophysiology of RLS/PLMD.

In contrast, Eisensher et al. [106] showed similar striatal dopamine transporter and D2 receptor binding in drug-naïve and levodopa-treated patients with RLS and in controls, suggesting a normal striatal DA transporter and receptor density in RLS. Similarly, the ^{123}I-IBMZ SPECT study by Tribl et al. [107] found no differences in striatal to frontal D2-receptors occupancy between 14 good treatment responders PLMS patients (with or without RLS) and 10 sex- and age-matched controls. The authors have theorized the existence of an abnormal dopaminergic system elsewhere, perhaps in the diencephalospinal part.

Cervenka et al. [108] showed the involvement of the dopamine system in the extrastriatal and striatal brain regions in the pathophysiology of RLS. They also reported higher D2-receptor availability in the thalamus, insula, and anterior cingulate cortex in 16 drug-naïve

RLS patients compared to 16 matched controls. Since the anterior cingulate cortex is part of medial nociceptive system [109,110], the authors hypothesized that RLS might be a somatosensory processing disorder. As confirmation of this hypothesis, opioid receptor agonists significantly improve RLS symptoms [111].

Moreover, cerebral iron metabolism has been implicated in the pathogenesis of PLMD/RLS [112]. Iron is an important cofactor for tyrosine hydroxylase, which is linked to dopamine synthesis, and is also implicated in the functioning of D2-receptors [67]. In 5 RLS patients compared to 5 healthy controls, Allen et al. [112] showed a lower iron concentration in the substantia nigra and putamen. This reduction was positively correlated with symptoms severity. More recently, another study by Earley at al. [113] reported a lower mean iron concentration across several brain regions, including the substantia nigra, red nucleus, globus pallidus, putamen, caudate nucleus, frontal white matter, dentate nucleus, pons, thalamus, and prefrontal cortex in patients with early-onset RLS, but not with late-onset RLS compared to controls. This suggests the involvement of impaired iron metabolism in the pathophysiology of RLS, which may affect the dopamine system.

Sleepwalking

Sleepwalking, or somnambulism, is a parasomnia consisting of a series of complex behaviors usually initiated during arousals from slow wave sleep, commonly culminating in walking with an altered state of consciousness and impaired judgment [20].

To date, only one functional neuroimaging study has explored regional brain function associated with sleepwalking. Using a SPECT with ^{99m}Technetium ethylene-cysteinate dimer (^{99m}Tc-ECD) one night before and one night during a sleepwalking episode in a man with a history of sleepwalking, Bassetti and colleagues [114] demonstrated increased blood flow in the cerebellar vermis and posterior cingulate cortex, and a decline in the frontoparietal association cortices during sleepwalking.

The loss of frontoparietal function might reflect unconsciousness, while the preserved thalamocingulate blood flow might correlate with the persistence of motor generators in the sleepwalking behavior. These interesting data are worthy of further investigation.

REM Sleep Behavior Disorder

REM sleep behavior disorder (RBD) is characterized by the absence of the normal skeletal muscle atonia during REM sleep, with the appearance of elaborate motor activity associated with dream mentation [115]. The exact pathogenesis of RBD remains uncertain. The disease may be idiopathic, although it is predominantly associated with neurodegenerative pathologies that are mostly characterized by synucleinopathies such as Parkinson's disease [116,117], multiple system atrophy [118,119], and Levy body dementia [120], for which it could be a precursor [117,120].

In 1979, Sakai and colleagues, using a feline experimental model of RBD, demonstrated the existence of a link between lesions in the mesopontine tegmentum with the disappearance of muscle atonia during REM sleep and the appearance of dream-enactment behavior [121].

In 1989, Culebras and colleagues reported similar results in men by using MRI in 6 patients with RBD, 3 of whom had lesions affecting the dorsal mesopontine tegmentum [122].

More recently, a ^{123}I-IMP SPECT study by Shirakawa et al. [123] found a decrease in the rCBF of the pons and superior frontal regions in 20 patients with RBD compared to 7 healthy subjects. In addition, patients were also subjected to MRI measurement, although no correlations were reported between decreased CBF and frontal lobe atrophy.

In 2006, Mazza and colleagues [124] conducted a ^{99m}Tc-ECD SPECT on 8 RBD patients and 9 age-matched controls that confirmed decreased perfusion in the frontal cortex (Brodmann Areas [BAs] 4, 6, 10, 43, 44, 47 and left BAs 9, 46) in patients. In addition, they observed decreased activity in the temporo-parietal cortices (bilateral BAs 13, 22, 43, and left BAs 7, 19, 20, 21, 39, 40, 41, 42), in contrast to increased activity in the pons and putamen bilaterally, and in the right hippocampus. The latter finding is in line with a MRI VBM study by Scherfler et al. [125], who reported increases of gray matter densities in the bilateral hippocampus and adjacent parahippocampal gyrus.

A ^{1}H-MRS single-case study conducted by Miyamoto et al. [126] revealed an increased choline/creatine ratio in the brainstem of a 69-year-old-man with RBD, supporting the hypothesis of mesopontine neuronal dysfunction in idiopathic RBD. In contrast, Iranzo et al. [127] did not observe any differences in N-acetylaspartate/creatine, choline/creatine or myoinosito/creatine ratios in the pontine tegmentum and midbrain between patients and controls.

Recently, the MRI study based on diffusion-tensor imaging (DTI) by Unger and colleagues [128] reported changes in the integrity of the brainstem (pons, substantia nigra), fornix, right visual stream, and left superior temporal lobe in a group of 12 RBD patients, suggesting involvement of both brainstem and cortical areas in the pathophysiology of RBD. In particular, this study reported decreases of axial diffusivity, which is a parameter assumed to indicate axonal loss, in the substantia nigra and pons, as well as decreases of fractional anisotropy and increases of radial diffusivity, assumed to be correlates of demyelization, in the cortical areas previously mentioned.

Scherfler and colleagues [125], in their DTI study, reported significant fractional anisotropy decreases in the tegmentum of the midbrain and rostral pons, and increases of mean diffusivity within the pontine reticular formation overlapping with a cluster of decreased fractional anisotropy in the midbrain. These results fit with neural and myelin damage in the pontomesencephalic tegmentum. No marked gray or white matter atrophy was identified by VBM in this particular brainstem area, and no DTI-related changes were found in cortical areas.

Using SPECT to study the striatal postsynaptic D2- receptors and the striatal presynaptic dopamine transporters in 8 patients with idiopathic subclinical RBD (i.e., REM sleep with the absence of skeleton muscle atonia, but without behavioral manifestations), 8 patients with idiopathic clinically-manifest RBD, 8 patients with Parkinson's disease, and 11 controls, Eisensehr et al. [129] found a progressive decrease in density of the presynaptic dopamine transporters from controls to patients with subclinical RBD, and from the latter to patients with clinical RBD and to patients with Parkinson's disease. This suggests the existence of a continuum of striatal dopaminergic dysfunction in the pathophysiological mechanisms of idiopathic RBD.

Another study by Albin et al. [130] observed reduced dopamine transporter binding in all striatal nuclei, with the greatest reduction in the posterior putamen.

Similarly, significant reduction in striatal ^{11}C-dihydrotetrabenazine (^{11}C-DTBZ, a monoamine vesicular transporter inhibitor used as an *in vivo* marker for dopamine nerve terminals) binding characterized 13 patients with multiple system atrophy [118]compared to healthy controls. Since striatal ^{11}C-DTBZ uptake in the multiple system atrophy group inversely correlated with the severity of the absence of REM atonia, it has been suggested that decreased nigrostriatal dopaminergic projections might contribute to RBD in multiple system atrophy. Moreover, the same group showed decreased ^{123}I-iodobenzovesamiol (^{123}I-IBVM, a radiotracer used as a marker for cerebral cholinergic neurons) binding in the thalamus.

Healthy adults reporting dream-enactment behavior have reduced CMRglu in the parietal, temporal, and posterior cingulated cortex, which are preferentially affected in patients with Alzheimer's disease and Levy body dementia, in addition to several other regions such as the anterior cingulate cortices [131]. These data suggest that dream-enactment behavior is a possible risk factor for the development of these neurodegenerative diseases.

To date, it is not clear if these abnormal structural and functional brain changes, mainly in the mesopontine tegmentum and dopamine neurotransmission, are involved in the pathophysiology of RBD or may instead reflect the consequence of drug-treatment or adaptation to pathological conditions.

Depressive Disorders

Patients with depressive disorders are known to have several sleep disturbances [132]. Depression is the most frequent diagnosis in patients suffering from insomnia [133]. This link has also been widely confirmed by functional neuroimaging studies on brain function during sleep. A PET study by Ho and colleagues [134] showed whole-brain CMRglu increase during NREM sleep in 10 patients with depression compared to 12 healthy subjects. The greatest increases were observed in the pons, amygdale, hippocampus, and posterior cingulate, temporal, and occipital cortices. During NREM sleep, the same study also showed a significant CMRglu reduction in the prefrontal and anterior cingulate cortices, caudate nucleus, and medial thalamus.

More recently, other studies confirmed an increased brain activity in patients with depression during NREM sleep, also showing a higher CMRglu in the insula and cerebellum [135,136]. Nofzinger et al. [136] reported higher activity measured with CMRglu in 24 patients with depression compared to 14 controls during REM sleep in several brain regions, including the frontal, parietal, premotor and sensorimotor cortices, and the insula, ventral pallidum, and midbrain reticular formation.

These data suggest that hyperarousal might also be applied to the insomnia that occurs in patients with depression, providing indications for a link between depressive disorders and insomnia on the basis of a supposed neurophysiological mechanism underlying both sleep and mood regulation. In particular, hyperarousal in depression can be related to dysfunction in a network between limbic and posterior cortical regions, while the decreased medial frontal and striatal metabolism might be a hallmark of depression [137].

Neuroimaging studies have also provided several potential biological links between depression and OSAS by demonstrating overlaps of structural and functional deficits in the hippocampus, anterior cingulate, and frontal cortices, which consistently showed abnormal structure and/or function in patients affected by OSAS [75].

Schizophrenia

Phenomenological similarities between dreams and hallucinations noted by clinical investigators [138] inspired several studies focused on sleep in patients affected by schizophrenia, who often manifest prominent sleep disturbances [139,140].

To date, only a few neuroimaging studies have explored the relationship between some aspects of sleep and the neuropathophysiology of schizophrenia.

A PET study by Weiler and colleagues [141] investigated the relationship between REM-sleep and schizophrenia. The authors assumed that brain regional metabolism during healthy REM sleep might resemble that of awake patients affected by schizophrenia, given some phenomenological similarities between neurocognition during dreaming and psychotic states. However, they found significant differences in CMRglu between 49 schizophrenics, 30 control subjects in the waking state, and 12 control subjects in REM sleep, discounting the possibilty that schizophrenia can represent an intrusion of REM sleep cognition into wakefulness. Moreover, they showed lower left caudate CMRglu in patients affected by schizophrenia with hallucinations and a significant decrease in callosal CMRglu in controls compared to patients with schizophrenia during the waking state, as well as in patients compared to controls during the REM state.

Later, Keshavan et al. [142] investigated the association between cerebral morphology as revealed by CT and sleep polysomnographic findings in psychotic patients. They reported that the third ventricle-brain, caudate, and anterior horn ratios were negatively associated with sleep maintenance, and positively correlated with rapid eye movement (REM) latency, suggesting a dysfunction of forebrain structures related to sleep disturbances in patients with schizophrenia and schizoaffective disorders.

Conclusion

The recent neuroimaging techniques have provided a wealth of data on the activity of the nervous system during sleep and about the morphological changes in patients with sleep disorders or sleep disturbances. These techniques can be used to further complement the numerous data obtained through EEG and polysomnography, allowing an ever-greater clarification on both the physiological sleep activity and the neurophysiopathology of sleep disorders. The available data mainly concern idiopathic insomnia, narcolepsy, obstructive sleep apnea syndrome, restless legs syndrome, and periodic limb movement disorder in sleep, sleepwalking, and REM sleep behavior disorder. Other important data were obtained from patients suffering from sleep disturbances related to depressive disorders and schizophrenia. Each of these syndromes has been correlated to specific patterns of brain activation, and in some cases to changes in brain morphometry (see Table 1).

Neuroimaging techniques are playing a leading role in scientific research focused on sleep disorders, and will probably contribute to future clarification in their nosography.

Table 1. Main neuroimaging findings in sleep disorders and sleep disturbances

Diagnosis	Reported brain morphological changes	Reported brain functional changes
Idiopathic Insomnia		Global increased cerebral metabolism ([18]FDG PET) from waking to NREM sleep.[24] Smaller CMRglu decline in the ascending reticular activating system, hypothalamus, thalamus, amygdala, hippocampus, and insular, anterior cingulate, and medial prefrontal cortices from waking to NREM sleep.[24] rCBF decrease (SPECT) in the frontal medial, occipital, and parietal cortices, and basal ganglia during NREM sleep.[28]
Narcolepsy	Gray matter loss (MRI VBM) in frontal and temporal areas, hypothalamus, ventral striatum, cerebellum (vermis), superior temporal gyrus, and right nucleus accumbens.[38-41]	Reduced neuronal function (^{1}H-MRS) in the hypothalamus,[44] and ventral pontine areas.[43] Reduced baseline activity during wakefulness ([18]FDG PET) in the bilateral precuneus, hypothalamus, and mediodorsal thalamic nuclei.[45,46] Lower brainstem and cerebellar rCBF ([18]FDG PET) during wakefulness, and increased rCBF in all other areas, particularly in the temporo-parietal regions, after sleep onset.[47] Increased blood flow (SPECT) in several cortical and subcortical regions including limbic areas, motor regions, brainstem and cingulated and orbitofrontal cortices during cataplexy.[51,53]

Diagnosis	Reported brain morphological changes	Reported brain functional changes
Obstructive Sleep Apnea Syndrome	Hippocampal atrophy.[78] Gray matter loss (MRI VBM) in the left hippocampus.[77] Gray matter loss (MRI VBM) in cerebral regions involved in different cognitive functions and in motor regulation of the upper airway.[75]	Reduced neuronal function (^{1}H-MRS) in the left hippocampus.[79] Decreased NAA/Cho ratio (^{1}H-MRS) in the left hippocampus and right frontal cortex in pediatric patients.[80] NAA/Cr and Cho/Cr ratios (^{1}H-MRS) significantly lower in the frontal white matter of OSAS patients compared to controls.[83] Lower brain white matter NAA/Cr ratio (^{1}H-MRS) in patients with moderate to severe OSAS compared to patients with mild OSAS and healthy subjects.[84] During cognitive tasks reduced activation (fMRI) of the dorsolateral prefrontal cortex,[85,86] and increased neural response in frontal lobe, cingulated, thalamus, cerebellum, precuneus and temporoparietal junction.[86,87] Abnormal brain fMRI responses to experimentally induced respiratory and cardiovascular stresses affecting the cerebellum, insula, cingulated and motor cortices.[94-97]
Restless Legs Syndrome and Periodic Limb Movement Disorder	Bilateral gray matter increase (MRI VBM) in the pulvinar.[100]	Increased fMRI activation in the cerebellum, thalamus, red nuclei and brainstem reticular formation during periodic limb movements with sensory leg discomfort.[101] Reduced striatal 123I-IBZM binding (SPECT) in PLMD patients and increased binding after dopaminergic therapy.[102-104]

Table 1. (Continued)

Diagnosis	Reported brain morphological changes	Reported brain functional changes
Sleepwalking		Lower D2 receptors occupancy (SPECT) in 10 drug-naïve patients affected by both PLMS and RLS compared to 10 age-matched healthy controls.[105] Higher D2-receptor availability (PET) also in the thalamus, insula, and anterior cingulate cortex in 16 drug-naïve RLS patients compared to 16 matched controls.[108] Lower MRI-determined iron concentration in the substantia nigra and putamen. This reduction was positively correlated with symptoms severity.[112] Diminished MRI-determined mean iron concentration across several brain regions, including substantia nigra, red nucleus, globus pallidus, putamen, caudate nucleus, frontal white matter, dentate nucleus, pons, thalamus, prefrontal cortex, in patients with early-onset RLS.[113] Increased blood flow (SPECT) in the cerebellar vermis and posterior cingulate cortex and hypoperfusion in the frontoparietal association cortices.[114]

Diagnosis	Reported brain morphological changes	Reported brain functional changes
REM Sleep Behavior Disorder	Lesions affecting the dorsal mesopontine tegmentum.[122] Increases of gray matter densities (MRI VBM) in the bilateral hippocampus and the parahippocampal gyrus.[125] MRI with DTI technique reported changes in the integrity of the brainstem (pons, substantia nigra), fornix, right visual stream, and left superior temporal lobe.[128] Fractional anisotropy decreases in the tegmentum of the midbrain and rostral pons, and increases of mean diffusivity within the pontine reticular formation overlapping with a cluster of decreased fractional anisotropy in the midbrain.[125]	Decreased blood flow (SPECT) in the pons and superior frontal regions.[123] Increased activity (SPECT) in the pons, putamen and right hippocampus.[124] Progressive SPECT decrease in density of the presynaptic dopamine transporters from controls to patients with subclinical RBD, and from the latter to patients with clinical RBD.[129] Reduced dopamine transporter binding (PET) in all striatal nuclei, with greatest reduction in the posterior putamen.[130]
Sleep disturbances in Depressive Disorders		Whole-brain PET CMRglu increase during NREM sleep in 10 depressed patients compared to 12 healthy subjects, in the pons, amygdale, hippocampus, and posterior cingulate, temporal, and occipital cortices. Significant CMRglu reduction during NREM sleep in the prefrontal and anterior cingulate cortices, caudate nucleus and medial thalamus.[134] Increased metabolism (^{18}F-FDG PET) across several cortical and subcortical regions (parietal, prefrontal, supplementary motor and posterior cingulated

Table 1. (Continued)

Diagnosis	Reported brain morphological changes	Reported brain functional changes
		cortices, insula, thalamus, ventral pallidum and ascending reticular activating system) during NREM and REM sleep compared to presleep wakefulness.[135,136]
Sleep disturbances in Schizophrenia	CT-determined third ventricle-brain ratios, caudate ratios, and anterior horn ratios negatively associated with sleep maintenance and positively correlated with REM latency.[142]	Lower PET-determined left caudate CMRglu in patients affected by schizophrenia with hallucinations and a significant decrease in callosal CMRglu in controls compared to patients during the waking state, and in patients as compared to controls during the REM state.[141]

Legend: ^{1}H-MRS: Single Voxel Proton Magnetic Resonance Spectroscopy; ^{18}F-FDG: ^{18}F-Fluorodeoxi-Glucose; CMRglu: Cerebral Metabolic Rate of Glucose consumption; Cho: Choline; Cr: Creatine; CT: Computed Tomography; fMRI: functional Magnetic Resonance Imaging; MRI: Magnetic Resonance Imaging; NAA: N-acetyl aspartate; NREM: Non-Rapid-Eye-Movement; PET: Positron Emission Tomography; REM: Rapid-Eye-Movement; SPECT: Single-Photon Emission Computed Tomography; VBM: Voxel-Based Morphometry.

References

[1] Braun AR, Balkin TJ, Wesenten NJ, Carson RE, Varga M, Baldwin P, Selbie S, Belenky G, Herscovitch P. Regional cerebral blood flow throughout the sleep-wake cycle. An H2(15)O PET study. *Brain.* 1997;120(Pt 7):1173-97.

[2] Dang Vu TT, Desseilles M, Peigneux P, Laureys S, Maquet P. Sleep and sleep states: PET activation patterns. In: Squire LR, ed. Encyclopedia of neuroscience. Oxford: Academic Press, 2009: 955-61.

[3] Madsen PL, Holm S, Vorstrup S, Friberg L, Lassen NA, Widschiodtz G. Human regional cerebral blood flow during rapid-eye-movement sleep. *J Cereb Blood Flow Metab.* 1991;11(3):502-7.

[4] Maquet P, Dive D, Salmon E, Sadzot B, Franco G, Poirrier R, von Frenckell R, Franck G. Cerebral glucose utilization during sleep-wake cycle in man determined by positron emission tomography and [^{18}F]2-fluoro-2-deoxy-D-glucose method. *Brain Res.* 1990;513(1):136-43.

[5] Maquet P, Péters J, Aerts J, Delfiore G, Degueldre C, Luxen A, Franck G. Functional neuroanatomy of human rapid-eye-movement sleep and dreaming. *Nature.* 1996;383(6596):163-6.

[6] Maquet P, Philips C. Functional brain imaging of human sleep. *J Sleep Res.* 1998;7(Suppl 1):42-7.

[7] Maquet P. Functional neuroimaging of normal human sleep by positron emission tomography. *J Sleep Res.* 2000;9(3):207-31.

[8] Nofzinger EA, Buysse DJ, Miewald JM, Meltzer CC, Price JC, Sembrat RC, Ombao H, Reynolds CF, Monk TH, Hall M, Kupfer DJ, Moore RY. Human regional cerebral glucose metabolism during non-rapid eye movement sleep in relation to waking. *Brain.* 2002;125(Pt 5):1105-15.

[9] Andersson JL, Onoe H, Hetta J, Lidström K, Valind S, Lilja A, Sundin A, Fasth KJ, Westerberg G, Broman JE, Watanabe Y, Långström B. Brain networks affected by synchronized sleep visualized by positron emission tomography. *J Cereb Blood Flow Metab.* 1998;18(7):701-15.

[10] Kajimura N, Uchiyama M, Takayama Y, Uchida S, Uema T, Kato M, Sekimoto M, Watanabe T, Nakajima T, Horikoshi S, Ogawa K, Nishikawa M, Hiroki M, Kudo Y, Matsuda H, Okawa M, Takahashi K. Activity of midbrain reticular formation and neocortex during the progression of human non-rapid eye movement sleep. *J Neurosci.* 1999;19(22):10065-73.

[11] Maquet P, Degueldre C, Delfiore G, Aerts J, Péters JM, Luxen A, Franck G. Functional neuroanatomy of human slow wave sleep. *J Neurosci.* 1997;17(8):2807-12.

[12] Saint-Cyr JA, Taylor AE, Nicholson K. Behavior and the basal ganglia. *Adv Neurol.* 1995;65:1-28.

[13] Szirmai I, Vastagh I, Szombathelyi E, Kamondi A. Strategic infarcts of the thalamus in vascular dementia. *J Neurol Sci.* 2002;203-204:91-7.

[14] Maquet P, Laureys S, Peigneux P, Fuchs S, Petiau C, Phillips C, Aerts J, Del Fiore G, Degueldre C, Meulemans T, Luxen A, Franck G, Van Der Linden M, Smith C, Cleeremans A. Experience-dependent changes in cerebral activation during human REM sleep. *Nat Neurosci.* 2000;3(8):831-6.

[15] Maquet P, Ruby P, Maudoux A, Albouy G, Sterpenich V, Dang-Vu T, Desseilles M, Boly M, Perrin F, Peigneux P, Laureys S. Human cognition during REM sleep and the activity profile within frontal and parietal cortices: a reappraisal of functional neuroimaging data. *Prog Brain Res.* 2005;150:219-27.

[16] LeDoux JE. Emotion circuits in the brain. *Annu Rev Neurosci.* 2000;23:155-84.

[17] Malik S, McGlone F, Dagher A. State of expectancy modulates the neural response to visual food stimuli in humans. *Appetite.* 2011;56(2):302-9.

[18] Vuilleumier P. How brains beware: neural mechanisms of emotional attention. *Trends Cogn Sci.* 2005;9(12):585-94.

[19] Zald DH. The human amygdala and the emotional evaluation of sensory stimuli. *Brain Res Brain Res Rev.* 2003;41(1):88-123.

[20] American Academy of Sleep Medicine. International classification of sleep disorders 2nd ed: diagnostic and coding manual. Westchester, IL: *American Academy of Sleep Medicine*, 2005.

[21] Guilleminault C. Medical and Neurological Disorders. In Guilleminault C, editor. Principles and Practices of Sleep Medicine. Third edition. Philadelfia: W.B. Saunders Co., 2000] pp. 997-1122.

[22] Bonnet MH, Arand DL. Hyperarousal and insomnia. *Sleep Med Rev.* 1997;1(2):97-108.

[23] Perlis ML, Merica H, Smith MT, Giles DE. Beta EEG activity and insomnia. *Sleep Med Rev.* 2001;5(5):365-76.

[24] Nofzinger EA, Buysse DJ, Germain A, Price JC, Miewald JM, Kupfer DJ. Functional neuroimaging evidence for hyperarousal in insomnia. *Am J Psychiatry.* 2004;161(11):2126-8.

[25] Thomas M, Sing H, Belenky G, Holcomb H, Mayberg H, Dannals R, Wagner H, Thorne D, Popp K, Rowland L, Welsh A, Balwinski S, Redmond D. Neural basis of alertness and cognitive performance impairments during sleepiness. I. Effects of 24 h of sleep deprivation on waking human regional brain activity. *J Sleep Res.* 2000;9(4):335-52.

[26] Drummond SP, Brown GG. The effects of total sleep deprivation on cerebral responses to cognitive performance. *Neuropsychopharmacology.* 2001;25(5):S68-73.

[27] Smith MT, Perlis ML, Chengazi VU, Pennington J, Soeffing J, Ryan JM, Giles DE. Neuroimaging of NREM sleep in primary insomnia: a Tc-99-HMPAO single photon emission computed tomography study. *Sleep.* 2002;25(3):325-35.

[28] Smith MT, Perlis ML, Chengazi VU, Soeffing J, McCann U. NREM sleep cerebral blood flow before and after behavior therapy for chronic primary insomnia: preliminary single photon emission computed tomography (SPECT) data. Sleep Med. 2005;6(1):93-4.

[29] Daniels LE. Narcolepsy. *Medicine.* 1934;13:1-122.

[30] Dauvilliers Y, Arnulf I, Mignot E. Narcolepsy with cataplexy. *Lancet.* 2007;369(9560):499-511.

[31] Plazzi G, Serra L, Ferri R. Nocturnal aspects of narcolepsy with cataplexy. *Sleep Med.* 2008;12(2):109-128.

[32] Mignot E, Lammers GJ, Ripley B, Okun M, Nevsimalova S, Overeem S, Vankova J, Black J, Harsh J, Bassetti C, Schrader H, Nishino S. The role of cerebrospinal fluid hypocretin measurement in the diagnosis of narcolepsy and other hypersomnias. *Arch Neurol.* 2002;59(10):1553-62.

[33] Peyron C, Faraco J, Rogers W, Ripley B, Overeem S, Charnay Y, Nevsimalova S, Aldrich M, Reynolds D, Albin R, Li R, Hungs M, Pedrazzoli M, Padigaru M, Kucherlapati M, Fan J, Maki R, Lammers GJ, Bouras C, Kucherlapati R, Nishino S, Mignot E. A mutation in a case of early onset narcolepsy and a generalized absence of hypocretin peptides in human narcoleptic brains. *Nat Med.* 2000;6(9):991-7.

[34] Baumann CR, Bassetti CL. Hypocretins (orexins): clinical impact of the discovery of a neurotransmitter. *Sleep Med Rev.* 2005;9(4):253-68.

[35] Bassetti C, Aldrich MS, Quint DJ. MRI findings in narcolepsy. *Sleep.* 1997;20(8):630-1.

[36] Frey JL, Heiserman JE. Absence of pontine lesions in narcolepsy. *Neurology.* 1997;48(4):1097-9.

[37] Plazzi G, Montagna P, Provini F, Bizzi A, Cohen M, Lugaresi E. Pontine lesions in idiopathic narcolepsy. *Neurology.* 1996;46(5):1250-4.

[38] Brenneis C, Brandauer E, Frauscher B, Schocke M, Trieb T, Poewe W, Högl B. Voxel-based morphometry in narcolepsy. *Sleep Med.* 2005;6(6):531-6.

[39] Kaufmann C, Schuld A, Pollmacher T, Auer DP. Reduced cortical gray matter in narcolepsy: preliminary findings with voxel-based morphometry. *Neurology.* 2002;58(12):1852-5.

[40] Draganski B, Geisler P, Hajak G, Schuierer G, Bogdahn U, Winkler J, May A. Hypothalamic gray matter changes in narcoleptic patients. Nat Med. 2002 Nov;8(11):1186-8] *Nat Med.* 2004;10(4):435.

[41] Buskova J, Vaneckova M, Sonka K, Seidi Z, Nevsimalova S. Reduced hypothalamic gray matter in narcolepsy with cataplexy. *Neuro Endocrinol Lett.* 2006;27(6):769-72.

[42] Overeem S, Steens SC, Good CD, Ferrari MD, Mignot E, Frackowiak RS, van Buchem MA, Lammers GJ. Voxel-based morphometry in hypocretin-deficient narcolepsy. *Sleep.* 2003;26(1):44-6.

[43] Ellis CM, Simmons A, Lemmens G, Williams SC, Parkes JD. Proton spectroscopy in the narcoleptic syndrome. Is there evidence of a brainstem lesion? *Neurology.* 1998;50(2):S23-6.

[44] Lodi R, Tonon C, Vignatelli L, Iotti S, Montagna P, Barbiroli B, Plazzi G. In vivo evidence of neuronal loss in the hypothalamus of narcoleptic patients. *Neurology.* 2004;63(8):1513-5.

[45] Joo EY, Tae WS, Kim JH, Kim BT, Hong SB. Glucose hypometabolism of hypothalamus and thalamus in narcolepsy. *Ann Neurol.* 2004;56(3):437-40.

[46] Joo EY, Hong SB, Tae WS, Kim JH, Han SJ, Cho YW, Yoon CH, Lee SI, Lee MH, Lee KH, Kim MH, Kim BT, Kim L. Cerebral perfusion abnormality in narcolepsy with cataplexy. *Neuroimage.* 2005;28(2):410-6.

[47] Meyer JS, Sakai F, Karacan I, Derman S, Yamamoto M. Sleep apnea, narcolepsy, and dreaming: regional cerebral hemodynamics. *Ann Neurol.* 1980;7(5):479-85.

[48] Asenbaum S, Zeithofer J, Saletu B, Frey R, Brücke T, Podreka I, Deecke L. Technetium-99m-HMPAO SPECT imaging of cerebral blood flow during REM sleep in narcoleptics. *J Nucl Med.* 1995;36(7):1150-5.

[49] Bassetti C, Aldrich MS. Narcolepsy. Neurol Clin. 1996;14(3):545-71.

[50] Sturzenegger C, Bassetti CL. The clinical spectrum of narcolepsy with cataplexy: a reappraisal. *J Sleep Res.* 2004;13(4):395-406.

[51] Hong SB, Tae WS, Joo EY. Cerebral perfusion changes during cataplexy in narcolepsy patients. *Neurology.* 2006;66(11):1747-9]

[52] Schwartz S, Ponz A, Poryazova R, Werth E, Boesiger P, Khatami R, Bassetti CL. Abnormal activity in hypothalamus and amygdala during humour processing in human narcolepsy with cataplexy. *Brain.* 2008;131(Pt 2):514-22.

[53] Chabas D, Habert MO, Maksud P, Tourbah A, Minz M, Willer JC, Arnulf I. Functional imaging of cataplexy during status cataplecticus. *Sleep.* 2007;30(2):153-6.

[54] Murillo-Rodriguez E, Arias-Carrion O, Zavala-Garcia A, Sarro-Ramirez A, Huitron-Resendiz S, Arankowsky-Sandoval G. Basic sleep mechanisms: an integrative review. *Cent Nerv Syst Agents Med Chem.* 2012;12(1):38-54.

[55] Sudo Y, Suhara T, Honda Y, Nakajima T, Okubo Y, Suzuki K, Nakashima Y, Yoshikawa K, Okauchi T, Sasaki Y, Matsushita M. Muscarinic cholinergic receptors in human narcolepsy: a PET study. *Neurology.* 1998;51(5):1297-302.

[56] Aldrich MS, Hollingsworth Z, Penney JB. Dopamine-receptor autoradiography of human narcoleptic brain. *Neurology.* 1992;42(2):410-5.

[57] Kish SJ, Mamelak M, Slimovitch C, Dixon LM, Lewis A, Shannak K, DiStefano L, Chang LJ, Hornykiewicz O. Brain neurotransmitter changes in human narcolepsy. *Neurology.* 1992;42(1):229-34.

[58] Eisensehr I, Linke R, Tatsch K, von Lindeiner H, Kharraz B, Gildehaus FJ, Eberle R, Pollmacher T, Schuld A, Noachtar S. Alteration of the striatal dopaminergic system in human narcolepsy. *Neurology.* 2003;60(11):1817-9.

[59] Hublin C, Launes J, Nikkinen P, Partinen M. Dopamine D2-receptors in human narcolepsy: a SPECT study with 123I-IBZM. *Acta Neurol Scand.* 1994;90(3):186-9.

[60] MacFarlane JG, List SJ, Moldofsky H, Firnau G, Chen JJ, Szechtman H, Garnett S, Nahmias C. Dopamine D2 receptors quantified in vivo in human narcolepsy. *Biol Psychiatry.* 1997;41(3):305-10.

[61] Rinne JO, Hublin C, Partinen M, Ruottinen H, Ruotsalainen U, Någren K, Lehikoinen P, Laihinen A. Positron emission tomography study of human narcolepsy: no increase in striatal dopamine D2 receptors. *Neurology.* 1995;45(9):1735-8]

[62] Staedt J, Stoppe G, Kögler A, Riemann H, Hajak G, Rodenbeck A, Mayer G, Steinhoff BJ, Munz DL, Emrich D, Rüther E. [^{123}I] IBZM SPET analysis of dopamine D2 receptor occupancy in narcoleptic patients in the course of treatment. *Biol Psychiatry.* 1996;39(2):107-11.

[63] Rinne JO, Hublin C, Någren K, Helenius H, Partinen M. Unchanged striatal dopamine transporter availability in narcolepsy: a PET study with [11C] -CFT. *Acta Neurol Scand.* 2004;109(1):52-5.

[64] Ellis CM, Monk C, Simmons A, Lemmens G, Williams SC, Brammer M, Bullmore E, Parkes JD. Functional magnetic resonance imaging neuroactivation studies in normal subjects and subjects with the narcoleptic syndrome. Actions of modafinil. *J Sleep Res.* 1999;8(2):85-93.

[65] Howard RJ, Ellis C, Bullmore ET, Brammer M, Mellers JD, Woodruff PW, David AS, Simmons A, Williams SC, Parkes JD. Functional echoplanar brain imaging correlates of amphetamine administration to normal subjects and subjects with the narcoleptic syndrome. *Magn Reson Imaging.* 1996;14(9):1013-6.

[66] Bradley TD, Floras JS. (Eds). Sleep Apnea: Implications for Cardiovascular and Cerebrovascular Disease. Dekker, New York, 2000.

[67] Kryger MH, Roth T, Dement WC, editors. Principles and practice of sleep medicine. Fourth ed: W.B. Saunders Company, 2005. pp. 1517.

[68] Perkin RM, Downey R, MacQuarrie J. Sleep-disordered breathing in infants and children. *Respir Care Clin N Am.* 1999;5(3):395-426.

[69] Aloia MS, Arndt JT, Smith L, Skrekas J, Stanchina M, Millman RP. Examining the construct of depression in obstructive sleep apnea syndrome. *Sleep Med* 2005;6:115-21.

[70] Brown WD. The psychosocial aspects of obstructive sleep apnea. *Semin Respir Crit Care Med.* 2005;26(1):33-43.

[71] Beebe DW, Groesz L, Wells C, Nichols A, McGee K. The neuropsychological effects of obstructive sleep apnea: a meta-analysis of norm-referenced and case-controlled data. *Sleep.* 2003;26(3):298-307.

[72] Engleman H, Joffe D. Neuropsychological function in obstructive sleep apnoea A review. *Sleep Med Rev.* 1999;3:59-78.

[73] Lanfranchi P, Somers VK. Obstructive sleep apnea and vascular disease. *Respir Res.* 2001;2(6):315-9

[74] Kawahara S, Akashiba T, Akahoshi T, Horie T. Nasal CPAP improves the quality of life and lessens the depressive symptoms in patients with obstructive sleep apnea syndrome. *Intern Med.* 2005;44(5):422-7.

[75] Macey PM, Henderson LA, Macey KE, Alger JR, Frysinger RC, Woo MA, Harper RK, Yan-Go FL, Harper RM. Brain morphology associated with obstructive sleep apnea. *Am J Respir Crit Care Med.* 2002;166(10):1382-7.

[76] Morrell MJ, McRobbie DW, Quest RA, Cummin AR, Ghiassi R, Corfield DR. Changes in brain morphology associated with obstructive sleep apnea. *Sleep Med.* 2003;4(5):451-4.

[77] O'Donoghue FJ, Briellmann RS, Rochford PD, Abbott DF, Pell GS, Chan CH, Tarquinio N, Jackson GD, Pierce RJ. Cerebral structural changes in severe obstructive sleep apnea. *Am J Respir Crit Care Med.* 2005;171(10):1185-90]

[78] Gale SD, Hopkins RO. Effects of hypoxia on the brain: neuroimaging and neuropsychological findings following carbon monoxide poisoning and obstructive sleep apnea. *J Int Neuropsychol Soc.* 2004;10(1):60-71.

[79] Bartlett DJ, Rae C, Thompson CH, Byth K, Joffe DA, Enright T, Grunstein RR. Hippocampal area metabolites relate to severity and cognitive function in obstructive sleep apnea. *Sleep Med.* 2004;5(6):593-6.

[80] Halbower AC, Degaonkar M, Barker PB, Earley CJ, Marcus CL, Smith PL, Prahme MC, Mahone EM. Childhood obstructive sleep apnea associates with neuropsychological deficits and neuronal brain injury. *PLoS Med.* 20063(8):e301.

[81] Bonelli RM, Cummings JL. Frontal-subcortical circuitry and behavior. *Dialogues Clin Neurosci.* 2007;9(2):141-51.

[82] Aloia MS, Arnedt JT, Davis JD, Riggs RL, Byrd D. Neuropsychological sequelae of obstructive sleep apnea-hypopnea syndrome: a critical review. *J Int Neuropsychol Soc.* 2004;10(5):772-85.

[83] Alchanatis M, Deligiorgis N, Zias N, Amfilochiou A, Gotsis E, Karakatsani A, Papadimitriou A. Frontal brain lobe impairment in obstructive sleep apnoea: a proton MR spectroscopy study. *Eur Respir J.* 2004;24(6):980-6.

[84] Kamba M, Suto Y, Ohta Y, Inoue Y, Matsuda E. Cerebral metabolism in sleep apnea. Evaluation by magnetic resonance spectroscopy. *Am J Respir Crit Care Med.* 1997;156(1):296-8.

[85] Thomas RJ, Rosen BR, Stern CE, Weiss JW, Kwong KK. Functional imaging of working memory in obstructive sleep-disordered breathing. *J Appl Physiol.* 2005;98(6):2226-34]

[86] Castronovo V, Canessa N, Ferini Strambi L, Aloia MS, Consonni M, Marelli S, Iadanza A, Bruschi A, Falini A, Cappa SF. Brain activation changes before and after PAP treatment in obstructive sleep apnea. *Sleep.* 2009;32(9):1161-72.

[87] Ayalon L, Ancoli-Israel S, Klemfuss Z, Shalauta MD, Drummond SP. Increased brain activation during verbal learning in obstructive sleep apnea. *Neuroimage.* 2006;31(4):1817-25.

[88] McMahon JP, Foresman BH, Chisholm RC. The influence of CPAP on the neurobehavioral performance of patients with obstructive sleep apnea hypopnea syndrome: a systematic review. *WMJ.* 2003;102(1):36-43.

[89] Jalbert F, Lacassagne L, Bessard J, Dekeister C, Paoli JR, Tiberge M. Oral appliances or maxillomandibular advancement osteotomy for severe obstructive sleep apnoea in patients refusing CPAP. *Rev Stomatol Chir Maxillofac.* 2012;113(1):19-26]

[90] Ficker JH, Feistel H, Möller C, Merkl M, Dertinger S, Siegfried W, Hahn EG. [Changes in regional CNS perfusion in obstructive sleep apnea syndrome: initial SPECT studies with injected nocturnal 99mTc-HMPAO. *Pneumologie.* 1997;51(9):926-30.

[91] Tonon C, Vetrugno R, Lodi R, Gallassi R, Provini F, Iotti S, Plazzi G, Montagna P, Lugaresi E, Barbiroli B. Proton magnetic resonance spectroscopy study of brain metabolism in obstructive sleep apnoea syndrome before and after continuous positive airway pressure treatment. *Sleep.* 2007;30(3):305-11.

[92] Hashimoto K, Ono T, Honda E, Maeda K, Shinagawa H, Tsuiki S, Hiyama S, Kurabayashi T, Ohyama K. Effects of mandibular advancement on brain activation during inspiratory loading in healthy subjects: a functional magnetic resonance imaging study. *J Appl Physiol.* 2006;100(2):579-86.

[93] Lim W, Bardwell WA, Loredo JS, Kim EJ, Ancoli-Israel S, Morgan EE, Heaton RK, Dimsdale JE. Neuropsychological effects of 2-week continuous positive airway pressure treatment and supplemental oxygen in patients with obstructive sleep apnea: a randomized placebo-controlled study. *J Clin Sleep Med.* 2007;3(4):380-6.

[94] Harper RM, Macey PM, Henderson LA, Woo MA, Macey KE, Frysinger RC, Alger JR, Nguyen KP, Yan-Go FL. fMRI responses to cold pressor challenges in control and obstructive sleep apnea subjects. *J Appl Physiol.* 2003;94(4):1583-95.

[95] Henderson LA, Woo MA, Macey PM, Macey KE, Frysinger RC, Alger JR, Yan-Go F, Harper RM. Neural responses during Valsalva maneuvers in obstructive sleep apnea syndrome. *J Appl Physiol.* 2003;94(3):1063-74.

[96] Macey PM, Macey KE, Henderson LA, Alger JR, Frysinger RC, Woo MA, Yan-Go F, Harper RM. Functional magnetic resonance imaging responses to expiratory loading in obstructive sleep apnea. *Respir Physiol Neurobiol.* 2003;138(2-3):275-90.

[97] Macey KE, Macey PM, Woo MA, Henderson LA, Frysinger RC, Harper RK, Alger JR, Yan-Go F, Harper RM. Inspiratory loading elicits aberrant fMRI signal changes in obstructive sleep apnea. *Respir Physiol Neurobiol.* 2006;151(1):44-60.

[98]   Allen RP, Picchietti D, Hening WA, Trenkwalder C, Walters AS, Montplaisi J. Restless Legs Syndrome Diagnosis and Epidemiology workshop at the National Institutes of Health; International Restless Legs Syndrome Study Group. Restless legs syndrome: diagnostic criteria, special considerations, and epidemiology. A report from the restless legs syndrome diagnosis and epidemiology workshop at the National Institutes of Health. *Sleep Med.* 2003;4(2):101-19.

[99]   Stiasny K, Oertel WH, Trenkwalder C. Clinical symptomatology and treatment of restless legs syndrome and periodic limb movement disorder. *Sleep Med Rev.* 2002;6(4):253-65.

[100] Etgen T, Draganski B, Ilg C, Schröder M, Geisler P, Hajak G, Eisensehr I, Sander D, May A. Bilateral thalamic gray matter changes in patients with restless legs syndrome. *Neuroimage.* 2005;24(4):1242-7.

[101] Bucher SF, Seelos KC, Oertel WH, Reiser M, Treknkwalder C. Cerebral generators involved in the pathogenesis of the restless legs syndrome. *Ann Neurol.* 1997;41(5):639-45.

[102] Staedt J, Stoppe G, Kögler A, Munz D, Riemann H, Emrich D, Rüther E. Dopamine D2 receptor alteration in patients with periodic movements in sleep (nocturnal myoclonus). *J Neural Transm Gen Sect.* 1993;93(1):71-4.

[103] Staedt J, Stoppe G, Kögler A, Riemann H, Hajak G, Munz DL, Emrich D, Rüther E. Nocturnal myoclonus syndrome (periodic movements in sleep) related to central dopamine D2-receptor alteration. *Eur Arch Psychiatry Clin Neurosci.* 1995;245(1):8-10.

[104] Staedt J, Stoppe G, Kögler A, Riemann H, Hajak G, Munz DL, Emrich D, Rüther E. Single photon emission tomography (SPET) imaging of dopamine D2 receptors in the course of dopamine replacement therapy in patients with nocturnal myoclonus syndrome (NMS). *J Neural Transm Gen Sect.* 1995;99(1-3):187-93.

[105] Michaud M, Soucy JP, Chabli A, Lavigne G, Montplaisir J. SPECT imaging of striatal pre- and postsynaptic dopaminergic status in restless legs syndrome with periodic leg movements in sleep. *J Neurol.* 2002;249(2):164-70.

[106] Eisensehr I, Wetter TC, Linke R, Noachtar S, von Lindeiner H, Gildehaus FJ, Trenkwalder C, Tatsch K. Normal IPT and IBZM SPECT in drug-naive and levodopa-treated idiopathic restless legs syndrome. *Neurology.* 2001;57(7):1307-9.

[107] Tribl GG, Asenbaum S, Happe S, Bonelli RM, Zeitlhofer J, Auff E. Normal striatal D2 receptor binding in idiopathic restless legs syndrome with periodic leg movements in sleep. *Nucl Med Commun.* 2004;25(1):55-60.

[108] Cervenka S, Palhagen SE, Comley RA, Panagiotidis G, Cselényi Z, Matthews JC, Lai RY, Halldin C, Farde L. Support for dopaminergic hypoactivity in restless legs syndrome: a PET study on D2-receptor binding. Brain. 2006;129(Pt 8):2017-28.

[109] Price DD. Psychological and neural mechanisms of the affective dimention of pain. *Science.* 2000;288(5472):1769-71.

[110] Rainville P, Duncan GH, Price DD, Carrier B, Bushnell MC. Pain affect encoded in human anterior cingulate but not somatosensory cortex. *Science.* 1997;277(5328):968-71.

[111] Walters AS. Review of receptor agonist and antagonist studies relevant to the opiate system in restless legs syndrome. *Sleep Med.* 2002;3(4):301-4.

[112] Allen RP, Barker PB, Wehrl F, Song HK, Earley CJ. MRI measurement of brain iron in patients with restless legs syndrome. *Neurology*. 2001;56(2):263-5.

[113] Earley CJ, P BB, Horska A, Allen RP. MRI-determined regional brain iron concentrations in early- and late-onset restless legs syndrome. *Sleep Med.* 2006;7(5):458-61.

[114] Bassetti C, Vella S, Donati F, Wielepp P, Weder B. SPECT during sleepwalking. *Lancet.* 2000;356(9228):484-5.

[115] Schenck CH, Bundlie SR, Ettinger MG, Mahowald MW. Chronic behavioral disorders of human REM sleep: a new category of parasomnia. *Sleep*. 1986;9(2):293-308.

[116] Gagnon JF, Bédard MA, Fantini ML, Petit D, Panisset M, Rompré S, Carrier J, Montplaisir J. REM sleep behavior disorder and REM sleep without atonia in Parkinson's disease. *Neurology*. 2002;59(4):585-9.

[117] Schenck CH, Bundlie SR, Mahowald MW. Delayed emergence of a parkinsonian disorder in 38% of 29 older men initially diagnosed with idiopathic rapid eye movement sleep behaviour disor-der. *Neurology*. 1996;46(2):388-93.

[118] Gilman S, Koeppe RA, Chervin RD, Consens FB, Little R, An H, Junck L, Heumann M. REM sleep behavior disorder is related to striatal monoaminergic deficit in MSA. *Neurology*. 2003;61(1):29-34]

[119] Plazzi G, Corsini R, Provini F, Pierangeli G, Martinelli P, Montagna P, Lugaresi E, Cortelli P. REM sleep behavior disorders in multiple system atrophy. *Neurology*. 1997;48(4):1094-7.

[120] Fantini ML, Ferini-Strambi L, Montplaisir J. Idiopathic REM sleep behavior disorder: toward a better nosologic definition. *Neurology*. 2005;64(5):780-6]

[121] Sakai K, Sastre JP, Salvert D, Touret M, Tohyama M, Jouvet M. Tegmentoreticular projections with special reference to the muscular atonia during paradoxical sleep in the cat: an HRP study. *Brain Res.* 1979;176(2):233-54.

[122] Culebras A, Moore JT. Magnetic resonance findings in REM sleep behavior disorder. *Neurology*. 1989;39(11):1519-23]

[123] Shirakawa S, Takeuchi N, Uchimura N, Ohyama T, Maeda H, Abe T, Ishibashi M, Ohshima Y, Ohshima H. Study of image findings in rapid eye movement sleep behavioural disorder. *Psychiatry Clin Neurosci.* 2002;56(3):291-2.

[124] Mazza S, Soucy JP, Gravel P, Michaud M, Postuma R, Massicotte-Marquez J, Decary A, Montplaisir J. Assessing whole brain perfusion changes in patients with REM sleep behavior disorder. *Neurology*. 2006;67(9):1618-22.

[125] Scherfler C, Frauscher B, Schocke M, Iranzo A, Gschliesser V, Seppi K, Santamaria J, Tolosa E, Högl B, Poewe W; SINBAR (Sleep Innsbruck Barcelona) Group. White and gray matter abnormalities in idiopathic rapid eye movement sleep behavior disorder: a diffusion-tensor imaging and voxel-based morphometry study. *Ann Neurol.* 2011;69(2):400-7]

[126] Miyamoto M, Miyamoto T, Kubo J, Yokota N, Hirata K, Sato T. Brainstem function in rapid eye movement sleep behavior disorder: the evaluation of brainstem function by proton MR spectroscopy (1H-MRS). *Psychiatry Clin Neurosci.* 2000;54(3):350-1.

[127] Iranzo A, Santamaria J, Pujol J, Moreno A, Deus J, Tolosa E. Brainstem proton magnetic resonance spectroscopy in idopathic REM sleep behavior disorder. *Sleep*. 2002;25(8):867-70.

[128] Unger MM, Belke M, Menzler K, Heverhagen JT, Keil B, Stiasny-Kolster K, Rosenow F, Diederich NJ, Mayer G, Möller JC, Oertel WH, Knake S. Diffusion tensor imaging in idiopathic REM sleep behavior disorder reveals microstructural changes in the brainstem, substantia nigra, olfactory region, and other brain regions. *Sleep.* 2010;33(6):767-73.

[129] Eisensehr I, Linke R, Tatsch K, Kharraz B, Gildehaus JF, Wetter CT, Trenkwalder C, Schwarz J, Noachtar S. Increased muscle activity during rapid eye movement sleep correlates with decrease of striatal presynaptic dopamine transporters. IPT and IBZM SPECT imaging in subclinical and clinically manifest idiopathic REM sleep behavior disorder, Parkinson's disease, and controls. *Sleep.* 2003;26(5):507-12.

[130] Albin RL, Koeppe RA, Chervin RD, Consens FB, Wernette K, Frey KA, Aldrich MS. Decreased striatal dopaminergic innervation in REM sleep behavior disorder. *Neurology.* 2000;55(9):1410-2.

[131] Caselli RJ, Chen K, Bandy D, Smilovici O, Boeve BF, Osborne D, Alexander GE, Parish JM, Krahn LE, Reiman EM. A preliminary fluorodeoxyglucose positron emission tomography study in healthy adults reporting dream-enactment behavior. *Sleep.* 2006;29(7):927-33.

[132] Tsuno N, Besset A, Ritchie K. Sleep and depression. *J Clin Psychiatry.* 2005;66(10):1254-9.

[133] Benca RM. Mood disorders. In: Kryger MH, Roth T, Dement WC, eds. Principles and practice of sleep medicine. 4th ed: Elsevier Saunders; 2005] pp. 1311-26.

[134] Ho AP, Gillin JC, Buchsbaum MS, Wu JC, Abel L, Bunney WE Jr. Brain glucose metabolism during non-rapid eye movement sleep in major depression. A positron emission tomography study. *Arch Gen Psychiatry.* 1996;53(7):645-52.

[135] Germain A, Nofzinger EA, Kupfer DJ, Buysse DJ. Neurobiology of non-REM sleep in depression: further evidence for hypofrontality and thalamic dysregulation. *Am J Psychiatry.* 2004;161(10):1856-63.

[136] Nofzinger EA, Buysse DJ, Germain A, Carter C, Luna B, Price JC, Meltzer CC, Miewald JM, Reynolds CF 3rd, Kupfer DJ. Increased activation of anterior paralimbic and executive cortex from waking to rapid eye movement sleep in depression. *Arch Gen Psychiatry.* 2004;61(7):695-702.

[137] Drevets WC, Price JL, Simpson JR Jr, Todd RD, Reich T, Vannier M, Raichle ME. Subgenual prefrontal cortex abnormalities in mood disorders. *Nature.* 1997;386(6627):824-7.

[138] Gillin JC, Wyatt RJ. Schizophrenia: perchance a dream? *Int Rev Neurobiol.* 1975;17:297-342.

[139] Hiatt JF, Floyd TC, Katz PH, Feinberg I.. Further evidence of abnormal non-rapid-eye-movement sleep in schizophrenia. *Arch Gen Psychiatry.* 1985;42(8):797-802.

[140] Zarcone Jr VP, Benson KL, Berger PA. Abnormal rapid eye movement latencies in schizophrenia. Arch Gen Psychiatry. 1987;44(1):45-48.

[141] Weiler MA, Buchsbaum MS, Gillin JC, Tafalla R, Bunney W. Explorations in the relationship of dream sleep to schizophrenia using positron emission tomography. *Neuropsychobiology.* 1990-1991;23(3):109-18.

[142] Keshavan MS, Reynolds CF 3rd, Ganguli R, Brar J, Houck P. Electroencephalographic sleep and cerebral morphology in functional psychoses: a preliminary study with computed tomography. *Psychiatry Res.* 1991;39(3):293-301.

Part IV.
Psychoeducation and Pharmacotherapies

In: Sleep Medicine
Editors: A. Del Casale, R. Brugnoli and P. Girardi

ISBN: 978-1-62808-515-0
© 2013 Nova Science Publishers, Inc.

Chapter XV

Psychoeducation in Sleep Medicine

Paolo Girardi, Antonio Del Casale, Chiara Brugnoli,
Lavinia De Chiara, Daniele Serata, Chiara Rapinesi
and Gloria Angeletti*
Sapienza University, School of Medicine and Psychology
NESMOS (Neuroscience, Mental Health and Sensory Organs) Department
Rome, Italy

Abstract

Insomnia is a frequent complaint that involves one-third of the adult population and is associated with a reduction in the quality of life, increased risk of medical and psychiatric comorbidities, and abuse of hypnotic medications.

Psychological and behavioral therapies are increasingly used in the last decades as they have been recognized to be valid and effective options in the treatment of chronic primary and secondary insomnia, with many advantages over pharmacological interventions, including fewer side effects and better maintenance of clinical progress over time.

Several non-pharmacological strategies, comprising the most widely known educational, behavioral and cognitive interventions, are described in terms of their effectiveness and recommendations. These therapies are suitable for adults of all ages and should be considered as first line intervention in the treatment of chronic insomnia.

Keywords: Sleep disorders, Sleep disturbance, Insomnia, Psychoeducation, Cognitive therapy, Sleep Hygiene, Behavioral Therapy

* Corresponding author: Prof. Paolo Girardi, "Sapienza" University, Rome. Email: paolo.girardi@uniroma1.it.

Introduction

Insomnia is a prevalent complaint in the general population. It may present as a primary disturbance or may be comorbid with another physical or mental illness [1].

In the most recent International Classification of Sleep Disorders [2], insomnia is diagnosed with the presence of sleep disorders, including difficulty falling asleep, difficulty staying asleep, or early wakening, during the better part of the night and persistent for at least one month, with worsened daytime functioning caused by these symptoms. The Diagnostic and Statistical Manual of Mental Disorders, 4th edition, text revision (DSM-IV TR), defines primary insomnia as a complaint lasting for at least one month, with difficulty in initiating and/or maintaining sleep or non-restorative sleep. Primary insomnia does not occur exclusively during the course of another sleep disorder or mental illness, and is not related to a general medical condition [3]. Secondary insomnia is relative to other conditions, including medical or psychiatric illnesses, substance abuse disorder or other sleep disorders.

Insomnia can be further classified according to temporal criteria in initial, middle, terminal-insomnia; lengthwise classifications divide insomnia as transient (<1 week), short term (1-3 weeks), and chronic (>3 weeks).

One-third of the general population suffers from insomnia symptoms, while 9-15% can experience insomnia symptoms with daytime consequences [4].

Among several treatment options available for the disorder, psychological and behavioral approaches deserve consideration in treating persistent insomnia since they are a valid option over pharmacological interventions.

Treatment mechanisms of cognitive and behavioral therapies for insomnia target the factors proposed by Spielman in his theoretical model, namely predisposing, precipitating, and perpetuating factors. Predisposing factors increase the individual's susceptibility to insomnia; precipitating factors trigger insomnia onset and mainly include acute stressors; perpetuating factors maintain sleep disturbances although the initial factors have resolved. Although some predisposing/precipitating factors may prompt the development of sleep disturbances, perpetuating factors (mainly behavioral and cognitive features and hyperarousal aspects) are involved in maintaining such disturbances in the long term, promoting the onset of chronic insomnia [5].

Behaviors can serve as perpetuating factors by altering homeostatic regulation and decreasing sleep drive. Cognitive processes underlying insomnia are related to increased worry and rumination about the inability to sleep, excessive effort focused on falling asleep, and daytime consequences of sleep deprivation. Cognitive and behavioral therapies, aiming at modifying learned negative sleep behaviors, distorted thoughts and attitudes, and sleep-related anxiety, work to affect these mediators and have a positive impact on sleep outcomes.

The available treatment strategies comprise educational (sleep hygiene), behavioral (stimulus control, relaxation therapy, sleep restriction), and cognitive therapies, which can be administered either separately or in combination.

Psychological and behavioral therapies present some advantages compared with medications. It is indeed documented that despite the tested efficacy and rapid clinical improvement gained with pharmacological treatment, non-pharmacological therapies are associated with less side effects. Currently, pharmacological therapy is overused and prescribed for long-term use on a regular basis, despite repeated recommendations for its short-term, intermittent use [6].

Cognitive behavioral therapy for insomnia (CBT-I) is the combination of cognitive, stimulus-control, and sleep-restriction therapies with or without relaxation therapy [7]. CBT-I is more effective than pharmacotherapy alone, and equal or superior to a combination of CBT and pharmacotherapy on most outcome measures [6]. Long-term follow up has shown that patients treated with psychological and behavioral therapies preserved better clinical gains over time compared to subjects treated with medications alone [8].

In brief, educational, psychological and behavioral therapies are safe, effective, and recommended treatments for chronic primary and secondary insomnia, and substantially produce greater benefit than pharmacotherapy. These treatments are suitable for adults of all ages with or without chronic use of hypnotic drugs, and should be considered as first-line interventions for patients affected by chronic insomnia [7].

Sleep Hygiene

Many behaviors can produce and perpetuate insomnia, such as bad or irregular sleep habits, excessive napping, and other activities that are incompatible with sleep. These practices are under the individual's behavioral control and produce a deleterious effect on sleep. They can be classified into two general categories: practices that produce increased arousal and habits that are inconsistent with sleep organization.

Arousal may be produced by commonly-used substances such as caffeine or nicotine. Alcohol ingestion may also interfere with sleep by producing arousal and sleep maintenance difficulties. Stress and excitement such as vigorous exercise close to bedtime and intense mental work late at night may lead to hyperarousal. Also, environmental factors can produce an increased arousal.

Watching the clock during an awakening in the middle of the night and other practices and behaviors that can interfere with regular timing and duration of sleep and wakeful periods also disturb physiological arousal. Sleep may become disrupted or variable when too much time is spent in bed, when there is excessive daily variation in bedtime, arising time, and amount of sleep, and when naps are taken during the day.

Basic information about sleep and sleep hygiene is usually provided as a core component of all treatments for insomnia.

"Sleep hygiene" is the term used to describe good sleep habits. It comprises the conditions and practices that promote continuous and effective sleep, and includes a set of guidelines and tips designed to enhance good sleep:

1) **Get regular**: By consistently going to bed and getting up at the same time, the body is conditioned to follow a regular pattern of sleep. This allows the body's natural clock to initiate and maintain sleep.

2) **Sleep when sleepy**: It is best to sleep when actually feel tired or sleepy, rather than spending too much time awake in bed.

3) **Avoid caffeine and nicotine**: It is best to avoid consuming any caffeine or cigarettes for at least 4-6 hours before going to bed. These substances act as stimulants and interfere with the ability to fall asleep.

4) **Avoid alcohol**: It is good to avoid alcohol for at least 4-6 hours before going to bed. Contrary to common practice, an alcoholic drink before bedtime can actually make sleep worse. Though it may cause drowsiness, alcohol fragments the stages of sleep and makes it more disrupted.

5) **Avoid heavy meals before sleep**: A healthy, balanced diet will help to sleep well, but timing is important. A heavy meal soon before bed can interrupt sleep. However, a very empty stomach at bedtime can be distracting, so it can be useful to have a light snack or a warm glass of milk before going to sleep.

6) **Arrange a dark, confortable, quiet sleep environment**: It is very important that the bed and bedroom are quiet and confortable for sleeping. It is good to provide curtains or an eye mask to block early morning light and earplugs if there is noise outside the room.

7) **Exercise every day, not too close to bedtime**: Regular exercise helps with good sleep, but it is recommended to not do strenuous physical activity in the 4 hours before bedtime.

8) **No clock-watching**: Many people who struggle with sleep tend to watch the clock too much. Frequently checking the clock during the night can cause waking up and reinforces negative thoughts.

9) **Use the bedroom only for sleeping and intimacy**: It is better to not use the bed for anything other than sleeping and intimacy, so that the body comes to associate the bed with sleep. Electronic devices must be removed because they are disruptive to sleep. The bedroom cannot be used for work and similar stimulating activities.

10) **Use a sleep diary**: This worksheet can be a useful way of making sure one has the right facts about sleep, rather than making assumptions.

11) **Do not take naps**: It is best to avoid taking naps during the day, to make sure to be tired at bedtime. If this cannot be avoided, make sure it is for less than one hour and before 3 pm.

12) **Sleep rituals**: Daily sleep rituals prior to going to bed allow unwinding and mentally preparing for sleep. These rituals should include quiet activities such as reading, listening to relaxing music, or even taking a warm bath.

This form of behavioral intervention aims to make patients more aware of health practices and environmental factors that may be either detrimental or beneficial for sleep. Although sleep hygiene education is always suggested and can often improve sleep disorders, insufficient evidence is available for this treatment to be an option as a single therapy, and it is often included with other forms of behavioral interventions [9].

Stimulus Control

Stimulus control occurs when an organism acts in one way in the presence of a given stimulus and in another way in its lack.

Table 1. Sleep Hygiene

Sleep Hygiene Rules	
Get regular	By consistently going to bed and getting up at the same time, the body is conditioned to follow a regular pattern of sleep. This allows the body's natural clock to initiate and maintain sleep.
Sleep when sleepy	It is best to sleep when actually feel tired or sleepy, rather than spending too much time awake in bed.
Avoid caffeine and nicotine	It is best to avoid consuming any caffeine or cigarettes for at least 4-6 hours before going to bed. These substances act as stimulants and interfere with the ability to fall asleep.
Avoid alcohol	It is good to avoid alcohol for at least 4-6 hours before going to bed. Contrary to common practice, an alcoholic drink before bedtime can actually make sleep worse. Though it may cause drowsiness, alcohol fragments the stages of sleep and makes it more disrupted.
Avoid heavy meals before sleep	A healthy, balanced diet will help to sleep well, but timing is important. A heavy meal soon before bed can interrupt sleep. However, a very empty stomach at bedtime can be distracting, so it can be useful to have a light snack or a warm glass of milk before going to sleep.
Arrange a dark, confortable, quiet sleep environment	It is very important that the bed and bedroom are quiet and confortable for sleeping. It is good to provide curtains or an eye mask to block early morning light and earplugs if there is noise outside the room.
Exercise every day, not too close to bedtime	Regular exercise helps with good sleep, but it is recommended to not do strenuous physical activity in the 4 hours before bedtime.
No clock-watching	Many people who struggle with sleep tend to watch the clock too much. Frequently checking the clock during the night can cause waking up and reinforces negative thoughts.
Use the bedroom only for sleeping and intimacy	It is better to not use the bed for anything other than sleeping and intimacy, so that the body comes to associate the bed with sleep. Electronic devices must be removed because they are disruptive to sleep. The bedroom cannot be used for work and similar stimulating activities.
Use a sleep diary	This worksheet can be a useful way of making sure one has the right facts about sleep, rather than making assumptions.
Do not take naps during the day	It is best to avoid taking naps during the day, to make sure to be tired at bedtime. If this cannot be avoided, make sure it is for less than one hour and before 3 pm.
Sleep rituals	Daily sleep rituals prior to going to bed allow unwinding and mentally preparing for sleep. These rituals should include quiet activities such as reading, listening to relaxing music, or even taking a warm bath.

With regards to sleep, several behaviors can be considered as stimulus control related. Stimulus control treatment is a behavioral technique in which instructions are given to patients, so to develop new permanent sleeping habits with the goal to associate the act of going to bed with restoring sleep [10-12].

This treatment began from a learning analysis that considered falling asleep as an instrumental act produced for reinforcement. Stimuli associated with sleep become discriminative stimuli for the occurrence of reinforcement. Inadequate stimulus control may lead to difficulties in falling asleep, or in falling back to sleep after wakening [13].

Patients affected by insomnia often engage in activities at bedtime that are incompatible with falling asleep, like watching television, snacking or worrying. Even long periods of being awake in bed predispose to alertness and a wakened state.

The main objective for stimulus-control therapy is to train the insomniac to reassociate the bed and bedroom with sleep and to reestablish a consistent sleep-wake schedule. The focus of the instructions is primarily on sleep onset. For sleep maintenance problems, the instructions are to be followed after awakening when patient has difficulty falling back to sleep. These rules are to be followed even after the insomniac recovers good sleep:

1) **Do not use the bed for any activity except sleep. Sexual activity is the only exception to this rule**. The goal is to have activities associated with arousal out of the bedroom, and to break up patterns that are associated with disturbed sleep.

2) **If you are not able to fall asleep within 20 or 30 minutes after lying in the bed, get up and move to a quiet place and relax until you feel sleepy. Then go back to bed. Repeat the procedure if necessary**. These instructions help to associate the bed with sleep, and avoid frustration and arousal associated with the inability of falling asleep. This also helps to cope with insomnia: patients can take control of their problem by getting out of bed and engaging in other activities.

3) **Set your alarm clock and wake up at the same time every morning, regardless of how much sleep you got during the night**. Many insomniacs have irregular sleep rhythms because they try to make up the lack of sleep by sleeping late or napping the day after. These rules enable consistent sleep rhythms and help maintaining the circadian cycling.

4) **No naps during daytime**. Irregular napping can disrupt sleep patterns, and causes the loss of advantage of the sleep lost in the previous night.

Since all these instructions are to be followed by patients at home, constituting self-managed treatment, adherence to treatment is crucial. Adherence can be improved by discussing directly and providing a rationale about each rule, with both patients and their partners. Stimulus control therapy is recommended and effective in the treatment of chronic insomnia, and can be administered either as a single therapy or in combination with other behavioral therapies [9].

Sleep Restriction

Sleep restriction is another behavioral therapy that is effective and recommended in the treatment of chronic insomnia. According to this method, the amount of time spent in bed is reduced to reflect the actual amount of sleep the patient is getting each night. The aim is to consolidate sleep by increasing the chance that patients will fall asleep once they are in bed [5].

Sleep deprivation produced by limiting the amount of time spent in bed leads to increased desire to sleep (sleep drive), and to a deeper and less fitful sleeping.

Patients affected by insomnia often claim they only get few hours of good sleep: the majority of the night is spent flitting in and out of wakefulness, trying hopelessly to fall asleep. This leads to poor "sleep efficiency" (the sleep time ratio during which the patient is actually asleep), and to a restless sleep due to fragmentation of sleep stages.

According to the instructions for sleep restriction therapy, sleep capacity is estimated with the help of a sleep diary, filled by patients in the previous two weeks. In this time the patient will collect the average amount of time in which he/she is actually asleep (Total Sleep Time, TST). Time allowed in bed (Total Time in Bed, TIB) is approximates the mean TST to achieve >85% sleep efficiency (TST/TIB x 100). This means that bedtime hours will be restricted to the total hours of actual sleep reported on the log, although the prescribed sleep window is always a minimum of 4.5 hours.

Typically, wake up time is held constant, while time to bed is delayed. It is important to consider that daytime sleepiness may be experienced at the beginning of treatment, and to discuss with the patient how wakefulness can be maintained until the scheduled bedtime.

Time allowed in bed can be adjusted weekly by looking at the sleep efficiency: when patient's sleep becomes more efficient, the therapist can allow increments in the amount of time elapsed in bed. If sleep efficiency has been over 85-90% during the last 7 nights, an additional 15 or 30 minutes of time in bed is allowed. If sleep efficiency is <80%, time in bed can be further decreased by 15-20 minutes. The process takes several weeks of diligent dedication to alter sleep patterns in order to see a result. Frequent contacts with the therapist are necessary to reduce drop-out rates [9].

Relaxation Training

Relaxation training comprises different behavioral techniques aimed at reducing somatic tension or intrusive thoughts at bedtime that interfere with sleep. Standard relaxation training consist of a variety of procedures, such as progressive muscle relaxation, guided imagery, abdominal breathing, and other techniques designed to lower somatic and cognitive arousal states connected with disrupted sleep. It is effective and recommended in the treatment of chronic insomnia [9].

Several data have suggested that insomnia is associated with hyperarousal [14,15], which is a quantitative disorder of consciousness marked by increased tension and alertness, reduced pain tolerance, anxiety, exaggerated startle responses, and fatigue. When this condition becomes chronic, it seems to underlie insomnia. According to Bonnet and Arand, insomnia is a primary physiological disorder of hyperarousal that can be measured and treated [16].

Relaxation training refers to sleep-related anxiety and bedtime arousal that can disrupt sleep.

Among the different strategies comprised in this method, "progressive muscle relaxation", developed by Edmund Jacobson in 1938 [17] and presented in manual form by Bernstein and Borkovec in 1973 [18], is one of the most widely used and researched. This technique involves methodical tensing and relaxing different muscle groups throughout the body, until a whole-body state of relaxation is obtained. The sequence of instruction is the following: *"Beginning on the muscles in your face, contract your muscles gently for one to two seconds and then relax. Repeat several times. Use the same technique for other muscle groups, in the following sequence: jaw and neck, shoulders, upper arms, lower arms, finger, chest, abdomen, buttock, thighs, calves, and feet. Repeat this cycle for 45 minutes, if necessary"*. Initially, the method may be performed in a clinical setting, but it is important to teach relaxation as a portable skill, allowing the patient to perform sessions on a daily basis in their home.

Another relaxation technique is "abdominal deep breathing", wherein the patient's attention is focused on breathing to overcome the underlying anxiety. The patient is asked to deeply breath from the nose, hold their breath for few seconds, then slowly exhale and repeat the sequence for 10 or 15 times before going to bed.

Finally, "guided imagery training" focuses the patient's attention on a relaxing imaginary journey with pleasurable and calming images. The patient, usually with the help of a live voice or a tape, is asked to walk through the sequence quietly to induce feelings of peace and reduce anxiety.

Biofeedback

Similar to relaxation training, biofeedback therapy is best characterized as a relaxation procedure, insomuch as there is usually a combination of these two techniques. Biofeedback uses various types of non-invasive monitors to have objective markers of the level of relaxation, in order to seek reduction in somatic arousal. Although biofeedback is primarily used to treat conditions such as high body pressure, headaches, and chronic pain, scientific clinical studies have reported its safety and effectiveness for treatment of chronic insomnia, for which it is a recommended therapy [9].

There are three types of biofeedback: electromyography (EMG), neurofeedback (EEG), and sensorimotor rhythm (SMR) EEG.

EMG biofeedback provides information about muscular activity. This technique gives visual and auditory feedback about the electrical activity (related to muscle tension) of particular groups of muscles, which is detected by the use of electrodes placed on the skin directly over the muscle that is being measured. Using this feedback, the patient can learn to voluntarily relax or tense his/her musculature.

EEG biofeedback is a self-regulation method in which the EEG is recorded and the patient receives instant feedback (auditory and/or visually) on brain cortical activity. Patients use the feedback to change the signal presented on screen using several different mental strategies, thus they can learn to influence specific brain signals.

Sensorimotor rhythm biofeedback is used to strengthen a 12- to 14-Hz EEG rhythm from the sensorimotor cortex. This frequency range (named sensorimotor rhythm) is known to be abundant during light non-rapid eye movement sleep, and is overlapping with the sleep spindle frequency band. Early findings have indicated that instrumental conditioning of these oscillations during wakefulness can influence subsequent sleep, increasing subjective sleep quality and reducing sleep onset latency [13].

Cognitive Therapy

Many people with insomnia report that mental events prevent them from sleeping. Cognitive aspects of insomnia include dysfunctional thinking, heightened anxiety about sleep, cortical arousal, sleep misperception, automaticity, and attentional processing.

Common cognitive errors found in insomnia patients are the misattribution of all their personal failing to their lack of sleep, some unrealistic expectations about the amount of time they have to sleep, and selective recall of a bad and wakeful night. Cognitive therapies attempt to restructure these faulty thoughts, replacing them with more adaptive and functional opinions.

"Paradoxical intention" and "cognitive restructuring" are two possible cognitive interventions. The former is a prescription requiring patients to perform behaviors that are outwardly incompatible with the goal for which they are seeking therapeutic assistance. For example, to reduce the anticipatory anxiety about sleep performance, which can inhibit sleep onset, patients are requested to get into bed and try to remain awake as long as possible, rather than to focus on trying to fall asleep. This intention can help in decreasing performance anxiety at bedtime due to the inability to fall asleep and excessive concern about negative outcomes associated with sleep loss [19].

Paradoxical intention tend to be most effective with patients who are resistant to therapeutic suggestions, because it subverts the target responses to a conventional program (aimed at helping individuals fall asleep more rapidly) and interrupt the cycle of "performance anxiety - failure to perform - increased performance anxiety" inadvertently supported by other techniques. This cognitive therapy was found to be effective and is recommended in the treatment of chronic insomnia with sleep initiation difficulties [9,20].

Cognitive restructuring is directed at changing maladaptive attitudes and beliefs about sleep. Negative, stressful thoughts can exacerbate insomnia by triggering negative emotions such as anxiety or frustration, which mobilize the stress response, strengthening the wakefulness system. Individuals with insomnia can experience increased worry and rumination about their inability to fall asleep, and about the effect of sleep loss on daytime performance. Moreover, they tend to overestimate how long they take to fall asleep and to underestimate their real amount of sleep. Cognitive restructuring involves challenging negative sleep thoughts, and replacing them with more rational substitutes.

These processes require some effort and accurate information to patients, because such thoughts are typically automatic and are sometimes difficult to eradicate. Thus, accurate education about sleep and insomnia must be provided to patients in order to be able to recognize and challenge negative thoughts regarding it; afterwards, patients will be asked to consider alternative ways of thinking to replace inaccurate and dysfunctional thoughts. With regular applications of this process, patients will become accustomed to this skill and can begin to overcome their insomnia.

While there is extensive evidence for the effectiveness of cognitive therapy in combination with other therapies, only limited evidence is available to recommend this as a single therapy [9].

Cognitive Behavioral Therapy for Insomnia (CBT-I)

According to this method, the therapist can resort to several behavioral and cognitive techniques in a multimodal approach, which is generally considered most effective. Cognitive therapy seeks to change the patient's dysfunctional beliefs and unrealistic expectations about sleep, as well as problematic behavior that precipitates and perpetuates insomnia symptoms.

Table 2. Main cognitive and behavioral treatments in sleep disorders / disturbances

Techniques	Description	Recommendations
Sleep Hygiene	General guidelines about healthy lifestyle practices that improve sleep and minimize sleep disturbance	Sleep regulation
Stimulus Control	A set of instructions designed to re-associate the bed and bedroom with rapid sleep onset and to develop a stable sleep-wake cycle	Chronic insomnia Sleep maintenance problems
Sleep Restriction	The method curtails time in bed to the actual amount of sleep time. This is aimed to achieve greater sleep continuity and to enhance sleep drive. When sleep continuity substantially improves, time in bed is gradually increased.	Chronic insomnia Sleep maintenance problems
Relaxation Training	Clinical procedures designed to lower somatic and cognitive arousal states that interfere with sleep.	Patients displaying elevated levels of arousal Chronic insomnia Sleep onset problems
Biofeedback	This technique trains the patient to control selected physiologic variables through visual or auditory feedback, in order to reduce somatic arousal	Chronic insomnia
Cognitive Therapy	Psychological methods aimed at challenging and changing unrealistic expectations and dysfunctional beliefs about sleep and insomnia, and at eliminating "performance anxiety" connected with falling asleep	Chronic insomnia
CBT-I	Combination of cognitive therapy coupled with behavioral treatments (stimulus control, sleep restriction),with or without relaxation therapy, in a multimodal approach	Chronic insomnia Insomnia Comorbid with depression, chronic pain, cancer and other medical and psychiatric illness Chronic insomnia in older adults
Multicomponent therapy (without cognitive therapy)	Utilizes various combinations of behavioral techniques (stimulus control, sleep restriction, relaxation), and sleep hygiene education	Chronic insomnia Chronic insomnia in older adults Insomnia comorbid with other medical or psychiatric conditions

Legend: CBT-I: Cognitive-behavioral Therapy for Insomnia.

CBT-I was developed as a psychological intervention to target these perpetuating and precipitating factors of insomnia, and each of its components involves distinct skills and strategies intended to target specific mechanisms of insomnia [21]. CBT-I is a short-term treatment and adopts a multicomponent approach, where the first-line components consist of stimulus control and sleep restriction, while sleep hygiene, cognitive restructuring, and relaxation therapy are considered adjunctive intervention.

The treatment is delivered over the course of 4-8 sessions that occur weekly for 30-60 minutes each. In current clinical practice it is usually necessary to refer to specialist clinicians to deliver this treatment, and there is evidence of equivalent treatment benefits of this therapy when implemented by trained primary care physicians [22] or nurse practitioners [23].

The American Academy of Sleep Medicine practice parameters recommend this therapy as standard treatment for insomnia based on strong empirical support of effectiveness. CBT-I improves quantity and quality of sleep parameters and diminishes the level of hyperarousal in patients with primary insomnia; it is also effective for insomnia that is comorbid with medical or psychiatric conditions [9].

Trials comparing CBT-I with hypnotic medications reveal comparable efficacy immediately after treatment, but longer lasting effects at follow-up were compared to medication [6, 24].

One disadvantage of CBT-I is the unavailability of trained CBT-I therapists in many healthcare settings. For this reason, recently the interest has focused on self-help treatments for insomnia, including internet-delivered [25] and book formats [26] to reach the majority of sleep disordered persons who do not promptly seek a face to face treatment. These kinds of therapies were found to be effective in improving global insomnia symptoms and daily sleep measures, although the results were restricted to patients without severe depression. Other unsupported self-help may be too complicated for many patients, preventing adherence to the intervention. Thus, a supported (with an additional therapist support) or advanced (with performed internet programming) architecture may encourage more patients and enhance the efficacy of treatment.

Multicomponent Therapy (without Cognitive Therapy) and Brief Behavioral Treatment for Insomnia

This treatment incorporates several behavioral components (such as stimulus control, relaxation, and sleep restriction) for treating insomnia. Typically, sleep hygiene education is a part of multicomponent therapy. Although CBT-I is now considered the standard treatment for insomnia, it has limited use due to the shortage of specially trained clinicians and the duration and intensity of the treatment.

To overcome these difficulties, a brief, manual behavioral treatment program called "Brief behavioral treatment for insomnia" (BBTI) was developed by Troxel and colleagues [27] for encouraging behavioral treatment for insomnia in primary care practices. The core components of BBTI are principles of stimulus control and sleep restriction therapies, and the interventions involve two in-person sessions and two telephone sessions, delivered in a concise, brief and efficacious format. Both multicomponent therapy and BBTI are effective and recommended in the treatment of chronic primary insomnia.

Several randomized controlled trials have compared the effects of multicomponent interventions (without cognitive therapy) with single interventions, confirming that multicomponent interventions are effective in the management of long-term insomnia [8]. In summary, BBTI is considered as a simple, efficacious, and durable intervention for chronic insomnia in older adults [28] and comorbid insomnia [29], and is a promising intervention in treating patients with residual depression and refractory insomnia [29].

Conclusion

Psychological and behavioral therapies are effective treatment options for the management of chronic primary insomnia, insomnia associated with other psychiatric or medical conditions, and older adults with insomnia. Additional evidence has shown that cognitive and behavioral interventions can facilitate hypnotic drug interruption in patients who are chronic hypnotic drug users, with a reduction in side effects and costs at follow-up [30].

Although many single therapies are considered effective and are recommended in the treatment of chronic insomnia, there is still little information that establishes the relative efficacy of each intervention, and usually the trend is to combine multiple treatments composed of two or more cognitive and behavioral therapies. There is some evidence showing a greater effect of progressive muscle relaxation upon sleep-onset problems, and a greater benefit of stimulus control plus sleep restriction combination in sleep maintenance difficulties [31]. At any rate, among the psychological and behavioral strategies, CBT-I should be considered as a first-line intervention for chronic insomnia, showing, with its multicomponent approach, a greater ability to address the various perpetuating factors involved in the development of chronic insomnia [1], as well as a significantly greater and more durable benefit than cognitive and behavioral strategies associated with pharmacotherapy or pharmacotherapy alone [6,24].

To overcome the difficulties in finding specifically trained physicians, new strategies in administering CBT have been developed and analyzed. Self-help treatments, including computerized CBT, delivered with an internet format, or written manuals, with or without additional telephone consultations, appears to be promising options in the stepped care model for insomnia, showing a moderate effect in the short-term treatment of chronic insomnia [26,32]. Group therapy, or CBT administered by adequately trained primary care nurses or physicians, can be an adjunctive and clinically-effective option in the treatment of chronic insomnia, and represent an opportunity for patients with cost-effective benefits.

References

[1]   Morin CM, Bootzin RR, Buysse DJ, Edinger JD, Espie CA, Lichstein KL. Psychological and behavioral treatment of insomnia: update of the recent evidence (1998-2004). *Sleep*. 2006;29(11):1398-414.

[2]   American Academy of Sleep Medicine. International classification of sleep disorders, 2nd ed: Diagnostic and coding manual. American Academy of Sleep Medicine, Westchester, IL: 2005.

[3]   American Psychiatric Association. Diagnostic and statistical manual of mental disorders. American Psychiatric Association, Washington, DC: 2000.

[4]   Ohayon MM. Epidemiology of insomnia: what we know and what we still need to learn. *Sleep Med Rev.* 2002;6:97-111.

[5]   Spielman AJ, Caruso LS, Glovinsky PB. A behavioral perspective on insomnia treatment. *Psychiatr Clin North Am.* 1987;10(4):541-53

[6]   Jacobs GD, Pace-Schott EF, Stickgold R, Otto MW. Cognitive behavior therapy and pharmacotherapy for insomnia: a randomized controlled trial and direct comparison. *Arch Intern Med.* 2004;164(17):1888-96.

[7]   Schutte-Rodin S, Broch L, Buysse D, Dorsey C, Sateia M. Clinical guideline for the evaluation and management of chronic insomnia in adults. *J Clin Sleep Med.* 2008;4(5):487-504.

[8]   Morin CM, Bootzin RR, Buysse DJ, Edinger JD, Espie CA, Lichstein KL. Psychological and behavioral treatment of insomnia:update of the recent evidence (1998-2004). *Sleep.* 2006;29(11):1398-414.

[9]   Morgenthaler T, Kramer M, Alessi C, Friedman L, Boehlecke B, Brown T, Coleman J, Kapur V, Lee-Chiong T, Owens J, Pancer J, Swick T; American Academy of Sleep Medicine. Practice parameters for the psychological and behavioral treatment of insomnia: an update. An american academy of sleep medicine report. *Sleep.* 2006;29(11):1415-9.

[10]   Bootzin RR. A Stimulus Control treatment for Insomnia. *Proceedings of the American Psychological Association.* 1972;395-396.

[11]   Bootzin RR. Effects of self-control procedures for insomnia. In: R. B. Stuart (Ed.), Behavioral self-management: Strategies, techniques and outcomes. New York, Brunner Mazel: 1977.

[12]   Bootzin RR, Nicassio P. Behavioral treatments for insomnia. In: M. Hersen, R. M. Eisler, & P. M. Miller (Eds.), Progress in behavior modification (Vol. 6, pp. 1-45). New York, Academic Press: 1978.

[13]   Bootzin RR, Epstein D, Wood JM: Stimulus control instructions. In: P. J. Hauri (ed): Case Studies in Insomnia (Chap. 2, pp. 19-28). New York: Plenum Medical Book Company: 1991.

[14]   Bonnet MH. Hyperarousal and insomnia. *Sleep Med Rev.* 2010;14(1):33.

[15]   Monroe LJ. Psychological and physiological differences between good and poor sleepers. *J Abnorm Psychol.* 1967;72:255-64.

[16]   Bonnet MH, Arand DL. Hyperarousal and Insomnia: State of the science. *Sleep Med Rev.* 2010;14(1):9-15.

[17]   Jacobson E. Progressive relaxation (2nd ed.). Chicago: University of Chicago Press: 1938.

[18]   Bernstein DA, Borkovec TD. Progressive relaxation training: a manual for the helping professions. Champaign, IL: Research Press: 1973.

[19]   Ascher LM, Efran JS. Use of paradoxical intention in a behavioral program for sleep onset insomnia. *J Consult Clin Psychol.* 1978;46(3):547-50.

[20] Broomfield NM, Espie CA. Initial insomnia and paradoxical intention: An experimental investigation of putative mechanisms using subjective and actigraphic measurement of sleep. *Behav Cogn Psychoth.* 2003;31:313-24.

[21] Schwartz DR, Carney CE. Mediators of cognitive-behavioral therapy for insomnia: a review of randomized controlled trials and secondary analysis studies. *Clin Psychol Rev.* 2012;32(7):664-75.

[22] Baillargeon L, Demers M, Ladouceur R. Stimulus-control: nonpharmacologic treatment for insomnia. *Can Fam Physician.* 1998;44:73-9.

[23] Espie CA, Inglis SJ, Tessier S, Harvey L. The clinical effectiveness of cognitive behaviour therapy for chronic insomnia: implementation and evaluation of a sleep clinic in general medical practice. *Behav Res Ther.* 2001;39:45-60.

[24] Mitchell MD, Gehrman P, Perlis M, Umscheid CA. Comparative effectiveness of cognitive behavioral therapy for insomnia: a systematic review. *BMC Fam Pract.* 2012;13:40.

[25] Ström L, Pettersson R, Andersson G. Internet-based treatment for insomnia: a controlled evaluation. *J Consult Clin Psychol.* 2004;72:113-20.

[26] Lancee J, van den Bout J, van Straten A, Spoormaker VI. Internet-delivered or mailed self-help treatment for insomnia?: a randomized waiting-list controlled trial. *Behav Res Ther.* 2012;50(1):22-9.

[27] Troxel WM, Germain A, Buysse DJ. Clinical management of insomnia with brief behavioral treatment (BBTI). *Behav Sleep Med.* 2012;10(4):266-79.

[28] Buysse DJ, Germain A, Moul DE, Franzen PL, Brar LK, Fletcher ME, Begley A, Houck PR, Mazumdar S, Reynolds CF 3rd, Monk TH. Efficacy of brief behavioral treatment for chronic insomnia in older adults. *Arch Intern Med.* 2011;171(10):887-95.

[29] Watanabe N. [Clinical efficacy of psychotherapy targeted for insomnia in comorbid depression]. *Seishin Shinkeigaku Zasshi.* 2012;114(2):158-66.

[30] Morgan K, Dixon S, Mathers N, Thompson J, Tomeny M. Psychological treatment for insomnia in the management of long-term hypnotic drug use: a pragmatic randomised controlled trial. *Br J Gen Pract.* 2003;53(497):923-8.

[31] Waters WF, Hurry MJ, Binks PG, Carney CE, Lajos LE, Fuller KH, Betz B, Johnson J, Anderson T, Tucci JM. Behavioral and hypnotic treatments for insomnia subtypes. *Behav Sleep Med.* 2003;1(2):81-101.

[32] Cheng SK, Dizon J. Computerised cognitive behavioural therapy for insomnia: a systematic review and meta-analysis. *Psychother Psychosom.* 2012;81(4):206-16.

In: Sleep Medicine
Editors: A. Del Casale, R. Brugnoli and P. Girardi

ISBN: 978-1-62808-515-0
© 2013 Nova Science Publishers, Inc.

Chapter XVI

Pharmacotherapies in Sleep Medicine

Luigi Ferini-Strambi[*] *and Sara Marelli*
Department of Clinical Neurosciences, Sleep Disorders Center,
Università Vita-Salute San Raffaele, Milan, Italy

Abstract

Research to evaluate and formulate treatments for insomnia is often complicated by the fact that insomnia is usually of multifactorial etiology. Benzodiazepine receptor agonists represent the mainstay of hypnotic therapy. Sedating antidepressants are commonly used 'off-label' to treat insomnia, despite limited efficacy data and potential significant safety concerns. Melatoninergic compounds, as ramelteon and agomelatine, may represent a possible alternative in treating insomnia. Orexin antagonists are the most promising new agents for the treatment of insomnia, with encouraging results in preliminary clinical trials.

In narcolepsy, treatment is targeted at symptom management. Currently, sodium oxybate, amphetamines, methylphenidate, modafinil, and armodafinil are the only medications approved by the FDA for the treatment of narcolepsy. Although treatment of EDS in narcolepsy may have a mild beneficial effect on cataplexy, most wake-promoting agents/stimulants do not provide sufficient relief from cataplexy. Most medications used for the treatment of cataplexy have REM sleep suppressant properties and/or increase aminergic (especially by blocking the norepinephrine transporter) transmission. Tricyclic antidepressant agents and serotonin reuptake inhibitors have been successfully used for decades for the treatment of cataplexy. More recently, sodium oxybate, has been found to be highly efficacious for the treatment of cataplexy in narcolepsy, and is also effective for the treatment of EDS as well as improving sleep quality in narcoleptic patients.

It is increasingly evident that narcolepsy is autoimmune and that an upper airway infection, may be related to H1N1 influenza, triggers narcolepsy. Trials using intravenous immunoglobulins in recent onset cases had conflicting results, and not once was the disease fully reversed. Another intriguing aspect is that for narcolepsy/hypocretin deficiency cases the most logical intervention would be to use a hypocretin receptor agonist during the day.

---

[*] Email: ferinistrambi.luigi@hsr.it.

In restless legs syndrome (RLS), a pharmacological treatment should be limited to those patients who suffer from clinically relevant RLS symptoms including intermittent RLS with impaired sleep quality or quality of life. In the recently published European guidelines on management of RLS, rotigotine, ropinirole, pramipexole, gabapentin enacarbil, gabapentin and pregabalin are all considered effective for the short-term treatment for RLS. For the long-term treatment for RLS, rotigotine is considered effective, gabapentin enacarbil is probably effective, and ropinirole, pramipexole and gabapentin are considered possibly effective. However, it should be considered that trial results in RLS may lack broad generalizability. Recruited subjects had greater disease severity, frequency, and duration than reported by the estimated 1.5% of individuals in the general population described as "RLS sufferers".

Pharmacological Treatment Of Insomnia

Introduction

The goals of insomnia treatment are to improve quantitative and qualitative aspects of sleep, to reduce the distress and anxiety associated with poor sleep, and to improve the impaired daytime function [1].

Patients often try self-help strategies including reading, relaxation, and over-the-counter remedies such as alcohol, antihistamines, and natural products [2].

Insomnia treatment includes 2 broad categories, cognitive-behavioural treatment (CBT) and medication treatment. Patients often prefer nonpharmacologic approaches [3]. Moreover, it has been reported that CBT is effective for treating insomnia when compared with medications, and its effects seem to be more durable than medications [4].

The treatment of insomnia since antiquity to the 1960s has included several substances and medications such as alcohol, laudanum, bromides, chloral hydrate, paraldehyde, and barbiturates. Benzodiazepines (BDZs) have been used to treat insomnia, but the prolonged use of these drugs is thought to be related to severe withdrawal symptoms and potential dependency. These problems associated with daytime drowsiness have resulted in providers prescribing this class of medications less frequently to their patients. The benzodiazepine receptor agonists (zolpidem, zaleplon, zopiclone, altogether Z-drugs) which unlike BZD are used exclusively for the treatment of insomnia, were thought to have a lesser tendency to induce physical dependence and addiction than BZDs, and are therefore widely prescribed for the treatment of insomnia, particularly in elderly patients [5]. Nevertheless, safety issues are still a matter of concern [6, 7]

Antidepressants with sedating properties such as trazodone, amitriptyline, and mirtazapine are commonly prescribed to insomnia sufferers. These antidepressants, are used at "lower doses" for insomnia than their standard antidepressant doses [8]. The major problem with using these drugs as hypnotics is that there is limited information regarding the dose range along which they improve sleep and their safety at those doses.

Atypical antipsychotics such as olanzapine and quetiapine are also prescribed to patients with insomnia and also are associated with adverse effects that are not minor, such as dizziness, anticholinergic effects, and weight gain. Newer treatment options, which will be the focus of this chapter, include medications acting on the melatonin receptors or histamine receptors.

Benzodiazepines (BDZs)

BDZs have been the drugs of choice for the treatment of insomnia since their introduction approximately 50 years ago. They occupy benzodiazepine alpha receptors of the gamma-aminobutyric acid (GABA)$_A$ receptor complex, and occupation of the receptor results in opening the chloride ion channel and facilitation of the inhibitory action of GABA, which is a widely distributed, inhibitory neurotransmitter in the central nervous system (CNS). In contrast to the barbiturates and barbiturate derivatives, which the BDZs replaced have narrow therapeutic indices and act directly at the receptors on the GABA complex without the need for the presence of GABA. The hypnotic efficacy of BDZs has been well-documented using objective (nocturnal polysomnography) and subjective measures of sleep induction, maintenance, and duration in clinical trials, as well as in meta-analyses of trials using various compounds [9, 10].

Clinically important differences between specific BDZs result from their pharmacokinetic properties (Table 1). Most hypnotic BDZs have rapid absorption and onset of action. More slowly absorbed BDZs (eg, oxazepam, clorazepate) are less useful for insomnia. Elimination half-lives of hypnotic BDZs vary widely, with predictable clinical effects. For example, triazolam, with a short half-life, reduces sleep latency but has no significant effect on wakefulness after sleep onset; flurazepam and its metabolite have half-lives up to 120 hours, resulting in reduced wakefulness after sleep onset as well as increased daytime sleepiness.

Table 1. Benzodiazepine Receptor Agonist Drugs

	T_{max}h	Elimination half-Life, h	Usual Hypnotic Dose, mg
Benzodiazepines			
Triazolam	1-2	2-6	0.125-0.25
Temazepam	1-2	8-22	15-30
Estazolam	1.5-2	10-24	1-2
Quazepam	2-3	48-120	7.5-15
Flurazepam	1.5-4.5	48-120	15-30
Alprazolam	0.6-1.4	6-20	
Lorazepam	0.7-1	10-20	0.25-1
Clonazepam	1-2.5	20-40	0.5-3
Z-Drugs			
Zaleplon	1 (0.5-2)	1 (0.8-1.3)	5-20
Eszopiclone	1.5 (0.5-2)	6 (5-8)	1-3
Zolpidem	1.6 (0.5-1.5)	2.5 (1.6-4.5)	5-10

Pharmacokinetic differences can be used to clinical advantage. Patients with sleep-onset difficulties or morning sedation from hypnotics may benefit from a drug with a short half-life and patients with sleep maintenance difficulties may benefit from one with a longer half-life. The majority of efficacy studies have been short- and intermediate-term in duration, and given a paucity of controlled long-term data, and many uncontrolled clinical observations, tolerance development has remained an area of controversy. Tolerance is defined as the loss of effects with repeated use of a stable dose, or the need to increase a dose to maintain effects for repeated use.

Adverse reactions to BDZs in clinical practice and clinical trials are generally mild, short in duration, and occur in a minority of patients. Many of the adverse effects of BDZs are mediated by their desired pharmacological activity (i.e., sedation). In a study of hospital inpatients receiving hypnotics, the rate of adverse events was 1 in every 10,000 doses [11,12].

Falls in the elderly are often considered a special case of psychomotor impairment associated with BDZs, either due to elevated peak plasma concentrations or residual effects. However, data suggest that falls in the elderly is not a significant BDZ risk among insomniacs. Falls in the elderly are not unique to BDZs and when controlling for comorbid diseases are not independent risk factors [13]. Moreover, in a survey of the elderly living in community dwellings, the risk of fractures was associated with sleep problems after controlling for demographic variables and concurrent medical diseases [14]; among nursing home residents, the unique risk for falls was insomnia and not BDZs [15]. Thus, the risk of falls in the elderly associated with BDZs is actually less than untreated insomnia.

It is well known that an inability to remember information presented after drug administration, termed anterograde amnesia, is a characteristic of all BDZs [16]. It can be due to either attention failures and or both attention and consolidation failures in the memory process. The severity of amnesia is related to plasma concentration at the time of stimulus presentation, which is determined by dose and time since drug ingestion. Finally, it should be underlined that sleep itself is amnesic. People do not recall information presented during sleep, during brief awakenings from sleep, or during the sleep onset process. Words presented every minute during the sleep onset process are not remembered from the 5-minute time point on prior to electroencephalographic signs of sleep onset [17].

Although there have been reports of "global" amnesia (i.e., a total loss of memory for events during the previous 24 h when awake and functioning after taking BDZs), these have not been systematically verified or studied.

Additional concerns regarding BDZs include rebound insomnia, withdrawal, and dependence [18]. Rebound insomnia refers to an increase in sleep symptoms beyond baseline levels and is commonly observed during abrupt discontinuation, particularly for shorter-acting drugs. The most important determinant of rebound insomnia is dose. Clinical doses are rarely associated with rebound, whereas doses greater than the clinical dose are more likely to produce rebound. Rebound may be minimized by gradual dose reduction over weeks to months.

Withdrawal symptoms (ie, symptoms other than the initial one after discontinuation of the drug) can last for several weeks. Among individuals with no substance use history, BDZ self-administration represents therapy-seeking rather than drug-seeking behaviour. However, abuse may occur with BDZ hypnotics, particularly in individuals with a history of alcohol or other sedative abuse [19].

Z-Drugs

The Z-drugs include zolpidem, zaleplon, and eszopiclone. For the alpha receptor of the $GABA_A$ complex, 6 subtypes have been identified. All of the BDZs demonstrate similar affinity to the alpha 1, 2, 3, and 5 receptor subtypes. In contrast, zolpidem and zaleplon have a higher affinity for alpha 1 than the other subtypes. Eszopiclone shows a decreased preference for the alpha 1 subtype, having a greater affinity to alpha 2 and 3. Although knock-in genetic data from animal studies suggest differential effects associated with the different alpha receptor subtypes, this has not been directly demonstrated in human studies. However, based on the animal studies, it is hypothesized that alpha 1 mediates sleep promotion and amnesic effects, whereas alpha 2 and 3 are involved in anxiolytic and possibly antidepressant effects. In human studies, eszopiclone, which has alpha 2 and 3 affinities, has been shown to augment an antidepressant response in patients with insomnia comorbid with depression, as well as an anxiolytic response in patients with insomnia comorbid with generalized anxiety disorder (GAD) [20, 21].

Zolpidem and zaleplon have ultra short or short half-lives, whereas eszopiclone has an intermediate half-life. Zaleplon and zolpidem are specifically indicated for sleep induction, whereas eszopiclone is indicated for both sleep induction and sleep maintenance [22, 23].

Although Z-drugs have less adverse effects compared with BDZs, gastrointestinal problems such as diarrhea and stomach upset may occur in some patients, and in the case of eszopiclone, a transient metallic or unpleasant taste on awakening in the morning has been reported. In addition, perceptual difficulties, memory problems, confusion, and rarely sleepwalking have been observed in patients using Z-drugs. Reports of parasomnia-like episodes with associated amnesia have appeared in the literature. The behaviors reported have included sleep eating, sleep walking, sleep driving, and even violent behaviors [24-26]. The true incidence of these phenomena and the circumstances in which they occur is unclear because the rate of exposure in the population is unknown. Also, because there are no systematic, controlled data, what mediates these events is also unknown. Some authors reviewed the case report literature and underlined that the occurrence of parasomnia-like events was associated with high doses (i.e., doses much greater than the clinical dose), sleep deprivation, and co-ingestion of alcohol and other CNS depressant drugs [27].

Concerning tolerance with Z-drugs, some recent double-blind, placebo-controlled studies using self reports have shown eszopiclone is effective for 6 to 12 months of nightly use [23,28] and in a recent double-blind, placebo-controlled nocturnal polysomnography study, zolpidem remained effective for 8 months of nightly use [29]. Although several early studies suggested lower potential for rebound with Z-drugs compared with BDZs, rebound can occur with both.

Antidepressants

One analysis of data from a US national service tracking physician prescription activity in 2002 found that the most commonly used off-label drugs for the treatment of insomnia are antidepressants [8]. Trazodone, amitriptyline, and mirtazapine are the three most widely used antidepressants, that are used at "lower doses" for insomnia than their standard antidepressant doses. These drugs have complex and different neural receptor-binding profiles, however their commonality in having anti-histaminic and anti-serotonergic activity is thought to be responsible for their sedating effects [30].

In adults, the frequent prescription of sedating antidepressants for insomnia implies that prescribers believe these medications are more effective, or safer, or less prone to dependence or side effects when compared with classical hypnotic medications. However, the major problem with using antidepressants as hypnotics is that there is limited information regarding the dose range along which they improve sleep and their safety at those doses. There are no studies in primary insomnia with amitryptiline or mirtazapine, and there are only 3 studies with trazodone [31-33].

Montgomery and colleagues (1983) [31] found that trazodone (150 mg) failed to reduce sleep latency or increase total sleep time, although it did decrease wake after sleep onset for the 3-week study, in contrast, trazodone at a threefold lower dose (50 mg) reduced sleep latency and increased total sleep time, but the effect on total sleep time was present for only 1 week. Roth and colleagues (2011) [33] studied the effects of trazodone (50 mg) in sixteen primary insomniacs. Trazodone was administered to participants 30 min before bedtime for 7 days in a 3-week, within-subjects, randomized, double-blind, placebo-controlled design. Subjective effects, equilibrium (anterior/posterior body sway), short-term memory, verbal learning, simulated driving and muscle endurance were assessed the morning after days 1 and 7 of drug administration. Sleep was evaluated with overnight polysomnography. Trazodone produced small but significant impairments of short-term memory, verbal learning, equilibrium and arm muscle endurance across time-points. Relative to placebo across test days, trazodone was associated with fewer night-time awakenings, minutes of Stage 1 non-REM sleep and self-reports of difficulty sleeping. On day 7 only, slow wave sleep was greater with trazodone than with placebo. The authors concluded that although trazodone is efficacious for sleep maintenance difficulties, its associated cognitive and motor impairments may provide a modest caveat to health-care providers.

A retrospective study on sleep effects of trazodone in patients with dementia found that trazodone was among the antidepressants used with good tolerability in this sample, showing effectiveness in resolving sleep complaints and caregiver distress in 2/3 of the patients. "Effectiveness" was defined as improvement of the sleep complaint and reduction in distress of the caregiver as rated on the Neuropsychiatric Inventory Scale (Nighttime Behavior items). One third of patients terminated treatment with trazodone due to a lack of effectiveness but not due to adverse effects [34].

However, a variety of side effects by trazodone ranging from anti-cholinergic effects (i.e., dry mouth, urinary retention, and hallucinations) to orthostatic hypotension, priapism, cardiac arrhythmias, and conduction abnormalities have been reported [35].

Amitriptyline is a tricyclic antidepressant that inhibits reuptake of serotonin and norepinephrine, with cholinergic, histaminergic, and α_1-adreneregic receptor blockade. It has an elimination half-life of 20–30 hours. The typical antidepressant dosages are >75 mg.

There have been no data on the effects of amitriptyline on sleep in patients with primary insomnia and little data on sleep effects in patients with depression. In depressed patients, amitriptyline may improve objective sleep measures of total sleep time, sleep latency, early morning awakening, and total REM time [36].

Recently, one study with healthy male subjects investigated the impact of evening doses of 75 mg amitriptyline over 2 nights on nocturnal polysomnography (PSG) and day-time sleepiness measured by the multiple sleep latency test, in comparison to 10 mg escitalopram and placebo. While amitriptyline did reduce PSG-determined wake after sleep onset, compared with placebo, it also was associated with greater rates of periodic limb movements (PLMs) and a higher PLM-arousal index. In turn, amitriptyline was associated with increased daytime sleepiness compared with placebo, as reflected in shorter mean sleep latencies [37].

Mirtazapine is a tetracyclic piperazinoazepine with potent inhibition of 5-HT$_2$, 5-HT$_3$ and central α_2-adrenergic receptors, with minimal monoamine uptake. It has a half-life of 22–40 hours, and typical antidepressant dosage is >15 mg daily.

There have been no placebo-controlled randomized clinical trials of mirtazapine in primary insomniacs. Mirtazapine has been shown to reduce PSG-measured sleep latency and increase slow wave sleep and sleep efficiency in normal sleepers [38, 39].

In depressed insomniacs, 8 weeks of treatment produced greater reductions in PSG sleep latency and increased total sleep time as compared with fluoxetine, with no patient report described [40]. A recent study tested the effects of mirtazapine in depressed patients and found that patients experienced significant improvement of sleepiness and fatigue measures on subjective scales as well as the Multiple Sleep Latency Test (MSLT); however, there was no placebo comparison [41]. Antidepressants such as mirtazepine have also shown efficacy in treating disturbed sleep associated with hot flashes in perimenopausal women [42].

Side effects of bedtime mirtazapine 30 mg have been observed, include prolonged next-day motor reaction and impaired driving performance when compared with placebo, for acute but not chronic dosing [43]. Mirtazapine may also cause significant weight gain, as well as induce or worsen restless legs syndrome and/or PLMs [44].

Atypical Antipsychotics

The prescription of quetiapine for sleep difficulties in patients with psychiatric illness and dementia is common. In a retrospective cross-sectional study on the use of quetiapine for sleep in demented patients between January 2007 and December 2009, authors found that 43 of the 101 patients included in the study were prescribed quetiapine, "probably for sleep" [45].

In adolescents with autistic spectrum disorder and aggressive behavior, treatment with 25 mg twice a day (50 mg/d) for the first 4 days of treatment, titrated to a maximum of 150 mg/day based on physician judgment, significantly improved subjective sleep disturbances; a positive correlation was found between the improvements in aggression and sleep [46].

However, quetiapine and another atypical antipsychotic, such as olanzepine, are frequently used for the treatment of insomnia in nonpsychiatric patients. As with the antidepressants, these drugs affect multiple transmitter systems, but their sleep promoting effects are thought to be mediated by their antihistaminic activity. The concern for the use of these drugs, as with the other off-label drugs, is that there is limited information regarding efficacious and safe doses. Few open-label studies in primary or comorbid insomnia suggested improvement in self-reported sleep [47-49]. However, their safety is unknown. The risks of dopamine-associated movement disorders characteristic of typical antipsychotics are reduced with these atypical antipsychotics, but a metabolic disorder is a known risk [50].

A recent study evaluated the effect of quetiapine in primary insomnia in a randomized controlled trial. Quetiapine 25 mg at night led to non significant improvement of self-reported total sleep time and sleep latency in patients with primary insomnia [51].

Given the limited information regarding the dose range for the efficacy and safety of the atypical antipsychotics drugs, it is recommended they not be used as hypnotics. Adverse effects such as dizziness, weight gain, hyperglycemia, and anticholinergic effects must be considered [50].

Melatonin Agonists

Melatonin exhibits both hypnotic and chronobiotic properties and thus has been tried for inducing sleep and treating sleep disorders of children, adults, and elderly people. The results of melatonin action in insomnia have not been consistent probably due to its short half-life and ready metabolism after oral administration of fast release preparations. A prolonged released melatonin preparation was recently introduced and has shown good results in treating insomnia in elderly patients [52]. Interestingly, according to a recent consensus report of the British Association for Psychopharmacology on evidence-based treatment of insomnia, melatonin should be tried first in insomnia patients over 55 yr [53]. Another reason for the erratic effect of melatonin on sleep disturbances is probably the inadequate doses employed[54]. There are actually two melatonin agonists, ramelteon and agomelatine. Additionally, two melatonin agonists, tasimelteon and TIK-301, are going through clinical trials.

Neither ramelteon nor agomelatine can display the full spectrum of effects given by a very pleiotropic signaling molecule like melatonin [55]. Restriction of these agonists to membrane-bound receptors may be regarded as an advantage in terms of specificity.

Ramelteon binds to the MT1/MT2 receptor and has a rapid onset of action and a short half-life of less than three hours (half-life of its active metabolite is 2–5 hours) [56].

The suprachiasmatic nucleus (SCN), which contains both MT1 and MT2 receptors. The SCN receives input from the optic nerve in regard to the presence of light, and its output to CNS sleep/wake systems is an alerting, wake-promoting signal. The MT1 receptor is thought to attenuate the alerting signal of the SCN and thereby the occupation of the MT1 receptor decreases sleep latency. The MT2 receptor is thought to have phase-shifting properties, meaning it has the potential to alter the timing of sleep and wake [57].

Ramelteon has an FDA indication for sleep onset insomnia. This indication is supported by self-report and PSG studies showing that sleep onset is hastened along in a dosage range of 4 to 32 mg [58], although the indicated clinical dose is 8 mg.

Tolerance to sleep onset-inducing effects did not develop in the 6- to 12-month studies that have been conducted [59-60].

In the clinical trials of ramelteon (8 mg), the adverse events report included somnolence, fatigue, dizziness, and nausea, all occurring at rates <5 %. Given its short half-life, residual effects would not be expected and have not been observed, and at the clinical dose, rebound insomnia has not been shown [61, 62].

Agomelatine has been licensed by EMEA for the treatment of major depressive disorder (MDD). It has been hypothesized that agomelatine has a unique mechanism of action because its effects are mediated through MT1/MT2 melatonergic receptors and 5-HT2C serotonergic receptors, acting differently at different circadian phases of the day/night cycle. Through this dual action, agomelatine can promote and maintain sleep at night and helps to maintain alertness during daytime. Agomelatine given before sleep would have an immediate sleep promoting melatonergic effect that would prevail over its potentially anti-hypnotic 5HT2C antagonism [63].

The effectiveness of agomelatine in reducing the sleep complaints of depressed patients has been evaluated. Altered intra-night temporal distribution of REM sleep with increased amounts of early REM sleep is the specific EEG sleep patterns associated with depression. Hence, prevention of persistent sleep disturbances would help to reduce the risk of relapse or recurrence of depressive disorders. The treatment of depressive patients with agomelatine for

6 weeks increased the duration of NREM sleep without affecting REM sleep thereby causing improvements in both sleep quality and continuity [64]. In another study that compared the effect of agomelatine (25 mg) with venlafaxine, agomelatine promoted sleep earlier and scored higher on the 'criteria of getting into sleep' as assessed by the Leeds Sleep Evaluation Questionnaire [65]: the improved sleep quality was evident from first week of treatment with agomelatine, whereas venlafaxine did not produce any beneficial effect. This can be important clinically in as much as improvement in sleep disturbances often precede that of depressive symptoms. Moreover, agomelatine has been shown effective in reducing circadian rhythm disturbances seen in patients with MDD [66].

Agomelatine exhibits excellent safety and tolerability; however, it has been observed that some patients may show elevated transaminases [67].

Emerging Pharmacotherapies

Most of the approved hypnotics previously discussed act by enhancing or signaling the neurobiological mechanisms that control sleep. New emerging pharmacotherapies have begun to focus on antagonizing known wake neurobiological mechanisms, including histamine, serotonin, and orexin. Doxepin is a tricyclic antidepressant that inhibits reuptake of serotonin and norepinephrine, with cholinergic, histaminergic, and α_1-adreneregic receptor blockade. Typical antidepressant dosage is >75 mg daily. However, it is likely that at low doses under 10 mg, doxepin's main pharmacologic effect is histaminergic blockade, with little effect on serotonergic or adrenergic receptors. Some studies on doxepin at lower doses than typically used for antidepressant effect (1, 3, and 6 mg) were found to improve sleep as measured by PSG and patient self-report. Side effects of low-dose doxepin in primary insomniacs are similar to placebo [68, 69].

Orexin A and orexin B are hypothalamic neuropeptides that play critical roles in the maintenance of wakefulness. Loss of orexin neurons in humans is associated with narcolepsy, further suggesting the particular importance of orexin in the maintenance of the wakefulness state. These findings have encouraged pharmaceutical companies to develop drugs targeting orexin receptors as novel medications of sleep disorders, such as narcolepsy and insomnia. Suvorexant, a non-selective (dual) antagonist for orexin receptors, demonstrated promising results for the treatment of primary insomnia [70]. Interestingly, in healthy young men without sleep disorders, suvorexant promoted sleep with some evidence of residual effects at the highest doses [71].

Pharmacologic Treatment of Hypersomnias

Introduction

Narcolepsy and other syndromes associated with excessive daytime sleepiness (EDS) can be challenging to treat. According to the *Diagnostic and Statistical Manual of Mental Disorders, 5th edition* (DSM-5) currently being finalized, syndromes with primary hypersomnolence may be divided into 3 groups: 1) narcolepsy caused by hypocretin (orexin) deficiency, a disorder associated with Human Leukocyte Antigen (HLA) marker DQB1*06:02 and believed to be autoimmune (almost all cases with cataplexy), 2) Kleine-

Levin Syndrome (KLS), and 3) syndromes with EDS unexplained by hypocretin abnormalities (generally without cataplexy) [72]. This last group is the most challenging and the most frequent diagnosis. This diagnosis is only made after eliminating sleep deprivation, sleep apnea, disturbed nocturnal sleep, and psychiatric comorbidities as the primary cause of EDS.

The pharmacologic treatment of narcolepsy/hypocretin deficiency is well-codified, and includes sodium oxybate, stimulants, and/or antidepressants. Treatment for other syndromes with hypersomnolence is more challenging and less codified. Therapy should be preferably conservative (such as modafinil), but it may have to be more aggressive (high-dose stimulants, sodium oxybate) on a case-by-case, empirical trial basis. In these conditions it is important to challenge diagnosis and therapy over time, keeping in mind the possibility of tolerance and the development of stimulant addiction. Kleine-Levin Syndrome is usually best left untreated, although lithium can be considered in severe cases with frequent episodes.

Narcolepsy

In narcolepsy, treatment is targeted at symptom management. Even with optimum management, EDS and cataplexy are not always completely controlled.

Nonpharmacologic management should be considered in all patients. Good sleep habits with avoidance of sleep deprivation and/or irregular sleep patterns should be underlined. The scheduling of short naps (about 15 minutes) 2 to 3 times per day can help control EDS and improve alertness, but this is impractical in several settings. Patients and family members should also be warned about the potential dangers of sleepiness relative to driving or in other hazardous settings. However, lifestyle changes are rarely sufficient to adequately control the symptoms of narcolepsy and most patients require life-long medication to control symptoms.

Currently, sodium oxybate, amphetamines, methylphenidate, modafinil, and armodafinil are the only medications approved by the FDA for the treatment of narcolepsy (see table 2).

EDS has traditionally been treated with stimulants, such as methylphenidate or dextroamphetamine, but more recently, modafinil or armodafinil have become the first-line treatment [73].

Amphetamines are simple derivatives of catecholamines (dopamine, norepinephrine, epinephrine) that are made more lipophilic so that they enter the central nervous system easily. These compounds, first made available in 1935, mimic many of the catecholaminergic actions in the brain, primarily substituting for monoamines in presynaptic synapses and producing monoaminergic release.

Amphetamine derivatives not only affect adrenergic and dopaminergic synapses, but also to lesser extent serotoninergic synapses [74]. As a rule, amphetamine isomers of the D-type are more active than isomers of the L-type, and have more effects on dopaminergic synapses than on other monoaminergic synapses [75].

The main action responsible for the psychomotor stimulatory effects of these agents is on central dopamine systems. Most clinical studies of stimulant medications report objective improvements in somnolence in 65% to 85% of patients.

Side effects of amphetamines include peripheral release of norepinephrine, resulting in cardiac stimulation and vasoconstriction. Increased heart rate and blood pressure, palpitations, and sweating are common [76]. Nervousness, irritability and increased anxiety can occur in some patients. Mood may be temporarily enhanced, but the effect is generally not sustainable alone in patients with depression. At a high dose, an amphetamine may precipitate psychosis

[77], although most typically delusions are of the persecution subtype and are reversible with cessation of the medication.

Table 2. Current pharmacologic treatment for excessive daytime sleepiness associated with narcolepsy

Compound	Usual daily doses, mg	Half-life, h	Side effects/note
Methamphetamine	5-80	9-12	Irritability, mood changes, headache, palpitations, tremors, excessive sweating, insomnia
D-Amphetamine Sulfate	≤60	10-28	Irritability, mood changes, headache, palpitations, tremors, excessive sweating, insomnia
Methylphenidate HCl	≤80	2-4	Same as amphetamine; less reduction of appetite or increase in blood pressure
Mazindol	2-8	10-13	Reduction of appetite or increase in blood pressure
Modafinil	100-400	9-14[a]	No peripheral sympathomimetic action, headaches, nausea
Armodafinil	100-300	10-15[a]	Similar to those of modafinil
γ- Hydroxybutyrate; sodium oxybate	20-40 mg/kg/night	0.5-1	Overdose (a single dose of 60-100 mg/kg) induce dizziness, nausea, vomiting, confusion, agitation, epileptic seizures, hallucination, coma with bradycardia, and respiratory depression; evidence of withdrawal syndrome

The development of drug tolerance can also occur. Serious problems with long-term stimulant use are uncommon in narcoleptic patients. The risk of addiction with stimulant drugs is relatively low (<1% to 3% of cases), and is not higher than that in other patient groups; however, the risk is greater in patients taking high dosages of stimulants, in patients who have received long-term treatment with stimulants, and in those with an underlying psychiatric disorder.

Methylphenidate shares many of the actions of amphetamines, although it does not fully substitute for catecholamines at the level of the dopamine transporter. The compound, that became popular for use in narcolepsy in the 1950s, as an amphetamine is not fully specific for dopaminergic transmission, also affecting more mildly other monoamines. Methylphenidate has a short half-life, it is readily absorbed and enters the brain effectively, also producing rapidly increasing concentration in the brain and a sensation of rush. As for amphetamine, methylphenidate is addictive and can lead to drug-seeking behaviors and tolerance[78]. Methylphenidate has a similar side effect profile to amphetamines (e.g. cardiovascular effects, psychosis). Moreover, it also suppresses primarily non-REM sleep, promoting wakefulness, but also REM sleep. Thus, it is mostly effective on wakefulness and has minimal effects on cataplexy and other narcolepsy symptoms.

Selegiline, a monoamine oxidase B inhibitor, has produced statistically and clinically significant improvement in narcoleptic symptoms and polysomnographic measures in patients with narcolepsy, but is rarely used. The main advantage of this agent is its anticataplectic anticataleptic activity in addition to its relatively good alerting effect. However, the main disadvantage of selegine is having to maintain a diet low in tyramine [79].

Modafinil was developed and first used for the treatment of narcolepsy in France in the 1980s. Because it was rapidly shown that modafinil is pharmacologically distinct from amphetamine (but less so from methylphenidate) in some animal tests, and that abuse potential for the compound was low, the mode of action of modafinil was touted as totally different from other stimulants, and did not involve dopamine. However, in the last years animal studies and neuroimaging data in humans clearly indicated a primary dopaminergic mediation of modafinil in wake-promoting effects [80-81].

Modafinil is one of the few treatments that has been subjected to rigorous, double-blind, placebo-controlled studies in narcolepsy. Experience suggests that modafinil is effective for at least half of narcoleptic patients [82]. Because of the relatively low risk of addiction, modafinil can be more easily prescribed in patients without a clear, biochemically defined central hypersomnia syndrome, and is also easier to stop, if needed. Modafinil has an elimination half-life of 9 to 14 hours, permitting once-daily administration, although some patients prefer to have a second dose at midday. Usual doses of modafinil are 200 mg/d or 400 mg/d, but higher doses may be required in some patients [83]. The drug is well tolerated, with headache and nausea being the most common side effects. A long-acting isomeric form of modafinil, called armodafinil, has recently become available [74]. Armodafinil is the dextro-enantiomer component of modafinil. It has a similar therapeutic and side effect profile to modafinil but with the advantage of having a longer elimination half-life. Armodafinil has a T_{max} of about 2 hours and a half-life of about 10 to 14 hours compared with 3 to 4 hours with modafinil. Thus, it has a more prolonged effect during the day and may improve daytime sleepiness in the late afternoon and early evening in some patients with narcolepsy. Armodafinil has been shown to be effective and produces longer wakefulness than modafinil in patients with sleepiness caused by acute sleep loss [85].

Sodium oxybate, also called gamma hydroxybutyric acid (GHB), was first described 50 years ago when used as a general anesthetic agent. Unlike other anesthetic agents and sleep inducers, GHB was found to induce slow wave sleep and REM sleep, suggesting a very distinct mode of action and pharmacological profile. GHB inhibits the release of several neurotransmitters, including GABA, glutamate, and dopamine. Supraphysiologic concentrations seem necessary in order for GHB to bind to GABA(B) receptors, which are responsible for sleep induction and an increase in slow-wave sleep. Based on this observation and considering the fact that many patients with narcolepsy/hypocretin deficiency have disturbed nocturnal sleep, the compound was tried with the hypothesis that increased sleep, notably REM sleep, would reduce sleep pressure during the day and allow narcoleptic patients to be more awake [86].

Several double-blind studies have now demonstrated that GHB is effective on many narcolepsy symptoms [82] and the compound is FDA approved for the treatment of cataplexy and excessive daytime sleepiness in narcolepsy. The compound also has additional documented effects on all other symptoms of narcolepsy (disturbed nocturnal sleep, sleep paralysis, hypnagogic hallucinations). Not only does it have some effects on all symptoms, but a comparison of clinical trial effects on sleepiness, as measured subjectively (Epworth sleepiness scale) or objectively (MSLT or the Maintenance Test of Wakefulness (MWT), a variant of the MSLT most useful to assess whether patients can fight sleepiness) suggests that GHB is more effective than modafinil alone (400 mg) [87].

Because of its very short half-life (about 30 minutes) and a duration of action of only two to four hours, GHB typically needs to be administered twice during the night to fully consolidate a six to eight hour night. It is also a very low potency compound, requiring 6-9 g in adults per night to be effective, starting with a 4.5 g dose split into two (one at bedtime and another in the middle of the night). GHB adverse events include dizziness (23% incidence), headache (20%), nausea (16 %), pain (12%), somnolence (9%), sleep disorder (9%), confusion (7%), infection (7%), vomiting (6%), and enuresis (5%) with most described as mild or moderate in severity. Dizziness, nausea, vomiting, and enuresis may be dose-related [88]. Administration of GHB frequently leads to significantly decreased weight[89].

As narcolepsy/hypocretin deficiency is usually associated with weight gain (especially in children when the onset has been abrupt), weight loss may be actually a very useful effect. Weight loss, however, can be occasionally a problem in patients who have not had weight gain and who have pre-existing anorectic tendencies. More rarely, parasomnias, such as sleep-walking, night eating (also common in untreated patients) or expiratory groaning may occur, and these side effects are also dose-dependent [90].

Although treatment of EDS in narcolepsy may have a mild beneficial effect on cataplexy, most wake-promoting agents/stimulants do not provide sufficient relief from cataplexy. Most medications used for the treatment of cataplexy have REM sleep suppressant properties and/or increase aminergic (especially by blocking the norepinephrine transporter) transmission [73]. Tricyclic antidepressant agents (TCAs) and serotonin reuptake inhibitors (SSRIs) have been successfully used for decades for the treatment of cataplexy. More recently, sodium oxybate, as mentioned before, has been found to be highly efficacious for the treatment of cataplexy in narcolepsy, and is also effective for the treatment of EDS as well as improving sleep quality in narcoleptic patients.

TCAs were the first drugs discovered to have anticataplectic activity. This activity is generally attributed to TCA ability to block the presynaptic reuptake of catecholamines, thereby enhancing their postsynaptic activity. Several small open-label studies and several decades of use have demonstrated that REM-suppressing drugs, as desmethylimipramine, protriptyline, imipramine, and desipramine have beneficial anticataplectic effects; however, clomipramine remains the most efficacious and widely used, at doses of 10 to 75 mg daily [91]. Adverse events commonly associated with TCA therapy include nausea, anorexia, dry mouth, urinary retention, and tachycardia. Men may encounter decreased libido, impotency, or delayed ejaculation. An unusual property of TCAs is the rebound cataplexy phenomenon that occurs on abrupt discontinuation of TCA therapy. When severe, this is known as status cataplecticus and may be disabling for several days [92].

Like the TCAs, SSRIs also block the presynaptic reuptake of catecholamines, thereby increasing their activity; however, they are much more selective for serotonin than TCAs. Like the TCAs, the SSRIs also inhibit nocturnal REM sleep. Fluvoxamine, paroxetine, and fluoxetine have all been shown to have anticataplectic activity; however, fluoxetine seems to be the most commonly used of the SSRIs for the treatment of cataplexy [93]. As a class, the SSRIs are generally less efficacious than TCAs; however, they are safer and better tolerated than the older antidepressants. Reported adverse events include headache, nausea, weight gain, dry mouth, and delayed ejaculation. Other antidepressant medications have also been found to have some anticataplectic activity; these include monoamine oxidase inhibitors such as phenelzine and selegiline, and a norepinephrine/serotonine reuptake inhibitor such as venlafaxine [94]. As mentioned earlier, GHB taken at bedtime and again during the night increases slow-wave sleep, decreases light sleep (stage N1 sleep), and decreases the number of arousals. Other drugs have also been tried in the management of the fragmented sleep of narcoleptic patients. A study evaluating 0.25 mg of triazolam taken at bedtime showed improved sleep efficiency and overall sleep quality [95]. Other medications such as zolpidem, eszoplicone, or clonazepam have been used with in narcoleptic patients for improving sleep fragmentation. .

Kleine-Levin Syndrome (KLS)

Unsatisfactory therapeutic interventions have been attempted using different medications in KLS [96-97]. During episodes, the patients are not only sleepy but cognitively impaired. The administration of a stimulant compound may produce a paradoxical agitation, and thus is not indicated unless the episodes are mild (e.g., at a later phase of the disease when KLS is "burning out," typically after 30 years of age).

In most cases, notably when episodes are not too frequent (e.g., 1-3 times/year) the best approach is to do no harm and to let the patient sleep through the episodes undisturbed, asking for accommodation at school, etc. Depression is not a core feature of KLS, however some patients may become extremely upset during episodes, and it is important to monitor mood. Moreover, it is important to make sure the patient does not leave the house unattended, driving or putting themselves in dangerous situations during the episode. Reassurance regarding the long-term evolution of the condition is key.

If the episodes are severe and frequent (e.g., two weeks long, every 1-2 months), the only therapy that could be efficacious is lithium. An efficacy of lithium in 20 to 40 % of cases in preventing episodes and reducing severity has been reported [96]. When lithium is introduced, it is important to raise the dose until adequate blood levels (0.8-1.2 mEq/ml) are attained [97]. The effects of other mood stabilizers, such as valproic acid or carbamazepine are less well-documented. Antidepressants are not efficacious.

Emerging Therapies for Hypersomnias

It is increasingly evident that narcolepsy is autoimmune and that an upper airway infection, may be related to H1N1 influenza, triggers narcolepsy [98]. In the last years, patients are diagnosed closer and closer to disease onset. Thus, it is now possible to explore whether immune modulation near disease onset could rescue the disorder if caught early enough. Trials using intravenous immunoglobulins in recent onset cases had conflicting results, and not once was the disease fully reversed [99]. Since recent data suggest a T-cell rather than B-cell/antibody mediation [100], it may be that trials with newer medications targeting T-cells (e.g., alpha-4 integrin inhibitors blocking T-cell entry to the brain, such as natalizumab) would have more beneficial effects.

Another intriguing aspect is that for narcolepsy/hypocretin deficiency cases the most logical intervention would be to use a hypocretin receptor agonist (dual, or selective for receptor 2) during the day. Central administration of hypocretin-1 reverses narcolepsy in animal models [101], but unfortunately the hypocretin peptide does not cross the blood brain barrier. Thus, a centrally penetrating agonist is needed to be usable. Several molecules with hypocretin receptor antagonist properties have been successfully synthesized, one of which is awaiting FDA approval for the treatment of insomnia [102]; it is also likely that an agonist will be found and developed. Based on the fact that central administration of hypocretin-1 is strongly wake-promoting in rodents and dogs, it is likely that such compounds will be effective in narcolepsy and other hypersomnias. Whether or not they will have other desirable (e.g., antidepressant effects) or undesirable (addictive potential) effects will likely define their future therapeutic usefulness.

Finally, whereas a large number of safe hypnotics are available, clinicians have very few options for wake-promotion beside dopamine-acting compounds, such as modafinil and amphetamine-like stimulants. This is especially problematic for EDS patients without hypocretin deficiency. Adrenergic reuptake inhibitors and caffeine can be used, but these only have mild stimulant effects. Moreover, rapid development of tolerance makes caffeine ineffective for chronic treatment of EDS [103].

Benzodiazepine antagonist-like compounds could be potential therapies for a subset of EDS patients. Companies have been developing H3 antagonists (i.e., compounds that promote the release of the wake-promoting amine histamine). An H3 antagonist, thioperamide, has been found to produce significant wakefulness in narcoleptic mice [104]. However, whether or not these compounds will be particularly useful as wake-promoting agents in EDS population remain to be clarified [105].

Treatment of Sleep-Related Movement Disorders

Introduction

Sleep-related movement disorders represent a well established category of sleep disorders in the International Classification of Sleep Disorders, second edition (ICSD-2). This category includes restless legs syndrome (RLS), periodic limb movement disorder (PLMD), sleep-related leg cramps, sleep-related bruxism, sleep-related rhythmic movement disorders (RMDs), sleep-related movement disorder due to a drug or substance, and sleep-related movement disorder due to a medical condition. Some of these entities were previously categorized within the parasomnias or the wake-sleep transition disorders. All of these sleep-related movement disorders may cause fragmented sleep, insomnia, and/or excessive daytime sleepiness (EDS).

Restless Legs Syndrome (RLS)

Symptoms of RLS may greatly distress patients impeding falling asleep or causing awakenings or arousals, and are frequently associated with jerking or twitching movements of the legs and, especially during light sleep but sometimes also during relaxed wakefulness, by periodic limb movements in sleep (PLMS) or while awake (PLMW). RLS may occur secondary to other medical and neurological conditions, in particular during pregnancy and associated with uremia, but in most of the cases occurs as a primary condition, often familial. Aside from genetic factors, several data suggest that RLS is associated to some defect in the dopaminergic system and in iron regulation at the level of the central nervous system (CNS). The clearest evidence for dopamine system involvement is the pharmacological evidence acquired after the clinical observation of Akpinar of the beneficial effects of levodopa in RLS [106]. Evidence for an abnormality of iron metabolism also originated from clinical observations [107-108], recently confirmed [109-110] and was substantiated by pathological and metabolic studies suggesting a deficient regulation of iron stores at the CNS level [111]. These considerations are relevant to the treatment of RLS.

Concerning the non pharmacological treatment of RLS, there are very few and not well controlled studies. A randomized controlled 12-week trial evaluated the effectiveness of an exercise program on RLS [112]. Study participants were randomized to either exercise (conditioning program of aerobic and lower-body resistance training 3 days per week) or control groups. At the end of the 12 weeks, a significant improvement in RLS symptoms was observed in the exercise group compared to controls.

Exercise, including cycling for 45 minutes, was also effective in haemodialysis patients with RLS [113].

In the management of RLS, it is important to inform the patient to maintain a good sleep hygiene to prevent the development of insomnia that is frequently observed. Indeed, some patients go to bed later at night and remain active during hours when their symptoms make sleep difficult and some severe RLS patients may even change their working schedule for that purpose. Moreover, patients should avoid alcohol, caffeine and heavy meals in the evening since they may aggravate RLS symptoms. Improvement of RLS symptoms has been anecdotally reported by hot baths or applying something hot or cold, or keeping their mind alert by performing task requiring a large amount of concentration.

A proof-of-concept study on cognitive behavioral therapy tailored to RLS showed favorable results in both medicated and unmedicated RLS patients [114].

Both groups took part in eight group sessions on a weekly basis (session of 90 min each). Subjective ratings of RLS severity, as well as quality of life and mental health status of the patients, improved at the end of therapy and at follow-up 3 months later. These results suggest that psychological strategies may be included in an integrated treatment approach in RLS.

The high prevalence of RLS does not necessarily mean that all patients should be treated with pharmacological therapy. A pharmacological treatment should be limited to those patients who suffer from clinically relevant RLS symptoms including intermittent RLS with impaired sleep quality or quality of life [115-116].

All recent trials have focused the primary outcome measure on the International RLS Severity Scale (IRLS), that is 10-item scale, each item with a score of 0 to 4 (1 to 10 mild; 11 to 20 moderate; 21 to 30 severe; 31 to 40 very severe RLS) or polysomnographic sleep parameters (especially PLMS index).

In 2008, Trenkwalder and colleagues [117] underlined that, according to evidence-based medicine criteria, dopaminergic medications should be the first-line therapy in RLS (see table 3). Several open-label studies documented the short-term efficacy of levodopa given with a dopa-decarboxylase inhibitor. Dosages between 100 and 200 mg standard levodopa improve RLS symptoms. However, a possible side effect of levodopa is morning rebound, characterized by the presence of RLS symptoms occurring de novo as a consequence of evening or night time treatment. With levodopa, it is also possible to observe a rebound of PLMS in the last part of the night when levodopa is administered only at bedtime [116]. In rebound the reappearance of symptoms is compatible with the timing of withdrawal from medication: indeed, the plasma half-life of levodopa is very short (1-2 hours) and the beneficial effect rapidly decreases. The most frequent adverse effects of levodopa reported in a large controlled trial were nausea (10.4%), headache (9.3%), fatigue (4.4%), and nasopharyngitis (4.4%). However, the most relevant clinical side effect in the levodopa therapy is augmentation. Augmentation [118] is a phenomenon characterized by an earlier onset of symptoms by at least 4 hours or by an earlier onset between two and four hours plus at least one of the following compared to symptom status before treatment: a) shorter latency to symptoms when at rest; b) extension of symptoms to other body parts; c) greater intensity of symptoms; d) shorter duration of relief from treatment. Augmentation is probably triggered by intense dopaminergic stimulation of the D1 receptor compared with the D2 and D3 receptors, predominantly at the spinal level. Interestingly, iron deficiency and sleep deprivation may increase the risk of augmentation [119]. A recent study [120] that employed a specific scale for measuring the phenomenon (Augmentation Severity Rating Scale, ASRS) showed augmentation in 36 of 60 (60%) patients treated for six months with levodopa (median daily dose of 300 mg; range 50-500 mg). Increased severity of RLS and higher dosage of levodopa are associated with higher risk of developing augmentation.

Table 3. Therapies for Restless Legs Syndrome

Compound	Half-life, h	Initial dosage, mg	Dosage in RLS, mg	Max. dosage, mg
L-Dopa and Dopamine Agonist				
L-Dopa/Dopadecarbossilasi	2-3	50-100	200-400	600
Bromocriptina	3-8	1.25	2.5-5	7.5
Cabergolina	65	0.5	0.5-2	4
Lisuride	2-3	0.1	0.1-2	4
Pergolide	7-16	0.05	0.1-0.75	1.5
Dopamine Agonist NonErgot				
Pramipexole	8-12	0.125	0.125-0.5	0.75
Ropinirole	6	0.25	0.5-4	4
Rotigotine	5 (costant plasma levels because of patch application)	0.5 mg/24 h or 1 mg/24 h	0.5-3 mg/24 h	4 mg/24 h
Alpha-2-delta ligands				
Gabapentin	5-7	100	300-600	1200
Gabapentin Enacarbil	6-7	300	600-1200	1200
Pregabalin	6	25-50	75-300	450

Several double-blind controlled studies have shown that both ergoline (cabergoline, pergolide) and non-ergoline (ropinirole, pramipexole and rotigotine) dopamine agonists are able to control RLS symptomatology. However, retroperitoneal, pericardial and pleuropulmonary fibrosis are well known but rare complications of the treatment with ergolinic dopamine agonists. Some studies showed that pergolide and cabergoline have a similar risk of inducing valvular heart disease and cardiac-valve regurgitation [121-122].

In the last years the non-ergoline derivatives agonists have been extensively studied for the RLS treatment. Montplaisir and collegues[123] in a cross-over placebo-controlled study found that pramipexole was very effective in treating RLS and in suppressing PLMS. Other double-blind placebo-controlled studies confirmed the efficacy of pramipexole (median dose 0.35 mg/day) [124,125]. Some long-term follow-up studies of patients treated with pramipexole showed a sustained efficacy of the drug in more than 80% of RLS patients [116]. Augmentation with pramipexole was reported in open trials in 8.5 to 39% of patients [126].

Some randomized, placebo-controlled trials have shown that ropinirole is also effective to treat RLS[117]. In a flexible dose-titration polysomnographic trial, a mean dose of 1.8 mg ropinirole significantly reduced PLMS and improved sleep parameters [127]. A long-term open-label study showed that ropinirole (mean dose 1.90 mg/day) maintained the therapeutic efficacy in 82% of RLS patients [128].

Augmentation with ropinirole has been reported in 1.5% to 3% of patients [126].

In the absence of comparative trials of pramipexole versus ropinirole, a meta-analysis compared the efficacy and tolerability of the two dopamine agonists [129]. The direct meta-analysis confirmed superior efficacy for both treatments versus placebo in reducing RLS. Placebo comparisons showed a significantly higher incidence of nausea for pramipexole, whereas nausea, vomiting, dizziness and somnolence were significantly higher for ropinirole. The indirect comparison showed with a probability of >95%, a superior reduction in the mean IRLS score and significantly lower incidence of nausea, vomiting, and dizziness for pramipexole compared to ropinirole.

A first-night effect of pramipexole and ropinirole has been observed in RLS patients. A low dose of both drugs determines a significant effect on symptoms subjectively reported, as well as a significant improvement in PLMS [130-132].

Rotigotine is a new non-ergot agonist of D3, D2 and D1 dopamine receptors, with an almost 15-fold higher affinity for the D_2 receptor than for the D_1 receptor. In some placebo-controlled trials, transdermal rotigotine demonstrated significant improvement in RLS severity [133-135]. Transdermal 24-hour delivery of low-dose rotigotine (patch with 1 to 3 mg) may relieve the night-time and day-time symptoms of RLS: the efficacy and safety of long-term rotigotine treatment were also shown in 5-year extension study [136].

Concerning augmentation, the 5-year open-label extension study with rotigotine reported a clinically significant augmentation in 13% of patients: 5% were receiving a dose of rotigotine within the range approved by the European Medicines Agency (EMA; 1-3 mg/24 h) and 8% were receiving 4 mg/24 h rotigotine [137].

A low rate of typical dopaminergic side-effects have been observed in patients who receive rotigotine. Skin reactions, mostly mild or moderate, are frequently seen however in the application site of patch: the frequency increases with increasing rotigotine dose and can be minimized when changing the application site continuously [135].

Sleepiness associated with sudden onset of sleep was reported in patients with Parkinson's disease (PD) treated with dopamine agonists. In RLS patients, sleepiness might be seen during treatment with these medications but is much less problematic[116]; moreover, these compounds in RLS may, in contrast to PD, reduce the risk of sudden onset of sleep, probably for their beneficial effect on sleep [138].

Striatal and limbic dysregulation have been suggested in PD as putative factors in compulsive behaviors arising from dopamine agonists [139]. Recently, behavioral complications, such as pathological gambling and punding, have been reported also in some RLS cases under dopaminergic treatment [140-141]. Higher medication dose, young age of RLS onset, history of experimental drug use, female gender and a family history of gambling disorders have been reported as predisposing factors for developing impulse control behaviours in RLS with dopaminergic treatment [142].

Several open-label and controlled clinical trials evaluated the therapeutical effect of non-dopaminergic medications in RLS.

Opioids have long been known to successfully treat RLS [143]. Oxycodone administered at a mean daily dose of 11.4 mg both improved subjective ratings and decreased PLMS in 11 RLS patients, with evidence for decreased arousals and improve sleep efficiency [144]. A persistent effect of opioids was more recently reported in long-term follow-up studies [145-146]. Opioids may be prescribed to severe cases, especially to those unresponsive to other treatments [147]. It has been recently reported a case of successful long-term treatment of a patient with severe RLS using intrathecal morphine at dosages lower than those used in the treatment of chronic pain [148].

In the recently published European guidelines on management of RLS [149], the only non-dopaminergic medications that have been established as effective, according to adequately powered prospective, randomized, controlled, double-blind clinical trials in a representative population are calcium channel alpha-2-delta ligands. Rotigotine, ropinirole, pramipexole, gabapentin enacarbil, gabapentin and pregabalin are all considered effective for the short-term treatment for RLS. For the long-term treatment for RLS, rotigotine is considered effective, gabapentin enacarbil is probably effective, and ropinirole, pramipexole and gabapentin are considered possibly effective. Gabapentin enacarbil is currently the only one calcium channel alpha-2-delta ligand approved by the FDA for treatment of moderate to severe RLS.

Calcium channel alpha-2-delta ligands have been evaluated in several randomized, double-blind, placebo-controlled studies: they were effective in reducing RLS symptoms, and improving disease-specific quality of life [150].

A subjective improvement of RLS with gabapentin at doses of 300 to 2400mg a day has been reported in some open label trials and one placebo–controlled study [151].

A 14-day trial reported with gabapentin enacarbil a significant improvement in IRLS score and in CGI-I investigator and patient scores [152]: an improvement was also seen in wake after sleep onset and the number of awakenings, and there was an increase in sleep stages 3 and 4, and a decrease in stage 1 non-REM. A polysomnography crossover study found a dose of 1200 mg/day to significantly reduce the PLMS-arousals at week 4 compared with placebo [153].

One study finds gabapentin enacarbil to be efficacious at doses of 600 and 1200 mg/day [154]. In this study, gabapentin enacarbil 600 and 1200 mg/day significantly improved IRLS total scores at week 12 compared with placebo. The most commonly reported adverse events were somnolence (600 mg = 21.7%; 1200 mg = 18.0%; placebo = 2.1%) and dizziness (600 mg/day = 10.4%; 1200 mg/day = 24.3%; placebo = 5.2%). In all studies, the most common reported adverse events were somnolence and dizziness.

No specific data on augmentation have been provided for gabapentin enacarbil, although some authors did not find early markers of augmentation (e.g. an earlier onset of symptoms in the afternoon) [155].

In a 12-week study, pregabalin 150–450 mg/day (mean dose 337.50 mg/day) was found to significantly improve IRLS total score, CGI, sleep adequacy and sleep quantity [156]. In addition, there was an improvement in PLM index, and increased sleep stages 1 and 2 and slow-wave sleep. A 6-week study found that pregabalin (at least 150 mg/day) significantly reduced IRLS scores [157].

Other anticonvulsants, as carbamazepina and valproic acid, have been evaluated in RLS but seem to be less effective than calcium channel alpha-2-delta ligands.

Whilst there is evidence that patients with low ferritin plasma levels (<45 µg/l) benefit most from iron supplementation [149] it remains controversial whether patients with normal ferritin levels benefit to the same degree [158].

Finally, some aspects should be considered. All studies administered therapies daily rather than "as needed." Although the effectiveness, harms, and adherence to as-needed therapy are unknown, current recommendations note this as an option [159]. Evidence is lacking about the long-term effectiveness in, and applicability to, subjects with less-severe or less-frequent RLS symptoms. Trial results may lack broad generalizability. Exclusion criteria were many. Recruited subjects had greater disease severity, frequency, and duration than reported by the estimated 1.5% of individuals described as "RLS sufferers" [160].

Clinicians and patients should be aware of the large placebo response in clinical trials. Long-term observational studies reporting withdrawals due to loss of efficacy or adverse effects also suggest that pharmacologic treatment benefits are not sustained over time for many patients with RLS and that these treatments result in adverse effects leading to discontinuation[161]. Withdrawal from mostly dopamine agonist and levodopa treatment was common, occurring in 13% to 57% of subjects owing to either lack of efficacy or adverse effects. Long-term augmentation ranged from 2.5% to 60% and varied markedly by type of dopamine agonist, follow-up time, study design, and method used to ascertain augmentation. Little data exist on long-term adherence and adverse effects for alpha-2-delta ligands [150].

For individuals unable to initiate or tolerate dopamine agonist or alpha-2-delta ligands, or for whom these drugs have failed, recommended pharmacologic treatments include off-label opioids or sedative hypnotics. Unfortunately, there are no eligible studies evaluating these agents.

Periodic Limb Movement Disorder

PLMS represent a habitual motor accompaniment of RLS, found in over 80% of the cases on polysomnography. The recent finding that genes associated with RLS are highly associated with PLMS also indicates the close relationship between the two. PLMS, however, may also occur in normal individuals as a quasi-physiological age-related phenomenon, and associated to several other medical/neurological conditions. Therefore, their pathological relevance is still discussed [162-164]. PLMS are usually considered pathological only when they induce arousals and sleep fragmentation. The ICSD-2[165] allows a diagnosis of PLMD only when PLMS occur associated with a clinical sleep disturbance or a complaint of daytime fatigue. The decision to treat PLMD should consequently be based on the presence of clinical signs of disturbed sleep or its daytime consequences, and on polysomnographic evidence of a relevant PLMS index.

Most of the therapeutic trials in PLMD using medication have considered PLMS associated with RLS. Therefore, the best evidence comes from trials performed in primary RLS patients undergoing polysomnographic recordings. Very few trials have, however, been conduced specifically in PLMD. Dopaminergic agents come again as the drugs that have the best proofs of efficacy for suppressing PLMS, often at low dosages and after only a few days of use. Levodopa (mean dose 159/40 mg) in primary RLS reduced PLMS index by 27.8 events, and also reduced PLMS (at 200 mg/bedtime or 100 mg 5 times/day) in PLMD not associated to RLS or associated to narcolepsy or complete spinal lesions. Bromocriptine 7.5

mg and pergolide at dosages from 0.05 upwards to 1.5 mg also significantly decreased PLMS in primary RLS patients: pergolide caused a 79% reduction in PLMS index compared to 45% with levodopa [166]. Efficacy in reducing PLMS index in RLS patients was shown also with ropinirole (a mean dose 1.8 mg/day significantly improved PLMS index by 76.2% versus 14% on placebo) [127] and with pramipexole (significant reductions in PLMS index even at the initial dose of 0.125 mg, maximal effect at 0.5 mg) [167].

Recently, a prospective, placebo-controlled, single-blind, parallel group study was carried out in 46 drug-naive RLS patients [168]. Each patient underwent 2 consecutive full-night polysomnographic studies. The first night was the baseline night. Prior to the second night, 1 group received a single oral dose of 0.25 mg pramipexole, whereas a second group received a single oral dose of 0.5 mg clonazepam, and the remaining patients received placebo.

Pramipexole suppressed PLMS without affecting EEG instability (arousals), whereas clonazepam did the opposite, reducing EEG instability without effects on PLMS. This study demonstrates that a selective pharmacological approach can disconnect PLMS from arousal events, suggesting an indirect relation between each other. These results might weaken the hypothesis of a direct pathological role of PLMS in sleep disruption.

As concerns the other drugs used for treating RLS, oxycodone significantly reduced PLMS index by 34% in primary RLS [169], while short-term propoxyphene (at 100–200 mg before bedtime) reduced the number of arousals associated with the PLMS in PLMD, but not the PLMS index itself. Concerning benzodiazepines, triazolam 0.125 to 0.50 mg was ineffective while temazepam 30 mg and nitrazepam 2.5 to 10 mg were effective in reducing the PLMS index. Neither clonidine 0.5 mg nor valproate slow release 600 mg reduced PLMS index or the arousals associated with the PLMS, while gabapentin 1800 mg daily curtailed the PLMS index by 9.8 events. In a double-blind study, baclofen 20 to 40 mg suppressed the amplitude but not the total number of PLMS. Finally, in PLMD transdermal estradiol 2.5 g/day gel was ineffective either on PLMS index or on the number of the associated arousals [170].

The conclusive evidence for the PLMS is similar to that available for RLS, dopaminergic drugs appearing as the therapeutic agents best efficacious in reducing the PLMS. Remarkably, the dosages effective for PLMS are lower than those effective for RLS, and often act more quickly.

Sleep-Related Bruxism

Bruxism may be idiopathic but can also be precipitated by drugs. Instances are known when bruxism developed with the use of psychoactive medications, in particular neuroleptic drugs [171-172] and antidepressants, particularly selective serotonin reuptake inhibitors (SSRIs) [173] or recreational drugs [174]. However, use of SSRIs, neuroleptics, and other anti-dopaminergic medications trigger tooth grinding particularly while awake, and no tooth grinding during sleep has been reported with such medications [174]. Caffeine and tobacco smoking have been considered as triggering factors of sleep-related bruxism [175].

No intervention, pharmacological or not, has been demonstrated to definitively curtail sleep-related bruxism. Moreover, there are no controlled trials of medications for sleep-related bruxism, and most of the studies are open-label trials or case reports. Medications used for the treatment of sleep-related bruxism include dopaminergics such as bromocriptine and levodopa, on the basis of the rationale of abnormal striatal D2 receptor binding found upon brain single-photon emission computed tomography (SPECT) in patients with bruxism [176]. However, bromocriptine was ineffective when studied in controlled trials [177], while a controlled study revealed that levodopa reduced sleep bruxism motor activity by about 30% [178]. A controlled trial showed that amitryptiline was ineffective over a time period of four weeks [179]. Beneficial effects have been reported in selected cases with propranolol [180] and, in patients with iatrogenic bruxism related to SSRI or neuroleptic medications, buspirone [181], gabapentin [182], and propranolol [172] administration has been reported as effective. For short-term use, benzodiazepines such as diazepam [5 mg before bedtime or clonazepam 1 mg at bedtime [183] and muscle relaxants may be beneficial, but long-term use of benzodiazepines appears not to be warranted [184]. In an acute sleep laboratory study comparing clonidine and propranolol, clonidine was effective, but at a dose of 0.3 mg caused morning hypotension [185]. Propranolol did not decrease bruxism. Another more recent study showed the efficacy of clonidine compared to placebo in reducing sleep bruxism [186].

Finally, patients with severe sleep-related bruxism, primary or secondary to brain injury, may gain some benefit from botulinum toxin administration to the jaw muscles [187,188]. A recent evidence-based review on this topic [189] concluded that botulinum toxin injections at a dosage of <100 U are effective on bruxism and are safe to use.

References

[1]	Schutte-Rodin S, Broch L, Buysse D, et al. Clinical guideline for the evaluation and management of chronic insomnia in adults. *J Clin Sleep Med.* 2008;4(5):487-504.

[2]	Vincent N, Lionberg C. Treatment preference and patient satisfaction in chronic insomnia. *Sleep.* 2001;24(4):411-417.

[3]	Morin CM, LeBlanc M, Bélanger L, et al. Prevalence of insomnia and its treatment in Canada. *Can J Psychiatry.* 2011;56(9):540-548.

[4]	Mitchell MD, Gehrman P, Perlis M, et al. Comparative effectiveness of cognitive behavioral therapy for insomnia: a systematic review. *BMC Fam Pract.* 2012 May 25;13:40.

[5]	Hajak G, Müller WE, Wittchen HU, et al. Abuse and dependence potential for the non-benzodiazepine hypnotics zolpidem and zopiclone: a review of case reports and epidemiological data. *Addiction.* 2003 Oct;98(10):1371-8.

[6]	Finkle WD, Der JS, Greenland S, et al. Risk of fractures requiring hospitalization after an initial prescription for zolpidem, alprazolam, lorazepam, or diazepam in older adults. *J Am Geriatr Soc.* 2011 Oct;59(10):1883-90.

[7]	Greenblatt DJ, Roth T. Zolpidem for insomnia. *Expert Opin Pharmacother.* 2012 Apr; 13(6):879-93.

[8]	Walsh JK. Drugs used to treat insomnia in 2002: regulatory-based rather than evidence-based medicine. *Sleep* 2004;27:1441–1442.

[9]	Nowell PD, Mazumdar S, Buysse DJ, et al. Benzodiazepines and zolpidem for chronic insomnia: a meta-analysis of treatment efficacy. *JAMA* 1997;278:2170–2177.

[10]	Holbrook AM, Crowther R, Lotter A, et al. Meta-anlysis of benzodiazepine use in the treatment of insomnia. *Can Med Assoc J* 2000;162:225–233.

[11] Roth T, Roehrs T. Issues in the use of benzodiazepine therapy. *J Clin Psychiatry* 1992;53:S14–S18.

[12] Mendelson WB, Thompson C, Franko T. Adverse reactions to sedative/hypnotics: three years' experience. *Sleep* 1996;9:702–706.

[13] Ensrud KE, Blackwell T, Mangione CM, et al. Central nervous system active medications and risk for fractures in older women. *Arch Intern Med* 2003;163:949–957.

[14] Brassington GS, King AC, Bliwise DL. Sleep problems as a risk factor for falls in a sample of community-dwelling adults aged 64-99 years. *J Am Ger Soc* 2000;48:1234–1240.

[15] Avidan AY, Fries BE, James ML, et al. Insomnia and hypnotic use recorded in the minimum data set as predictors of fall and hip fractures in Michigan nursing homes. *J Am Ger Soc* 2005;53:955–962.

[16] Roehrs T, Roth T. Insomnia pharmacotherapy. *Neurotherapeutics.* 2012 Oct;9(4):728-38.

[17] Guillmineau C, Dement WC. Amnesia and disorders of excessive sleepiness. In: Drucker-Colin RR, McGaugh JL, eds. *Neurobiology of sleep and memory.* London: Academic Press, 1977.

[18] Buysse DJ. Insomnia. *JAMA.* 2013 Feb 20;309(7):706-16.

[19] Licata SC, Rowlett JK. Abuse and dependence liability of benzodiazepine-type drugs: GABA(A) receptor modulation and beyond. *Pharmacol Biochem Behav.* 2008; 90(1):74-89.

[20] Fava M, Schaefer K, Huang H, et al. A post hoc analysis of the effect of nightly administration of eszopiclone and a selective serotonin reuptake inhibitor in patients with insomnia and anxious depression. *J Clin Psychiat* 2011;72:473–479.

[21] Pollack M, Kinrys G, Krystal A, et al. Eszopiclone co-administered with escitalopram in patients with insomnia and comorbid generalized anxiety disorder. *Arch Gen Psychiat* 2009;65:551–562.

[22] Drover DR. Comparative pharmacokinetics and pharmacodynamics of short-acting hypnosedatives. *Clin Pharmacokinet* 2004; 43:227–238.

[23] Krystal AD, Walsh JK, Laska E, et al. Sustained efficacy of eszopiclone over 6 months of nightly treatment: results of a randomized, double-blind, placebo-controlled study in adults with chronic insomnia. *Sleep* 2003; 26:793–799.

[24] Lisko B, Pikalov A. Zaleplon overdose associated with sleepwalking and complex behavior. *J Am Acad Child Adolesc Psychiatry* 2004;43:927–928.

[25] Morgenthaler TI, Silber MH. Amnestic sleep-related eating disorder associated with zolpidem. *Sleep Med* 2002;3:323–327.

[26] Yang W, Dollear M, Muthukrishnan SR. One rare side effect of zolpidem – sleepwalking: a case report. *Arch Phys Med Rehabil* 2005;86:1265–1266.

[27] Roehrs TA, Roth T. Safety of insomnia pharmacotherapy. *Sleep Med Clinics* 2006;1:399–407.

[28] Walsh JK, Krystal AD, Amato DA, et al. Nightly treatment of primary insomnia with eszopiclone for six months: effects on sleep, quality of life, and work limitations. *Sleep* 2007;30:959–968.

[29] Randall S, Roehrs T, Roth T. Efficacy of eight months of nightly zolpidem: a prospective placebo controlled study. *Sleep* 2012 Nov 1;35(11):1551-7.

[30] Richelson E. The pharmacology of antidepressants at the synapse: focus on newer compounds. *J Clin Psychiatry* 1994;55(suppl A):34–39.

[31] Montgomery I, Oswald I, Morgan K, et al. Trazodone enhances sleep in subjective quality but not in objective duration. *Br J Clin Pharmacol* 1983;16:139–144.

[32] Walsh JK, Erman M, Erwin CW, et al. Subjective hypnotic efficacy of trazodone and zolpidem in DSM-III-R primary insomnia. *Hum Psychopharmacol* 1998:13:191–198.

[33] Roth AJ, McCall WV, Liguori A. Cognitive, psychomotor and polysomnographic effects of trazodone in primary insomniacs. *J Sleep Res.* 2011 Dec;20(4):552-8.

[34] Camargos E, Pandolfi M, Freitas M, et al. Trazodone for the treatment of sleep disorders in dementia: an open-label, observational and review study. *Arq Neuropsiquiatr.* 2011;69:44–9.

[35] Golden RN, Dawkins K, Nicholas L. Trazadone and nefazodone. In: Schatzberg A, Nemeroff C, eds. *The American Psychiatric Textbook Of Psychopharmacology.* Washington, DC: American Psychiatric Textbook, Inc., 2004:315–325.

[36] Kupfer DJ, Spiker DG, Coble P, et al. Amitriptyline and EEG sleep in depressed patients: I. *Drug effect Sleep.* 1978;1:149–59.

[37] Doerr J, Spiegelhalder K, Petzold F, et al. Impact of escitalopram on nocturnal sleep, day-time sleepiness, and performance compared to amitriptyline: a randomized, double-blind, placebo-controlled study in healthy male subjects. *Pharmacopsychiatry.* 2010;43:166–73.

[38] Ruigt GSF, Kemp B, Groenhout CM, et al. Effect of the antidepressant Org 3770 on human sleep. *Eur J Clin Pharmacol.* 1990;38:551–4.

[39] Aslan S, Isik E, Cosar B. The effects of mirtazapine on sleep: a placebo controlled, double-blind study in young healthy volunteers. *Sleep.* 2002;25:677–9.

[40] McCall C, McCall WV. What Is the Role of Sedating Antidepressants, Antipsychotics, and Anticonvulsants in the Management of Insomnia? Curr Psychiatry Rep. 2012 Oct;14(5):494-502.

[41] Shen J, Hossain N, Streiner D, et al. Excessive daytime sleepiness and fatigue in depressed patients and therapeutic response of a sedating antidepressant. *J Affect Disord.* 2011;134:421–6.

[42] Perez D, Loprinzi D, Barton DL. Pilot evaluation of mirtazapine for the treatment of hot flashes. *J Support Oncol.* 2004;2:50–6.

[43] Wingen M, Bothmer J, Langer S, et al. Actual driving performance and psychomotor function in healthy subjects after acute and subchronic treatment with escitalopram, mirtazapine, and placebo: a crossover trial. *J Clin Psychiatry.* 2005;66:436–43.

[44] Hoque R, Chesson AL Jr. Pharmacologically induced/exacerbated restless legs syndrome, periodic limb movements of sleep, and REM behavior disorder/REM sleep without atonia: literature review, qualitative scoring, and comparative analysis. *J Clin Sleep Med.* 2010 Feb 15;6(1):79-83.

[45] Dolder C, McKinsey J. Quetiapine for sleep in patients with dementia. *Consult Pharm.* 2010;25:676–9.

[46] Golubchik P, Sever J, Weizman A. A low-dose quetiapine for adolescents with autistic spectrum disorder and aggressive behavior: open-label trial. *Clin Neuropharmacol.* 2011;34:216–9.

[47] Wiegard M, Landry T, Bruckner T, et al. Quetiapine in primary insomnia: a pilot study. *Psychopharmacology* 2008;196:337–338.

[48] Juni C, Chana P, Tapia J, et al. Quetiapine for insomnia in Parkinson Disease: results from an open-label trial. *Clin Neuropharmacol* 2005;28:185–187.

[49] Estivill E, de la Fuente V, Segarra F, et al. The use of olanzapine in sleep disorders. An open trial with nine patients. *Rev Neurol* 2004;38:829–831.

[50] Cates ME, Jackson CW, Feldman JM, et al. Metabolic consequences of using low-dose quetiapine for insomnia in psychiatric patients. *Community Ment Health J* 2009;45:251–254.

[51] Tassniyom K, Paholpak S, Tassniyom S, et al. Quetiapine for primary insomnia: a double blind, randomized controlled trial. *J Med Assoc Thai.* 2010;93:729–34.

[52] Lemoine P, Zisapel N. Prolonged-release formulation of melatonin (Circadin) for the treatment of insomnia. *Expert Opin Pharmacother.* 2012 Apr;13(6):895-905.

[53] Wilson SJ, Nutt DJ, Alford C et al. British Association for Psychopharmacology consensus statement on evidence-based treatment of insomnia, parasomnias and circadian rhythm disorders. *J Psychopharmacol* 2010; 24:1577–1601.

[54] Cardinali DP, Srinivasan V, Brzezinski A, et al. Melatonin and its analogs in insomnia and depression. *J Pineal Res.* 2012 May;52(4):365-75.

[55] Hardeland R, Cardinali DP, Srinivasan V, et al. Melatonin-a pleiotropic, orchestrating regulator molecule. *Prog Neurobiol* 2011; 93:350–384.

[56] Morin CM, Hauri PJ, Espie CA, et al. Nonpharmacologic treatment of chronic insomnia. An American Academy of Sleep Medicine review. *Sleep* 1999; 22:1134–1156.

[57] Kato K, Hirai K, Nichiyama K, et al. Neurochemical properties of ramelteon [TAK-375], a selective MT1 and MT2 receptor agonist. *Neuropharmacology* 2005;48:301–310.

[58] Zammit G, Erman M, Wang-Weigand S, et al. Evaluation of the efficacy and safety of ramelteon in subjects with chronic insomnia. *J Clin Sleep Med* 2007;3:495–504.

[59] Mayer G, Wang-Weigand S, Roth-Schechter B, et al. Efficacy and safety of 6-month nightly ramelteon administration in adults with chronic primary insomnia. *Sleep* 2009;32:351–360.

[60] DeMicco M, Wang-Weigand S, Zhang J. Long-term therapeutic effects of ramelteon treatment in adults with chronic insomnia: a 1 year study. *Sleep* 2006;29(suppl):A234.

[61] Buysse DJ. Clinical pharmacology of other drugs used as hypnotics. In: Kryger MH, Roth T, Dement WC, eds. *Principles and Practices of Sleep Medicine. 5th ed.* St Louis, MO: Elsevier; 2011:492-509.

[62] Krystal AD. Pharmacologic treatment: other medications. In: Kryger MH, Roth T, Dement WC, eds. *Principles and Practices of Sleep Medicine. 5th ed.* St Louis, MO: Elsevier; 2011:916-930.

[63] Millan MJ. Multi-target strategies for the improved treatment of depressive states: conceptual foundations and neuronal substrates, drug discovery and therapeutic application. *Pharmacol Ther* 2006; 110:135–370.

[64] Quera Salva MA, Vanier B, Laredo J, et al. Major depressive disorder, sleep EEG and agomelatine: an open-label study. *Int J Neuropsychopharmacol* 2007; 10:691–696.

[65] Zupancic M, Guilleminault C. Agomelatine: a preliminary review of a new antidepressant. *CNS Drugs* 2006; 20:981–992.

[66] Kasper S, Hajak G, Wulff K, et al. Efficacy of the novel antidepressant agomelatine on the circadian rest-activity cycle and depressive and anxiety symptoms in patients with

major depressive disorder: a randomized, double-blind comparison with sertraline. *J Clin Psychiatry* 2010; 71:109–120.

[67] Carney RM, Shelton RC. Agomelatine for the treatment of major depressive disorder. *Expert Opin Pharmacother*. 2011;12(15):2411-9.

[68] Roth T, Rogowski R, Hull S, et al. Efficacy and safety of doxepin 1 mg, 3 mg, and 6 mg in adults with primary insomnia. *Sleep*. 2007;30:1555–61.

[69] Weber J, Siddiqui M, Wagstaff A. Low-dose doxepin: in the treatment of insomnia. *CNS Drugs*. 2010;24:713–20.

[70] Herring WJ, Snyder E, Budd K, et al. Orexin receptor antagonism for treatment of insomnia: a randomized clinical trial of suvorexant. *Neurology*. 2012 Dec 4;79(23):2265-74.

[71] Sun H, Kennedy WP, Wilbraham D, et al. Effects of suvorexant, an orexin receptor antagonist, on sleep parameters as measured by polysomnography in healthy men. *Sleep*. 2013 Feb 1;36(2):259-67.

[72] American Psychiatric Association. DSM-5 Development. In: DSM-5: The Future of Psychiatric Diagnosis. Available at: *http://www.dsm5.org/*.

[73] Didato G, Nobili L. Treatment of narcolepsy. *Expert Rev Neurother* 2009; 9 (6): 897–910.

[74] Robertson SD, Matthies HJ, Galli A. A closer look at amphetamine-induced reverse transport and trafficking of the dopamine and norepinephrine transporters. *Mol Neurobiol* 2009;39:73–80.

[75] Kanbayashi T, Honda K, Kodama T, Mignot E, Nishino S. Implication of dopaminergic mechanisms in the wake-promoting effects of amphetamine: a study of D- and L-derivatives in canine narcolepsy. *Neuroscience* 2000;99:651-659.

[76] Mitler MM, Hayduk R . Benefits and risks of pharmacotherapy for narcolepsy. *Drug Saf* 2002; 25:791–809.

[77] Guilleminault C. Amphetamines and narcolepsy: use of the Stanford database. *Sleep* 1993;16:199–201.

[78] Bogle KE, Smith BH. Illicit methylphenidate use: a review of prevalence, availability, pharmacology, and consequences. *Curr Drug Abuse Rev* 2009;2:157–176.

[79] Thorpy M. Therapeutic advances in narcolepsy. Sleep Med. 2007 Jun;8(4):427-40.

[80] Volkow ND, Fowler JS, Logan J, et al. Effects of modafinil on dopamine and dopamine transporters in the male human brain: clinical implications. *JAMA* 2009;301:1148–1154.

[81] Spencer TJ, Madras BK, Bonab AA, et al. A positron emission tomography study examining the dopaminergic activity of armodafinil in adults using [(1)(1)C]altropane and [(1)(1)C]raclopride. *Biological psychiatry* 2010;68:964–97.

[82] Mignot EM. A Practical Guide to the Therapy of Narcolepsy and Hypersomnia Syndromes. *Neurotherapeutics* 2012 Oct;9(4):739-52.

[83] Schwartz JR, Feldman NT, Bogan RK. Dose effects of modafinil in sustaining wakefulness in narcolepsy patients with residual evening sleepiness *J Neuropsychiatry Clin Neurosci* 2005; 17 (3): 405–412.

[84] Harsh JR, Hayduk R, Rosenberg R, et al. The efficacy and safety of armodafinil as treatment for adults with excessive sleepiness associated with narcolepsy *Curr Med Res Opin* 2006; 22(4): 761–774.

[85] Dinges DF, Arora S, Darwish M, et al. Pharmacodynamic effects on alertness of single doses of armodafanil in healthy subjects during a nocturnal period of acute sleep loss *Curr Med Res Opin* 2006; 22(1): 159–167.

[86] Broughton R, Mamelak M. The treatment of narcolepsy-cataplexy with nocturnal gamma-hydroxybutyrate. *Can J Neurol Sci* 1979;6:1–6.

[87] Xyrem MSG. A randomized, double blind, placebo-controlled multicenter trial comparing the effects of three doses of orally administered sodium oxybate with placebo for the treatment of narcolepsy. *Sleep* 2002;25:42–49.

[88] Wedin GP, Hornfeldt CS, Ylitalo LM. The clinical development of γ-hydroxybutyrate (GHB) *Curr Drug Saf* 2006; 1: 99–106.

[89] Husain AM, Ristanovic RK, Bogan RK. Weight loss in narcolepsy patients treated with sodium oxybate. *Sleep Med* 2009;10:661–663.

[90] Wallace DM, Maze T, Shafazand S. Sodium oxybate-induced sleep driving and sleep-related eating disorder. *J Clin Sleep Med* 2011;7:310–311.

[91] Chen SY, Clift SJ, Dahlitz MJ, et al. Treatment in the narcoleptic syndrome: self assessment of the action of dexamphetamine and clomipramine *J Sleep Res* 1995; 4: 113–118.

[92] Martinez-Rodriguez J, Iranzo A, Santamaria J, et al. Status cataplecticus induced by abrupt withdrawal of clomipramine. *Neurologia* 2002; 17: 113–116.

[93] Wise MS, Arand DL, Auger RR, Brooks SN, Watson NF; American Academy of Sleep Medicine. Treatment of narcolepsy and other hypersomnias of central origin. *Sleep.* 2007 Dec;30(12):1712-27.

[94] Lopez R, Dauvilliers Y. Pharmacotherapy options for cataplexy. *Expert Opin Pharmacother.* 2013 Mar 25. [Epub ahead of print].

[95] Thorpy MJ, Snyder M, Aloe FS, et al. Short-term triazolam use improves nocturnal sleep of narcoleptics. *Sleep* 1992; 15(3): 212–216.

[96] Arnulf I, Lin L, Gadoth N, et al. Kleine-Levin syndrome: a systematic study of 108 patients. *Ann Neurol* 2008;63:482–493.

[97] Arnulf I, Rico T, Mignot E. Diagnosis, disease course, and management of patients with Kleine-Levin syndrome. *Lancet Neurol* 2012;11:918–928.

[98] Han F, Lin L, Warby SC, et al. Narcolepsy onset is seasonal and increased following the 2009 H1N1 pandemic in China. *Ann Neurol* 2011;70:410–417.

[99] Knudsen S, Mikkelsen JD, Bang B, et al. Intravenous immunoglobulin treatment and screening for hypocretin neuron-specific autoantibodies in recent onset childhood narcolepsy with cataplexy. *Neuropediatrics* 2010;41:217–222.

[100] Hallmayer J, Faraco J, Lin L, et al. Narcolepsy is strongly associated with the T-cell receptor alpha locus. *Nat Genet* 2009;41:708–711.

[101] Mieda M, Willie JT, Hara J, et al. Orexin peptides prevent cataplexy and improve wakefulness in an orexin neuron-ablated model of narcolepsy in mice. *Proc Natl Acad Sci U S A* 2004;101:4649–4654.

[102] Hoever P, de Haas SL, Dorffner G, et al. Orexin receptor antagonism: an ascending multiple-dose study with almorexant. *J Psychopharmacol* 2012;26:1071–1080.

[103] Mitler MM, O'Malley MB. Wake-promoting medications: efficacy and adverse effects. In: Kryger MH, Roth T, Dement WC, eds. *Principles and Practice of Sleep Medicine. 4th ed.* Philadelphia: Elsevier Saunders, 2005:484–498.

[104] Shiba T, Fujiki N, Wisor JP, et al. Wake promoting effects of thioperamide, a histamine H3 antagonist in orexin/ataxin-3 narcoleptic mice. *Sleep* 2004; 27(suppl):A241.

[105] Inocente C, Arnulf I, Bastuji H, et al. Pitolisant, an inverse agonist of the histamine H3 receptor: an alternative stimulant for narcolepsy-cataplexy in teenagers with refractory sleepiness. *Clin Neuropharmacol* 2012;35:55–60.

[106] Akpinar S. Treatment of restless legs syndrome with levodopa plus benserazide. *Arch Neurol* 1982;39:739.

[107] Ekbom KA. Restless legs. *Acta Med Scand Suppl* 1945; 158:5–123.

[108] O'Keeffe ST, Gavin K, Lavan JN. Iron status and restless legs syndrome in the elderly. *Age Ageing* 1994; 23:200–203.

[109] Connnor JR, Wang XS, Patton SM, et al. Decreased transferring receptor express by neuromelanin cells in restless legs syndrome. *Neurology* 2004; 62:1563–1567.

[110] Allen RP, Auerbach S, Bahrain H, et al. The prevalence and impact of restless legs syndrome on patients with iron deficiency anemia. *Am J Hematol.* 2013 Apr;88(4):261-4.

[111] Salas RE, Gamaldo CE, Allen RP. Update in restless legs syndrome. *Curr Opin Neurol.* 2010 Aug;23(4):401-6.

[112] Aukerman MM, Aukerman D, Bayard M, et al. Exercise and restless legs syndrome: a randomized controlled trial. *J Am Board Fam Med* 2006; 19: 487-93.

[113] Giannaki CD, Sakkas GK, Hadjigeorgiou GM, et al. Non-pharmacological management of periodic limb movements during hemodialysis session in patients with uremic restless legs syndrome. *ASAIO J.* 2010 Nov-Dec;56(6):538-42.

[114] Hornyak M, Grossmann C, Kohnen R, et al. Cognitive behavioral group therapy to improve patients' strategies for coping with restless legs syndrome: a proof-of-concept trial. *J Neurol Neurosurg Psychiatry* 2008; 79:823-25.

[115] Trenkwalder C, Hogl B, Winkelmann J. Recent advances in the diagnosis, genetics and treatment of restless legs syndrome. *J Neurol* 2009; 256: 539-53.

[116] Ferini-Strambi L. Treatment options for restless legs syndrome. *Expert Opin Pharmacother.* 2009 Mar;10(4):545-54.

[117] Trenkwalder C, Hening WA, Montagna P, et al. Treatment of restless legs syndrome: An evidence-based review and implications for clinical practice. Mov Disord 2008; 23: 2267-2302.

[118] Garcia-Borreguero D, Allen RP, Kohnen R, et al. Diagnostic standards for dopaminergic augmentation of restless legs syndrome: report from World Association of Sleep Medicine-International Restless Legs Syndrome Study Group consensus conference at the Max Planck Institute. *Sleep Med* 2007; 8:520-530.

[119] Paulus W, Trenkwalder C. Less is more: pathophysiology of dopaminergic-therapy-related augmentation in restless legs syndrome. *Lancet Neurol* 2006; 5: 878-86.

[120] Högl B, García-Borreguero D, Kohnen R, et al. Progressive development of augmentation during long-term treatment with levodopa in restless legs syndrome: results of a prospective multi-center study. *J Neurol.* 2010 Feb;257(2):230-7.

[121] Zanetti R, Antonini A, Gatto G, et al. Valvular heart disease and the use of dopamine agonists for Parkinson's disease. *N Engl J Med* 2007; 356:39-46.

[122] Schade R, Andersohn F, Suissa S, et al. Dopamine agonists and the risk of cardiac-valve regurgitation. *N Engl J Med* 2007; 356:29-38.

[123] Montplaisir J, Nicolas A, Denesle R, et al. Pramipexole alleviates sensory and motor symptoms of restless legs syndrome. *Neurology* 1998;51:311-312.

[124] Oertel WH, Stiasny-Kolster K, Bergtholdt B, et al. Efficacy of pramipexole in RLS: a six-week, multicenter, randomized, double-blind study. *Mov Disord* 2007; 22: 213-219.

[125] Ferini-Strambi L, Aarskog D, Partinen M, et al. Effect of pramipexole on RLS symptoms and sleep: a randomized, double-blind, placebo-controlled trial. *Sleep Med.* 2008 Dec;9(8):874-81.

[126] Beneš H, García-Borreguero D, Ferini-Strambi L, et al. Augmentation in the treatment of restless legs syndrome with transdermal rotigotine *Sleep Med.* 2012 Jun;13(6):589-97.

[127] Allen R, Becker PM, Bogan R, et al. Ropinirole decreases periodic limb movements and improves sleep parameters in patients with restless legs syndrome. *Sleep* 2004;27:907-14.

[128] Garcia-Borreguero D, Grunstein R, Sridhar G, et al. A 52-week open-label study of the long-term safety of ropinirole in patients with restless legs syndrome. *Sleep Med* 2007; 8: 742-52.

[129] Quilici S, Abrams KR, Nicolas A, et al. Meta-analysis of the efficacy and tolerability of pramipexole versus ropinirole in the treatment of restless legs syndrome. *Sleep Med* 2008; 9:715-26.

[130] Manconi M, Ferri R, Zucconi M, et al. First night efficacy of pramipexole in restless legs syndrome and periodic leg movements. *Sleep Med* 2007; 8:491-97.

[131] Merlino G, Dolso P, Canesin P, et al. The acute effect of a low dosage of pramipexole on severe idiopathic restless legs syndrome: an open-label trial. *Neuropsychobiol* 2006; 54: 195-200.

[132] Saletu B, Gruber G, Saletu M, et al. Sleep laboratory studies in restless legs syndrome patients as compared with normals and acute effects of ropinirole. 1. Findings on objective and subjective sleep and awakening quality. *Neuropsychobiol* 2000; 41: 181-89.

[133] Stiasny-Kolster K, Kohnen R, Schollmayer E, et al. Patch application of the dopamine agonist rotigotine to patients with moderate to advanced stages of restless legs syndrome: a double-blind, placebo-controlled pilot study. *Mov Disord* 2004;19:1432-38.

[134] Oertel WH, Benes H, Garcia-Borreguero D, et al. Efficacy of rotigotine transdermal system in severe restless legs syndrome: a randomized, double-blind, placebo-controlled, six-week dose-finding trial in Europe. *Sleep Med* 2007;9:228-39.

[135] Trenkwalder C, Benes H, Poewe W, et al. Efficacy of rotigotine for treatment of moderate-to-severe restless legs syndrome: a randomised, double-blind, placebo-controlled trial. *Lancet Neurol* 2008;7:595-604.

[136] Dohin E, Högl B, Ferini-Strambi L, et al. Safety and efficacy of rotigotine transdermal patch in patients with restless legs syndrome: a post-hoc analysis of patients taking 1 - 3 mg/24 h for up to 5 years. *Expert Opin Pharmacother.* 2013 Jan;14(1):15-25.

[137] Oertel W, Trenkwalder C, Beneš H, et al, SP710 study group. Long-term safety and efficacy of rotigotine transdermal patch for moderate-to-severe idiopathic restless legs syndrome: a 5-year open-label extension study. *Lancet Neurol.* 2011 Aug;10(8):710-20.

[138] Moller C, Korner Y, Cassel W, et al. Sudden onset of sleep and dopaminergic therapy in patients with restless legs syndrome. *Sleep Med* 2006;7:333-39.

[139] Aarsland D, Alves G, Larsen JP. Disorders of motivation, sexual conduct, and sleep in Parkinson's disease. *Adv Neurol* 2005; 96:56-64.

[140] Evans AH, Stegeman JR. Punding in patients on dopamine agonists for restless leg syndrome. *Mov Disord* 2009; 24: 140-41.

[141] Schreglmann SR, Gantenbein AR, Eisele G, Baumann CR. Transdermal rotigotine causes impulse control disorders in patients with restless legs syndrome. *Parkinsonism Relat Disord.* 2012 Feb;18(2):207-9.

[142] Voon V, Schoerling A, Wenzel S, et al. Frequency of impulse control behaviours associated with dopaminergic therapy in restless legs syndrome. *BMC Neurol.* 2011 Sep 28;11:117.

[143] Oertel WH, Trenkwalder C, Zucconi M, et al. State of the art in restless legs syndrome: practice recommendations for treating restless legs syndrome. *Mov Disord* 2007; 22 (suppl. 18): S466-S475.

[144] Walters AS, Wagner ML, Hening WA, et al. Successful treatment of the idiopathic restless legs syndrome in a randomized double-blind trial of oxycodone versus placebo. *Sleep* 1993;16:327-32.

[145] Walters AS, Winkelmann J, Trenkwalder C, et al. Long-term follow-up on restless legs syndrome patients treated with opioids. *Mov Dis* 2001;6:1105-09.

[146] Ondo WG. Methadone for refractory restless legs syndrome. *Mov Disord* 2005; 20: 345-48.

[147] Nagandla K, De S. Restless legs syndrome: pathophysiology and modern management. *Postgrad Med J.* 2013 Mar 22. [Epub ahead of print].

[148] Hornyak M, Kaube H. Long-Term treatment of a patient with severe restless legs syndrome using intrathecal morphine. *Neurology.* 2012 Dec 11;79(24):2361-2.

[149] Garcia-Borreguero D, Ferini-Strambi L, Kohnen R, et al. European guidelines on management of restless legs syndrome: report of a joint task force by the European Federation of Neurological Societies, the European Neurological Society and the European Sleep Research Society *J Neurol.* 2012 Nov;19(11):1385-96.

[150] Wilt TJ, Macdonald R, Ouellette J, et al. Pharmacologic Therapy for Primary Restless Legs Syndrome: A Systematic Review and Meta-analysis. *JAMA Intern Med.* 2013, 4:1-10.

[151] Garcia-Borreguero D, Larrosa de la Liave Y, Verger K, et al. Treatment of restless legs syndrome with gabapentin. *Neurology* 2002;59:1573-79.

[152] Kushida CA, Walters AS, Becker P, et al. A randomized, double-blind, placebo-controlled, crossover study of XP13512/GSK1838262 in the treatment of patients with primary restless legs syndrome. *Sleep* 2009; 32: 159–168.

[153] Winkelman JW, Bogan RK, Schmidt MH, et al. Randomized polysomnography study of gabapentin enacarbil in subjects with restless legs syndrome. *Mov Disord* 2011; 26: 2065–2072.

[154] Lee DO, Ziman RB, Perkins AT, et al. A randomized, double-blind, placebo-controlled study to assess the efficacy and tolerability of gabapentin enacarbil in subjects with Restless Legs Syndrome. *JCSM* 2011; 7: 282–292.

[155] Ellenbogen AL, Thein SG, Winslow DH, et al. A 52-week study of gabapentin enacarbil in restless legs syndrome. *Clin Neuropharmacol* 2011; 34: 8–16.

[156] Garcia-Borreguero D, Larrosa O, Williams AM, et al. Treatment of restless legs syndrome with pregabalin. A double-blind, placebo-controlled study. *Neurology* 2010; 74: 1897–1904.

[157] Allen R, Chen C, Soaita A, et al. A randomized, double-blind, 6-week, dose-ranging study of pregabalin in patients with restless legs syndrome. *Sleep Med* 2010; 11: 512–519.

[158] Davis BJ, Rajput A, Rajput ML, et al. A randomized, double-blind placebo-controlled trial of iron in restless legs syndrome. *Eur Neurol* 2000; 43: 70–75.

[159] Silber MH, Ehrenberg BL, Allen RP, et al. Medical Advisory Board of the Restless Legs Syndrome Foundation. An algorithm for the management of restless legs syndrome. *Mayo Clin Proc.* 2004;79(7):916-922.

[160] Allen RP, Walters A, Montplaisir J, et al. Restless legs syndrome prevalence and impact : REST general population study. *Arch Intern Med* 2005;165:1286-92.

[161] Higgins JPT, ed, Green S, ed. Cochrane Handbook for Systematic Reviews of Interventions Version 5.1.0 [updated March 2011]. *The Cochrane Collaboration.* 2011.

[162] Mendelson WB. Are periodic leg movements associated with clinical sleep disturbance? *Sleep* 1996; 19:219–223.

[163] Hogl B. Periodic limb movements are associated with disturbed sleep. *Pro J Clin Sleep Med* 2007; 3: 12–14.

[164] Mahowald MW. Periodic limb movements are NOT associated with disturbed sleep. *Con J Clin Sleep Med* 2007; 3:15–17.

[165] American Academy of Sleep Medicine. *The International Classification of Sleep Disorders Diagnostic and Coding Manual. 2nd ed.* Westchester: American Academy of Sleep Medicine, 2005:193–195.

[166] Staedt J, Wassmuth F, Ziemann U, et al. Pergolide: treatment of choice in restless legs syndrome (RLS) and nocturnal myoclonus syndrome (NMS). A double-blind randomized crossover trial of pergolide versus L-Dopa. *J Neural Transm* 1997; 104:461–468.

[167] Partinen M, Hirvonen K, Jama L, et al. Efficacy and safety of pramipexole in idiopathic restless legs syndrome: a polysomnographic dose-finding study—the PRELUDE study. *Sleep Med* 2006; 7: 407–417.

[168] Manconi M, Ferri R, Zucconi M, et al. Dissociation of periodic leg movements from arousals in restless legs syndrome. *Ann Neurol.* 2012 Jun;71(6):834-44.

[169] Walters AS, Wagner ML, Hening WA, et al. Successful treatment of the idiopathic restless legs syndrome in a randomized double-blind trial of oxycodone versus placebo. *Sleep* 1993; 16:327–332.

[170] Polo-Kantola P, Rauhala E, Erkkola R, et al. Estrogen replacement therapy and nocturnal periodic limb movements: a randomized controlled trial. *Obstet Gynecol* 2001; 97:548–554.

[171] Micheli F, Fernandez Pardal M, Gatto M, et al. Bruxism secondary to chronic antidopaminergic drug exposure. *Clin Neuropharmacol* 1993; 16:315–323.

[172] Amir I, Hermesh H, Gavish A. Bruxism secondary to antipsychotic drug exposure: a positive response to propranolol. *Clin Neuropharmacol* 1997; 20:86–89.

[173] Gerber PE, Lynd LD. Selective serotonin-reuptake inhibitor-induced movement disorders. *Ann Pharmacother* 1998; 32:692–698.

[174] Winocur E, Gavish A, Voikovitch M, et al. Drugs and bruxism: a critical review. *J Orofac Pain* 2003; 17:99–111.

[175] Lavigne GL, Lobbezoo F, Rompre PH, et al. Cigarette smoking as a risk factor or an exacerbating factor for restless legs syndrome and sleep bruxism. *Sleep* 1997; 20:290–293.

[176] Lobbezoo F, Soucy JP, Montplaisir JY, et al. Striatal D2 receptor binding in sleep bruxism: a controlled study with iodine-123-iodobenzamide and single-photon-emission computed tomography. *J Dent Res* 1996; 75:1804–1810.

[177] Lavigne GL, Soucy JP, Lobbezoo F, et al. Double-blind, crossover, placebo-controlled trial of bromocriptine in patients with sleep bruxism. *Clin Neuropharmacol* 2001; 24:145–149.

[178] Lobbezoo F, Lavigne GJ, Tanguay R, et al. The effect of catecholamine precursor L-dopa on sleep bruxism: a controlled clinical trial. *Mov Disord* 1997; 12:73–78.

[179] Raigrodski AJ, Christensen LV, Mohamed SE, et al. The effect of four week administration of amitriptyline on sleep bruxism. A double-blind crossover clinical study. *Cranio* 2001; 19:21–25.

[180] Sjoholm TT, Lehtinen I, Piha SJ. The effect of propranolol on sleep bruxism: hypothetical considerations based on a case study. *Clin Auton Res* 1996; 6:37–40.

[181] Bostwick JM, Jaffee MS. Buspirone as an antidote to SSRI-induced bruxism in 4 cases. *J Clin Psychiatry* 1999; 60(12):857–860.

[182] Brown ES, Hong SC. Antidepressant-induced bruxism successfully treated with gabapentin. *J Am Dent Assoc* 1999; 130:1467–1469.

[183] Saletu A, Parapatics S, Saletu B, et al. On the pharmacotherapy of sleep bruxism: placebo-controlled polysomnographic and psychometric studies with clonazepam. *Neuropsychobiology* 2005; 51: 214–225.

[184] Montgomery MT, Nishioka GJ, Rugh JD, et al. Effect of diazepam on nocturnal masticatory muscle activity. *J Dent Res* 1986; 65:1980.

[185] Huynh N, Lavigne GJ, Lanfranchi PA, et al. The effect of 2 sympatholytic medications—propranolol and clonidine—on sleep bruxism: experimental randomized controlled studies. *Sleep* 2006; 29:307–316.

[186] Carra MC, Macaluso GM, Rompré PH, et al.Clonidine has a paradoxical effect on cyclic arousal and sleep bruxism during NREM sleep. *Sleep.* 2010 Dec;3(12):1711-6.

[187] Ivanhoe CB, Lai JM, Francisco GE. Bruxism after brain injury: successful treatment with botulinum toxin-A. *Arch Phys Med Rehabil* 1997; 78:1272–1273.

[188] Tan EK, Jankovic J. Treating severe bruxism with botulinum toxin. *J Am Dent Assoc* 2000; 131:211–216.

[189] Long H, Liao Z, Wang Y, et al. Efficacy of botulinum toxins on bruxism: an evidence-based review. *Int Dent J.* 2012 Feb;62(1):1-5.

Index

#

20th century, ix, 48

A

abuse, 19, 38, 51, 68, 158, 202, 206, 224, 231, 232, 233, 234, 237, 241, 243, 305, 322, 330
accelerometers, 257
access, 124, 232, 234, 240
accommodation, 332
accounting, 199
acetylcholine, 5, 8, 9, 100, 188, 195, 204, 233, 234, 236
acetylcholinesterase, 188
acid, 6, 7, 8, 135, 142, 143, 145, 149, 169, 205, 206, 207, 234, 235, 321, 330, 332, 337
ACTH, 188
activity level, 182, 186, 204
acute schizophrenia, 219
acute stress, 164, 165, 306
adaptation(s), 22, 24, 182, 197, 240, 286
adenocarcinoma, 144
adenoids, 80
adenosine, 237
adipocyte, 87
adiposity, 81
adjustment, 37, 38, 139
adolescents, 38, 49, 51, 72, 148, 154, 157, 161, 170, 174, 226, 239, 325, 342
adrenocorticotropic hormone, 188
adulthood, 38, 70, 179, 269
advancement(s), 91, 140, 148, 225, 282, 298
adverse effects, 150, 193, 197, 222, 243, 320, 322, 323, 324, 334, 338, 345
adverse event, 322, 326, 331, 337
aetiology, 188, 191, 218

affective disorder, 159, 160, 162, 183, 186, 188, 189, 210, 214, 215, 239
affective experience, 195
Africa, 241
African-American, 97, 132
aggregation, 82, 99, 109
aggression, 50, 194, 325
aggressive behavior, 325, 342
aging population, 52
agonist, 35, 198, 204, 207, 211, 299, 319, 332, 336, 338, 343, 346
agoraphobia, 168, 177
airways, 76, 77
alcohol abuse, 155, 235
alcohol consumption, 87, 130, 192, 234
alcohol dependence, 211, 235, 244
alcohol use, 19, 45, 68, 234, 235
alcoholism, 154
aldosterone, 87
alertness, 19, 20, 21, 22, 25, 40, 41, 46, 51, 68, 88, 91, 250, 276, 294, 310, 311, 326, 328, 345
algorithm, 37, 349
allele, 140
alpha activity, 9
alpha wave, 9, 11
alters, 92, 212
American Psychiatric Association, 28, 51, 72, 174, 209, 243, 317, 344
American Psychological Association, 317
amine, 333
amnesia, 64, 166, 322, 323
amphetamines, 241, 245, 319, 328, 329
amplitude, 9, 10, 11, 12, 78, 182, 184, 185, 250, 252, 257, 265, 339
amygdala, 5, 8, 33, 198, 239, 277, 282, 288, 294, 296
analgesic, 237, 242
anatomy, 80
anemia, 94, 96, 116, 144, 346

anger, 47, 164, 224
angiotensin II, 87
anisotropy, 285, 291
ankles, 103
anorexia, 331
antagonism, 237, 326, 344, 345
anterior cingulate cortex, 239, 280, 283, 290
anterograde amnesia, 63, 322
antibody, 332
anticholinergic, 67, 189, 196, 211, 320, 325
anticholinergic effect, 196, 320, 325
antidepressant(s), 35, 66, 99, 105, 125, 167, 172, 178, 180, 181, 189, 191, 195, 196, 197, 198, 201, 203, 206, 207, 208, 211, 212, 213, 214, 215, 231, 240, 319, 320, 323, 324, 325, 327, 328, 331, 333, 339, 342, 343
antidepressant medication, 105, 125, 212, 331
antiepileptic drugs, 169
antigen, 35
antihistamines, 9, 63, 320
antipsychotic, 161, 207, 217, 218, 219, 220, 223, 224, 228, 229, 325, 349
antipsychotic drugs, 217, 218, 219, 223, 224, 228
anxiety disorder, 30, 35, 49, 52, 68, 154, 155, 156, 159, 162, 163, 164, 165, 168, 170, 171, 172, 174, 175, 179
apathy, 49, 224
apnea, 40, 42, 44, 67, 75, 76, 77, 78, 80, 81, 82, 83, 84, 85, 86, 89, 90, 92, 107, 112, 116, 124, 125, 126, 127, 129, 130, 140, 166, 237, 259, 260, 261, 265, 268, 271, 280, 282, 295
apoplexy, 106
appetite, 194, 200, 329
appraisals, 194
Aristotle, vii, ix
arterial hypertension, 124, 125
artery, 106
articulation, 136
Asia, 79
Asian countries, 96
asparagus, 241
aspartate, 4, 233, 279, 281, 292
ASPD, 264
aspiration, 236
assault, 175, 216
assessment, 27, 29, 34, 35, 36, 45, 56, 89, 103, 120, 136, 146, 164, 165, 166, 167, 177, 214, 249, 257, 258, 261, 271, 345
assessment tools, 35, 36
asymmetry, 100
asymptomatic, 21, 38
ataxia, 48

atrophy, 48, 69, 80, 279, 280, 284, 285, 286, 289, 300
attitudes, 31, 306, 313
auditory stimuli, 10, 280
autism, 141
autoantibodies, 345
automaticity, 313
automobile, 131
autonomic activity, 64
autonomic nervous system, 13, 64
autopsy, 97
autosomal dominant, 20, 69, 94, 99, 118
autosomal recessive, 99
avoidance, 20, 22, 64, 66, 165, 168, 328
awareness, ix, 9, 10, 68

B

Bahrain, 116, 346
ban, 241
barbiturates, 320, 321
barriers, 258
basal forebrain, 5, 8, 9, 12, 41, 42, 233, 277
basal ganglia, 33, 90, 98, 100, 239, 277, 279, 282, 288, 293
base, 238
baths, 334
Beck Depression Inventory, 48
behavior modification, 317
behavior therapy, 53, 176, 180, 215, 294, 317
behavioral change, 168, 235
behavioral disorders, 300
behavioral manifestations, 64, 285
behaviors, 19, 64, 65, 69, 101, 155, 156, 169, 255, 264, 265, 306, 307, 309, 313, 323, 329
beneficial effect, 20, 319, 327, 331, 332, 333, 334, 336
benefits, 167, 206, 208, 315, 316, 338
benign, 63, 70
benzodiazepine, 235, 320, 321, 340, 341
beta wave, 250
beverages, 42, 103, 237
bible, ix, xi
bilateral, 289, 299
biofeedback, 139, 312
biological activities, 4
biological markers, 186, 198
biological processes, 240
biological rhythms, 201
biomarkers, 201, 211
biosynthesis, 197
bipolar disorder, 156, 157, 160, 213, 214, 215
bipolar illness, 156, 157

bleeding, 144

blindness, 23, 264

blood, 13, 14, 16, 33, 43, 45, 86, 87, 97, 98, 99, 106, 111, 112, 129, 172, 184, 193, 236, 279, 282, 284, 288, 290, 291, 328, 329, 332

blood flow, 13, 14, 33, 111, 279, 284, 288, 290, 291

blood pressure, 13, 14, 16, 43, 86, 87, 99, 106, 111, 112, 129, 184, 193, 282, 328, 329

bloodstream, 23

body fat, 109

body mass index (BMI), 43, 78, 80, 81, 83, 84, 89, 106, 123, 125, 127, 128, 130, 271

bone(s), 94, 138

bone resorption, 138

borderline personality disorder, 162

bradycardia, 329

brain activity, ix, 33, 92, 100, 101, 115, 139, 185, 186, 245, 276, 277, 279, 282, 286, 294

brain damage, 239

brain functions, 193

brain size, 192

brain stem, 277

brain structure, 33, 89, 275

brain wave patterns, x, 3

brainstem, 5, 12, 82, 93, 100, 101, 188, 276, 277, 279, 283, 285, 288, 289, 291, 295, 300, 301

breathing disturbances, 259

bruxism, 69, 72, 76, 95, 97, 99, 103, 104, 106, 115, 116, 117, 119, 120, 121, 135, 136, 137, 138, 141, 143, 145, 146, 147, 148, 254, 255, 266, 268, 333, 339, 340, 350

buccal mucosa, 138

C

caffeine, 22, 32, 67, 95, 140, 141, 142, 158, 231, 234, 236, 237, 243, 244, 307, 308, 309, 333, 334

calcium, 234, 337

caliber, 81

calorie, 68

cancer, 314

cannabinoids, 239, 241

cannabis, 231, 239, 240, 241

CAP, 33, 119, 120, 252, 270

capsule, 90, 241

carbamazepine, 207, 332

carbon, 85, 177, 280, 297

carbon dioxide, 85, 177

carbon monoxide, 280, 297

cardiac activity, 101

cardiac arrhythmia, 324

cardiovascular disease(s) CVD, 77, 105, 106, 109, 121, 123, 125, 193

cardiovascular system, 13, 78

care model, 316

case study(s), 48, 176, 285, 350

cataplexy, 8, 15, 27, 41, 46, 47, 48, 56, 57, 58, 164, 262, 263, 271, 277, 279, 288, 294, 295, 296, 319, 327, 328, 329, 330, 331, 345, 346

catatonic, 219

catecholamines, 236, 328, 329, 331

category a, 34

category d, 76

caucasians, 46

causal attribution, 29

causal relationship, 69, 138, 140, 203

CBP, 183

central nervous system (CNS), x, 14, 34, 39, 58, 62, 63, 139, 176, 184, 188, 191, 192, 199, 201, 205, 213, 227, 231, 236, 239, 240, 266, 298, 321, 323, 326, 328, 333, 334, 343, 344

central sleep apnea (CSA), 76, 77, 78, 79, 81, 82, 107, 109

cerebellum, 4, 278, 280, 281, 283, 286, 288, 289

cerebellum express clock genes, 4

cerebral blood flow, 16, 53, 277, 293, 294, 295

cerebral cortex, 8, 238, 244

cerebral function, 280

cerebral palsy, 149

cerebrospinal fluid, 47, 57, 98, 294

cerebrovascular disease, 78, 106, 280

challenges, 58, 107, 177, 181, 183, 282, 298

changing environment, 182

chaos, 215

chemical, 55, 193

chemoreceptors, 81

chemotherapy, 231, 240

Cheyne-Stokes respiration, 81, 107, 108, 109

Chicago, x, 71, 145, 146, 317

childhood, 18, 38, 63, 72, 80, 97, 107, 141, 147, 175, 218, 226, 269, 271, 345

children, 25, 37, 43, 45, 50, 61, 62, 64, 66, 67, 69, 70, 71, 72, 77, 78, 81, 83, 85, 97, 98, 107, 108, 109, 110, 116, 137, 138, 142, 143, 147, 148, 149, 150, 164, 170, 171, 174, 179, 263, 267, 280, 297, 326, 331

China, 345

chloral, 320

cholesterol, 78, 106

choline, 239, 244, 281, 285

chromosome, 99, 117, 118

chronic fatigue, 77, 78

chronic fatigue syndrome, 78

chronic heart failure (CHF), 79, 81, 108

chronic illness, 53

chronic kidney disease (CKD), 97, 116

chronic obstructive pulmonary disease, 237
chronobiology, 201
chronotherapy, 20
cigarette smoke, 236
circadian clock genes, 14, 160
circadian rhythm(s), v, x, xi, 4, 8, 14, 17, 18, 19, 21,
    23, 24, 54, 119, 120, 139, 157, 170, 171, 181,
    183, 186, 190, 198, 200, 201, 202, 204, 205, 210,
    213, 256, 264, 270, 271
Circadian Rhythm Sleep Disorders, v, 17, 19
circadian rhythmicity, 55
circulation, 81
citalopram, 171, 197
city, 135
classes, 217, 218, 222
classical conditioning, 32
classification, x, 10, 11, 15, 17, 28, 29, 44, 49, 51,
    59, 70, 83, 145, 204, 270, 294, 317
classroom, 42
clavicle, 254
clinical application, 85
clinical assessment, 115, 270
clinical depression, 105
clinical diagnosis, 55, 263, 265
clinical disorders, 43
clinical examination, 136
clinical presentation, 78, 108
clinical symptoms, 36, 93, 97, 124, 127, 194, 259
clinical syndrome, 69, 76
clinical trials, 65, 120, 319, 321, 322, 325, 326, 336,
    337, 338
closure, 9, 270
clozapine, 223, 224, 228, 229
clusters, 165
cocaine, 205, 214, 231, 234, 237, 238, 240, 241, 244
cocaine abuse, 238, 244
cocoa, 237
coding, x, 15, 71, 73, 145, 270, 294, 317
coefficient of variation, 137
coffee, 149, 237
cognition, 3, 33, 50, 88, 90, 112, 277, 287, 294
cognitive abilities, 88
cognitive activity, 32
cognitive deficit(s), 90, 93, 112, 222
cognitive dysfunction, 88, 89, 158, 193, 194, 222
cognitive effort, 239
cognitive function, 88, 90, 91, 154, 181, 182, 229,
    238, 280, 289, 297
cognitive impairment, 23, 49, 86, 89, 90, 93, 114,
    157, 206, 207, 217, 218
cognitive models, 31
cognitive performance, 90, 113, 150, 238, 294
cognitive process, 88, 89

cognitive tasks, 281, 289
cognitive therapy, 139, 313, 314, 316
cognitive-behavioral therapy, 318
collaboration, 272, 273
college students, 245
coma, 234, 329
commercial, 86
communication, 141
community(s), 52, 96, 105, 106, 108, 111, 116, 131,
    132, 176, 180, 218, 241, 322, 341
comorbidity, 48, 67, 86, 124, 125, 154, 174, 240
comparative analysis, 342
complement, 130, 287
complex behaviors, 63, 284
complexity, 41, 103, 118, 197
compliance, 114, 130, 133
complications, 38, 124, 132, 143, 144, 150, 268, 280,
    335, 336
composition, 89, 109, 235
compounds, 94, 222, 231, 237, 239, 240, 241, 244,
    281, 319, 321, 328, 333, 336, 342
compulsion, 232
compulsive behavior, 336
computed tomography, 33, 53, 54, 227, 294, 301,
    340, 350
computer, 254
concordance, 141, 200
conditioning, 31, 77, 312, 334
conduction, 324
conference, 346
conflict, 22
congestive heart failure, 30, 75, 79, 82, 86, 104, 107,
    131
connectivity, 119
consciousness, vii, ix, 47, 64, 67, 184, 262, 284, 311
consensus, 77, 138, 144, 198, 326, 343, 346
consolidation, 184, 193, 195, 322
consulting, 124
consumers, 235, 237, 238, 241
consumption, 42, 141, 142, 231, 235, 237, 241, 244,
    277, 292
contraceptives, 50
control group, 49, 220, 239, 334
controlled studies, 48, 119, 171, 323, 330, 334, 335,
    337, 350
controlled trials, 139, 167, 316, 318, 336, 339
controversial, 207, 279, 338
controversies, 71, 267
cor pulmonale, 78
cornea, 10
coronary artery disease, 106, 131
coronary heart disease, 121
corpus callosum, 90

correlation(s), 33, 86, 194, 219, 221, 222, 232, 240, 285
cortex, 4, 5, 9, 33, 92, 99, 100, 187, 211, 212, 239, 244, 258, 280, 282, 283, 284, 286, 290, 299, 301, 312
corticosteroids, 231, 240
cortisol, 18, 32, 34, 166, 179, 182, 183, 184, 185, 186, 188, 190, 193, 199, 229, 233
cost, 59, 75, 85, 102, 103, 154, 316
cotinine, 236
cough, 13
cough reflex, 13
coughing, 14, 103
counseling, 135, 143
cranial nerve, 254
creatine, 239, 279, 281, 285
creatinine, 279
Creutzfeldt-Jakob disease, 69
critical period, 212
criticism, 243
CRM, 254, 262
cross-sectional study, 30, 325
crystalline, 241
CSF, 47, 51, 57, 59, 98, 117, 263
cues, 4, 19, 21, 167, 183, 210
cure, 144, 204
cycles, 4, 9, 18, 19, 51, 77, 78, 184, 185, 201, 229, 234, 249, 252, 277
cycling, 50, 207, 252, 310, 334
cytokines, 32, 193
cytoplasm, 183

D

daily living, 101
data analysis, 44, 271
data processing, 257
data set, 341
database, 155, 344
deaths, 241
defects, 135, 136, 137, 138
deficiency, 15, 28, 57, 59, 94, 98, 116, 188, 189, 199, 211, 319, 327, 328, 330, 331, 332, 333, 335, 346
deficit, 78, 220, 280, 300
degradation, 183, 231, 236
delirium, 234
Delta, 159, 184
delta wave, 11, 199, 250, 252
delusions, 157, 161, 218, 224, 225, 276, 329
dementia, 22, 23, 65, 68, 69, 71, 89, 114, 125, 258, 265, 284, 286, 324, 325, 342
dental caries, 138

Department of Health and Human Services, 271
deposits, 108
depressants, 63
depressive symptomatology, 58, 209
depressive symptoms, 48, 155, 156, 193, 194, 201, 209, 212, 297, 327
deprivation, 39, 51, 98, 104, 156, 174, 189, 191, 192, 194, 195, 202, 203, 208, 209, 212, 215, 277, 311
depth, 10, 171
derivatives, 224, 239, 321, 328, 335, 344
desensitization, 193
destruction, 42, 95, 106, 138, 279
detachment, 138
detectable, 12
detection, 85, 89, 102, 103, 110, 111, 161, 225, 257, 259, 267, 271
detoxification, 243
developmental process, 191, 192
dexamethasone suppression test, 185
diabetes, 77, 89, 104, 105, 106, 107, 123, 124, 125, 128
Diagnostic and Statistical Manual of Mental Disorders, 28, 51, 67, 72, 165, 186, 243, 306, 327
diagnostic criteria, 28, 30, 49, 52, 53, 63, 64, 79, 96, 105, 115, 120, 135, 136, 137, 138, 139, 140, 147, 155, 164, 171, 202, 263, 264, 272, 299
Diagnostic Techniques, vi, 247
diaphoresis, 64
diarrhea, 323
dichotomy, 213
diet, 129, 144, 308, 309, 330
differential diagnosis, 30, 35, 36, 45, 63, 65, 68, 70, 93, 94, 96, 102, 103, 115, 156, 202, 265, 268, 269
diffusion, 236, 285, 300
diffusivity, 114, 285, 291
disability, 141, 186
discomfort, 94, 95, 103, 135, 136, 137, 138, 268, 283, 289
discriminative stimuli, 310
diseases, 23, 125, 129, 161, 181, 322
dissatisfaction, 29, 30, 36
dissociation, 65
distortions, 194, 211
distress, 27, 28, 36, 153, 164, 165, 167, 169, 170, 198, 234, 258, 320, 324, 333
distribution, 15, 33, 38, 80, 126, 127, 129, 130, 326
dizygotic, 141, 200
dizygotic twins, 141, 200
dizziness, 174, 320, 325, 326, 329, 331, 336, 337
dogs, 333
dominance, 202
dopamine, 6, 7, 8, 98, 100, 117, 119, 142, 169, 188, 205, 207, 233, 236, 245, 279, 283, 284, 285, 286,

291, 296, 299, 301, 325, 328, 329, 330, 333, 335, 336, 338, 344, 346, 347, 348

dopamine agonist, 335, 336, 338, 346, 347, 348

dopamine antagonists, 98

dopaminergic, 5, 9, 15, 41, 55, 94, 98, 99, 100, 117, 205, 214, 236, 237, 239, 240, 266, 279, 283, 285, 286, 289, 296, 299, 301, 328, 329, 330, 333, 334, 336, 337, 339, 344, 346, 347, 348

dorsal raphe nuclei, 185

dorsolateral prefrontal cortex, 281, 289

dosage, 324, 326, 327, 335, 340, 347

dosing, 325

double-blind trial, 348, 349

down syndrome, 141, 143

down-regulation, 235

drawing, 90

dream, ix, 63, 65, 66, 71, 164, 166, 194, 209, 210, 215, 216, 227, 228, 235, 264, 265, 284, 286, 301

dreaming, x, xi, 65, 185, 276, 279, 287, 293, 295

drug abuse, 62, 155, 156, 158, 202

drug addict, 232

drug addiction, 232

drug dependence, 232

drug discovery, 343

drug therapy, 67, 144

drug treatment, 178, 266, 280

DSM, 186

DSM-IV-TR, 165, 174, 232, 233

dysphoria, 182, 232, 240

dyspnea, 40, 70, 276

dysthymia, 156

dystonia, 70, 73, 269, 273

E

eating disorders, 68

economics, 76

ecstasy, 231, 237, 238, 241, 242

editors, 15, 16, 71, 229, 244, 297

education, 89, 92, 208, 308, 313, 314, 315

EEG activity, 9, 53, 100, 101, 184, 185, 254, 271, 294

EEG patterns, ix, 32, 228

ejaculation, 331

EKG, 104, 125, 256

elderly population, 105, 112, 121

electrocardiogram, 104, 253, 256

electrodes, 86, 254, 261, 267, 268, 269, 270, 312

electroencephalogram, vii, ix, 99, 182, 235, 249, 253, 272

electroencephalography, 50, 137, 178

electromyography, 36, 102, 136, 312

elementary school, 147

EMG, 9, 10, 11, 12, 45, 46, 103, 125, 136, 137, 143, 185, 249, 250, 252, 253, 254, 255, 256, 257, 261, 264, 265, 267, 268, 312

emission, 33, 53, 54, 294, 296, 299, 340, 350

emotion, 33, 154, 192, 194, 195, 262

emotion regulation, 154, 192

emotional distress, 21

emotional experience, 195, 224

emotional information, 195

emotional processes, 191

emotional responses, 193

emotional state, 232

empathy, 241

employment, 22

EMS, 113

enamel, 137

encephalitis, 82

encephalopathy, 69

endocrine, 4, 13, 16, 95

endocrinology, 117

endogenous depression, 192, 212

endophenotypes, 200, 212

endothelial dysfunction, 87

endurance, 324

energy, 83, 97, 105, 109, 182, 197, 200, 202, 237, 276

energy recovery, 276

enlargement, 83

entorhinal cortex, 93

enuresis, 67, 72, 255, 331

environment, 13, 14, 32, 34, 37, 46, 67, 103, 168, 182, 194, 231, 257, 258, 262, 268, 308, 309

environmental change, 182, 197

environmental effects, 244

environmental factors, 18, 141, 142, 200, 217, 218, 307, 308

environmental stimuli, 39, 47, 168, 193

environmental variables, 46

enzyme, 205

EOG, 9, 10, 11, 45, 125, 137, 185, 249, 250, 253, 254, 255, 257, 261

epidemic, 81

epidemiologic, 52, 159

epidemiology, 96, 108, 115, 116, 120, 176, 177, 178, 272, 299

epilepsy, ix, 62, 63, 70, 168, 261, 268, 269, 273

epinephrine, 328

equilibrium, 324

equipment, 36, 44, 103, 266

ERS, 111

erythropoietin, 98, 117

escitalopram, 172, 179, 180, 197, 324, 341, 342

esophagitis, 142, 144

esophagus, 142, 143, 144, 145
ethanol, 235
ethics, 125
ethnic groups, 47, 57
ethnicity, 108
ethylene, 284
etiology, 27, 31, 50, 57, 139, 159, 169, 171, 269, 319
euphoria, 238, 241, 242
Europe, 79, 141, 236, 239, 241, 244, 245, 347
European, 241, 245
European Monitoring Centre for Drugs and Drug Addiction (EMCDDA), 241, 245
event-related potential, 33
evoked potential, 102
evolution, 31, 53, 130, 332
examinations, 80, 125, 137, 266
excess body weight, 123
excitability, 118, 119
excitation, 34
exclusion, 35
excretion, 13, 34
execution, 100
executive function(s), 88, 89, 90, 113, 218, 281
exercise, 23, 70, 95, 182, 307, 308, 309, 334
experimental condition, 197
exposure, x, 19, 21, 22, 23, 24, 87, 165, 167, 170, 193, 233, 235, 323, 349
extensor, 255
extensor digitorum, 255
external environment, 182, 183
extinction, 166
extrapyramidal effects, 224
eye movement, x, xi, 3, 5, 10, 11, 12, 45, 46, 48, 62, 65, 139, 140, 157, 159, 161, 184, 185, 187, 193, 212, 213, 226, 250, 252, 265, 269, 272, 287, 301

F

facial muscles, 254
facial pain, 148
failure to thrive, 280
Fairbanks, 213
families, 99, 200, 213
family history, 82, 94, 266, 336
family members, 103, 200, 258, 328
family studies, 98
fat, 80, 81, 106, 108
FDA, 319, 326, 328, 330, 332, 337
FDA approval, 332
fear(s), 41, 49, 64, 70, 164, 165, 166, 168, 169, 172, 193, 204, 205
feelings, 58, 102, 155, 165, 174, 209, 312
ferritin, 98, 117, 338

fiber(s), 80, 109, 245
fibroblasts, 4
fibromyalgia, 78
fibrosis, 335
Finland, 30
first generation, 223
flexibility, 88
flexor, 118
flight(s), 19, 22, 24
fluctuations, 270
fluid, 67, 98
fluoxetine, 171, 197, 205, 214, 325, 331
fluvoxamine, 171
food, 18, 41, 68, 103, 137, 142, 294
food intake, 18
force, 267, 273, 348
Ford, 155, 159
forebrain, 5, 195, 287
formation, 12, 32, 183, 187, 233, 277, 283, 285, 286, 289, 291, 293
foundations, 343
fractures, 322, 340, 341
fragments, 191, 308, 309
France, 30, 123, 125, 330
Freud, vii, ix, xi
friction, 69
frontal cortex, 89, 185, 276, 281, 285, 289
frontal lobe, 70, 93, 269, 273, 281, 285, 289
functional changes, 276, 288, 289, 290, 291, 292
Functional Magnetic Resonance Imaging (fMRI), 34, 92, 275, 276, 279, 280, 281, 282, 283, 289, 292, 298
functional MRI, 34, 99

G

GABA, 6, 7, 8, 12, 34, 54, 100, 119, 169, 206, 224, 234, 235, 321, 330, 341
gambling, 336
ganglion, x, 18
gastric ulcer, 141
gastrin, 149
gastroesophageal reflux, 77, 135, 136, 146, 149, 150, 259
gastrointestinal tract, 149
gel, 339
gender differences, 124
gene expression, 181, 182, 183, 205, 240
gene transfer, 205
generalizability, 320, 338
generalized anxiety disorder, 163, 164, 165, 171, 179, 180, 323, 341

genes, 4, 99, 157, 161, 182, 183, 190, 199, 200, 201, 205, 214, 217, 218, 240, 338
genetic disease, 20
genetic factors, 333
genetic predisposition, 194
genetics, 57, 59, 202, 346
genome, 24
genomic regions, 118
genomics, 214
Germany, 30, 84, 140
gingival, 138
globus, 283, 284, 290
glucocorticoids, 185, 193
glucose, 13, 33, 131, 185, 193, 277, 293, 301
glucose regulation, 13
glutamate, 7, 234, 235, 330
glycine, 12, 101
glycogen, 205
grass, 242
gravity, 130
gray matter, 5, 7, 9, 12, 15, 55, 63, 89, 92, 239, 278, 280, 282, 283, 285, 289, 291, 295, 299, 300
group therapy, 346
group treatment, 176
growth, 13, 81, 182, 228, 229
growth hormone, 13, 182, 228, 229
guidelines, 56, 85, 86, 87, 110, 126, 136, 144, 150, 167, 209, 254, 267, 307, 314, 320, 337, 348
guilt, 49, 155

H

habituation, 234, 240
half-life, 206, 236, 237, 321, 323, 324, 326, 329, 330, 331, 334
hallucinations, 47, 49, 68, 157, 158, 164, 168, 218, 224, 241, 242, 262, 287, 292, 324
haplotypes, 190, 205
harmful effects, 237
Hawaii, 160
head trauma, 48
headache, 72, 77, 83, 138, 329, 330, 331, 334
health, 28, 30, 48, 53, 58, 75, 104, 105, 121, 154, 157, 159, 162, 167, 172, 180, 182, 244, 308, 324
health care, 30
health condition, 28, 30
health problems, 30
health risks, 182
health status, 154
heart disease, 78, 105, 346
heart failure, 78, 79, 107, 108, 109
heart rate, 13, 32, 86, 100, 139, 141, 177, 178, 254, 262, 328
heartburn, 142
heat loss, 13, 14, 33
height, 43
helplessness, 165
hemodialysis, 346
hemoglobin, 107
hemorrhage, 82
hepatic encephalopathy, 23
heredity, 139
heritability, 200
heroin, 231, 240
heterogeneity, 99, 109, 118, 186, 200
high blood pressure, 87, 129
hip fractures, 341
hippocampus, 4, 5, 12, 33, 34, 89, 92, 93, 205, 239, 277, 280, 281, 282, 285, 286, 287, 288, 289, 291
histamine, 6, 7, 8, 51, 55, 59, 100, 198, 320, 327, 333, 346
history, ix, 34, 42, 49, 62, 65, 66, 75, 76, 82, 84, 93, 94, 106, 115, 154, 155, 172, 186, 195, 200, 209, 233, 234, 235, 243, 254, 257, 258, 263, 265, 269, 284, 322, 336
homeostasis, 19, 55, 101, 198
homovanillic acid, 98
Hong Kong, 79, 108
hormone(s), 4, 5, 13, 16, 50, 130, 182, 183, 186, 193, 202, 207, 225, 233
hormone levels, 183
hospitalization, 340
hostility, 224
HPA axis, 193, 198, 212
human, vii, ix, x, 3, 15, 18, 24, 33, 46, 55, 57, 87, 145, 183, 195, 205, 211, 212, 227, 228, 241, 249, 276, 277, 279, 293, 294, 295, 296, 299, 300, 323, 342, 344
human brain, 33, 195, 344
Human Chronobiology, v, 3
human leukocyte antigen (HLA), 46, 50, 57, 277, 327
human subjects, 15
humidity, 181
hygiene, 20, 22, 23, 24, 42, 158, 208, 231, 242, 306, 307, 308, 314, 315, 334
hyperactivity, 192, 193, 205, 224, 276
hyperarousal, 27, 29, 32, 33, 34, 35, 38, 54, 163, 164, 165, 199, 224, 258, 276, 277, 286, 294, 306, 307, 311, 315
hyperglycemia, 325
hyperinsulinism, 87
hypersensitivity, 103, 137, 183
hypersomnia, 27, 29, 39, 40, 42, 43, 45, 49, 50, 58, 59, 63, 68, 83, 155, 156, 186, 199, 201, 232, 234, 235, 240, 241, 242, 243, 249, 253, 256, 263, 330

hypertension, 75, 77, 84, 86, 87, 105, 106, 111, 112, 123, 124, 130, 131
hyperthyroidism, 35
hypertrophy, 43, 81, 121, 129, 135, 136, 137, 138, 139, 239
hyperventilation, 177
hypnagogic hallucinations, 49, 50, 51, 68, 279, 330
hypnosis, 167
hypochondriasis, 38
hypoplasia, 43
hypotension, 107, 340
hypothalamus, x, 3, 4, 5, 6, 7, 8, 9, 15, 18, 21, 33, 41, 48, 55, 63, 100, 183, 190, 191, 211, 233, 277, 279, 288, 295, 296
hypothesis, 33, 100, 119, 143, 144, 156, 180, 188, 189, 190, 191, 192, 194, 195, 201, 203, 211, 213, 220, 276, 281, 283, 284, 285, 330, 339
hypoxemia, 40, 75, 76, 77, 78, 89, 112, 114, 280
hypoxia, 87, 89, 111, 114, 280, 297

I

iatrogenic, 68, 95, 340
ideal, 249
identification, 85, 164, 199, 200, 208, 209, 271
identity, 67
idiopathic, 27, 38, 40, 42, 43, 45, 50, 58, 59, 66, 68, 72, 77, 81, 94, 109, 116, 256, 263, 266, 275, 277, 278, 283, 284, 285, 287, 295, 299, 300, 301, 339, 347, 348, 349
illicit drug use, 232
illicit substances, 231
illusions, 241
image(s), 46, 300, 312
imagery, 167, 175, 311, 312
imitation, 283
immobilization, 102, 120
immune function, 32
immune modulation, 332
immunoglobulin, 345
impairments, 30, 88, 89, 91, 107, 222, 229, 236, 258, 275, 294, 324
improvements, 90, 93, 190, 204, 325, 327, 328
impulses, 80
impulsive, 245
impulsivity, 245
in transition, 70
in vivo, 34, 228, 286, 296
incidence, 18, 30, 78, 87, 96, 97, 116, 137, 140, 218, 225, 280, 323, 331, 336
incisors, 69, 83
independence, 190

individuals, 19, 21, 23, 30, 32, 45, 47, 48, 50, 51, 76, 77, 78, 88, 94, 105, 113, 141, 143, 156, 165, 169, 171, 182, 209, 215, 218, 219, 220, 223, 224, 232, 236, 238, 239, 240, 257, 258, 259, 267, 313, 320, 322, 338
induction, 141, 200, 211, 227, 234, 240, 283, 321, 323, 330
industrialized countries, 22
ineffectiveness, 207, 209
inevitability, 174
infancy, 38, 77, 149
infants, x, 10, 70, 71, 110, 202, 297
infarction, 82, 106
infection, 319, 331, 332
inferiority, 141
inflammation, 81, 87
information processing, 32, 91
informed consent, 125
ingestion, 185, 237, 307, 322, 323
inhaler, 236
inheritance, 50, 94, 99
inhibition, 34, 87, 100, 149, 184, 188, 198, 205, 236, 252, 324
inhibitor, 286, 329, 332, 334, 349
initiation, 31, 32, 38, 91, 98, 142, 143, 169, 197, 313
injections, 205, 340
injury, 62, 63, 71, 89, 149, 165, 172, 238, 255, 265, 273, 297, 340, 350
inositol, 239
insects, 49, 65
insulin, 13, 131, 193
insulin resistance, 13
integration, 85, 109
integrin, 332
integrity, 89, 93, 165, 193, 258, 285, 291
intelligence, 112
intercourse, 47
interface, 98
interference, 172
internal clock, 21
internal processes, 182
internalization, 159
International Classification of Diseases, 186
interneurons, 12
intervention, 153, 160, 166, 224, 255, 305, 308, 315, 316, 319, 332, 339
intimacy, 308, 309
intoxication, 232, 233, 234, 235, 237, 240, 241
intravenous immunoglobulins, 319, 332
intravenously, 241
introversion, 141
inversion, 224
iodine, 350

Iraq, 176
iron, 94, 96, 98, 116, 117, 284, 290, 300, 333, 335, 338, 346, 349
irritability, 37, 50, 51, 164, 171, 232, 237, 328
irritable bowel syndrome, 78
IRT, 67
isolation, 21, 167, 170, 182
isomers, 328
Israel, 15, 48, 52, 71, 110, 114, 116, 132, 145, 270, 271, 298
issues, 105, 115, 161, 227, 249, 253, 271, 275, 320
Italy, ix, 27, 30, 75, 140, 181, 217, 231, 239, 249, 305, 319

J

Japan, 46, 48, 121, 135
Jordan, 215
jumping, 65

K

kidney, 94, 97, 116
kidney transplantation, 94
knees, 262
Korea, 172

L

laboratory studies, 347
laboratory tests, 27, 34, 35
latency, 34, 37, 45, 48, 51, 56, 157, 159, 160, 166, 170, 171, 187, 190, 191, 192, 193, 194, 196, 197, 200, 202, 204, 209, 212, 213, 219, 220, 221, 222, 223, 225, 229, 234, 256, 258, 262, 263, 287, 292, 324, 335
later life, 191
laterodorsal tegmental nuclei, 4, 5, 9
LDL, 106
lead, 30, 38, 41, 63, 65, 69, 75, 76, 77, 80, 86, 94, 99, 156, 163, 164, 191, 199, 203, 231, 234, 241, 275, 280, 307, 310, 329
learned helplessness, 104, 182
learning, 4, 90, 182, 192, 195, 244, 281, 298, 310, 324
learning difficulties, 192
learning task, 281
legend, 6, 7
legs, 35, 93, 94, 95, 96, 102, 115, 116, 117, 118, 119, 120, 121, 145, 168, 266, 282, 299, 333, 346, 348, 349
leptin, 87

lesions, xi, 15, 55, 63, 80, 149, 284, 295, 338
libido, 331
lifestyle changes, 145, 328
lifetime, 62, 66, 163, 168, 174, 176, 200, 217, 218, 239
ligand, 28, 240, 279, 280, 283, 337
light, x, 4, 10, 13, 14, 18, 19, 20, 21, 22, 23, 24, 25, 30, 36, 43, 46, 70, 100, 136, 139, 140, 171, 181, 185, 204, 207, 208, 210, 211, 233, 308, 309, 312, 326, 332, 333
limbic system, 13, 14, 69, 185, 236
lithium, 63, 68, 157, 205, 206, 208, 215, 328, 332
localization, 15, 191
loci, 99, 118
locomotor, 8
locus, 4, 5, 6, 7, 8, 9, 12, 41, 99, 117, 118, 188, 191, 345
longitudinal study, 80, 138, 155, 228, 229
long-term memory, 32, 88
low risk, 330
lower esophageal sphincter, 142
lying, 43, 83, 94, 166, 174, 310
lymph, 81
lymph node, 81
lymphoid, 81
lymphoid tissue, 81

M

magnetic resonance, 33, 34, 54, 81, 89, 92, 93, 115, 239, 296, 298, 300
magnetic resonance imaging (MRI), 33, 34, 54, 81, 89, 92, 98, 117, 276, 278, 280, 283, 285, 288, 289, 290, 291, 292, 295, 296, 298, 300
magnetic resonance spectroscopy, 34, 54, 89, 93, 115, 239, 298, 300
major depression, 38, 39, 49, 105, 155, 156, 167, 177, 179, 198, 200, 212, 213, 215, 218, 226, 301
major depressive disorder, 30, 154, 156, 164, 166, 172, 226, 326, 344
majority, 12, 96, 168, 170, 202, 203, 209, 219, 220, 223, 252, 311, 315, 321
malaise, 51
malocclusion, 43, 139, 146
mammals, 14, 55, 182, 183, 192
man, 118, 129, 149, 213, 228, 284, 285, 293
management, 55, 59, 72, 107, 115, 136, 139, 146, 150, 157, 174, 176, 178, 198, 206, 208, 225, 257, 258, 316, 317, 318, 319, 320, 328, 332, 334, 337, 340, 345, 346, 348, 349
mandible, 138, 254
mania, 156, 157, 159, 160, 190, 200, 202, 203, 204, 205, 206, 207, 208, 209, 213, 214

manic, 156, 157, 160, 200, 201, 202, 203, 204, 205, 213, 214
manic episode, 156, 202, 203
manic symptoms, 156, 202, 204
manic-depressive illness, 160, 213
manipulation, 204, 208
marijuana, 245
Marx, 160, 213
Maryland, 243
MAS, 104
mass, 43
masseter, 100, 104, 121, 135, 136, 137, 138, 139, 148, 254, 268
mastoid, 254
matter, 44, 89, 92, 93, 236, 245, 279, 280, 281, 288, 289, 320
measurement(s), 41, 44, 85, 110, 113, 117, 126, 132, 140, 257, 271, 285, 294, 300, 318
median, 5, 7, 42, 335
mediation, 330, 332
medical history, 82, 95, 103
medication, ix, 19, 23, 31, 35, 36, 42, 64, 69, 95, 100, 106, 149, 206, 219, 220, 221, 233, 263, 265, 267, 282, 315, 320, 328, 329, 334, 336, 338
medicine, vii, 145, 146, 193, 212, 242, 334, 340
Mediterranean, 96
Mediterranean countries, 96
medulla, 12, 42
melanin, 5, 7
melatonin, x, 4, 13, 18, 19, 20, 21, 22, 25, 171, 179, 186, 198, 206, 207, 224, 233, 320, 326, 343
mellitus, 124, 129
membranes, 237
memory, 32, 47, 63, 67, 83, 88, 89, 91, 92, 93, 113, 114, 124, 182, 184, 193, 194, 195, 211, 218, 222, 227, 239, 280, 322, 323, 324, 341
memory formation, 32
memory function, 222
memory performance, 89, 91, 114, 280
memory processes, 239
menarche, 50
menopause, 31, 130
mental ability, 22, 182
mental activity, 29, 94
mental disorder, x, 29, 52, 64, 71, 153, 160, 174, 182, 191, 193, 199, 236, 263, 265, 267, 317
mental health, x, 28, 104, 334
mental illness, 186, 306
mental retardation, 21, 141, 143, 148
mental state, 220
mentally impaired, 19, 23
meridian, 156

meta-analysis, 88, 112, 166, 170, 174, 178, 179, 189, 192, 211, 219, 226, 276, 297, 318, 336, 340
metabolic, 292, 343
metabolic changes, 92, 239
metabolic disorder, 325
metabolic syndrome, 182
metabolism, 13, 14, 16, 33, 98, 115, 117, 131, 182, 185, 187, 284, 286, 287, 288, 291, 293, 298, 301, 326, 333
metabolites, 51, 239, 297
meter, 253
meth, 241
methadone, 240
methamphetamine, 237, 245, 329
methodology, 79, 86
methylphenidate, 319, 328, 329, 330, 344
Mexico, 242
mice, 57, 205, 333, 345, 346
microstructure, 33, 53, 252, 258, 270
midbrain, 5, 8, 41, 63, 100, 187, 282, 285, 286, 291, 293
migraines, 50
misuse, 241
MMA, 100
moclobemide, 196
models, 12, 15, 27, 31, 32, 36, 47, 87, 97, 188, 192, 193, 211, 332
moderating factors, 219
modifications, 93, 240, 280
molecules, 224, 235, 241, 332
monoamine oxidase inhibitors, 66, 331
monozygotic twins, 141, 200
mood change, 259, 329
mood disorder, 35, 39, 58, 68, 154, 156, 157, 159, 171, 172, 174, 181, 183, 187, 190, 193, 194, 195, 202, 280, 301
mood states, 186
morbidity, 75, 76, 160, 186
morphine, 242, 337, 348
morphological abnormalities, 139
morphology, 93, 114, 226, 227, 287, 297, 301
morphometric, 276
mortality, 186, 225
motivation, 4, 39, 41, 46, 47, 51, 197, 218, 348
motor activity, 36, 41, 65, 99, 100, 103, 186, 213, 269, 284, 340
motor behavior, 65, 70, 264, 270, 275
motor control, 262, 282
motor neurons, 12
movement disorders, 23, 50, 69, 76, 93, 136, 207, 266, 269, 271, 273, 325, 333, 349
mucosa, 236
multidimensional, 30, 43, 44

multiple factors, 39
multiple sclerosis, 48, 82, 109
Multiple Sleep Latency Test (MSLT), 28, 45, 46, 48, 51, 55, 56, 83, 185, 201, 255, 256, 257, 262, 263, 270, 325, 330
muscarinic receptor, 188, 189
muscle contraction, 95, 100
muscle relaxant, 139, 340
muscle relaxation, 311, 316
muscles, 47, 70, 80, 82, 87, 95, 100, 102, 103, 104, 137, 138, 139, 143, 254, 261, 262, 265, 267, 268, 272, 282, 312, 340
muscular dystrophy, 82
music, 308, 309
mutant, 205
mutation, 20, 57, 295
myasthenia gravis, 82
myelin, 285
myocardial infarction, 13, 106, 131
myoclonus, 69, 103, 116, 120, 273, 299, 349
myogram, 249, 253
mythology, ix, xi

N

narcotics, 82
National Health and Nutrition Examination Survey, 107
National Institute of Mental Health, 155
National Institutes of Health, 29, 52, 115, 120, 272, 299
natural evolution, 243
nausea, 326, 329, 330, 331, 334, 336
negative effects, 81, 234
negative emotions, 164, 313
negative mood, 194, 236
negative outcomes, 313
neocortex, 12, 293
nerve, 8, 13, 14, 15, 16, 75, 86, 109, 245, 286
nerve fibers, 245
nervous system, 14, 39, 62, 184, 287, 321, 333, 341
neural function, 281
neural network(s), 8
neurobiology, 15, 55, 231, 243
neurodegenerative diseases, 65, 235, 244, 286
neurogenesis, 34, 193
neurogenic bladder, 67
neuroimaging, vii, x, 33, 54, 75, 89, 92, 118, 239, 275, 276, 277, 278, 279, 280, 281, 283, 284, 286, 287, 288, 293, 294, 297, 330
neuroleptic drugs, 339
neuroleptics, 339
neuromuscular diseases, 82

neurons, 4, 5, 6, 7, 8, 9, 12, 15, 42, 55, 57, 82, 101, 185, 188, 190, 191, 197, 211, 233, 236, 240, 277, 279, 286, 327
neuropathy, 80, 143
neuropeptides, 8, 277, 327
neurophysiology, vii, 171
neuropsychological tests, 88, 89
neurosarcoidosis, 48
neuroscience, 293
neurotoxicity, 235
neurotransmission, 98, 185, 188, 196, 234, 235, 237, 286
neurotransmitter(s), 3, 8, 12, 34, 139, 140, 142, 169, 188, 197, 212, 233, 295, 296, 321, 330
New Zealand, 30
nicotine, 42, 155, 158, 231, 236, 243, 244, 307, 308, 309
Niemann-Pick disease, 59
night terrors, 71, 265
nightmares, 64, 66, 71, 79, 156, 164, 165, 166, 167, 168, 169, 175, 176, 209, 255, 265
nigrostriatal, 100, 286
nitric oxide, 87, 118
nitric oxide synthase, 87, 118
nocturia, 109
non-institutionalized, 105
non-smokers, 236, 239
norepinephrine, 167, 169, 199, 207, 237, 319, 324, 327, 328, 331, 332, 344
normal children, 97
normal distribution, 51
North America, 96
NPS, 8
nuclei, 3, 4, 5, 7, 8, 9, 12, 14, 41, 190, 279, 282, 283, 285, 288, 289, 291
nucleus, 4, 5, 6, 7, 8, 9, 12, 14, 15, 42, 99, 183, 191, 207, 236, 278, 282, 284, 286, 288, 290, 291
nucleus tractus solitarius, 42
nurses, 316
nursing, 16, 116, 204, 322, 341
nursing home, 116, 322, 341

O

obesity, 75, 76, 77, 78, 80, 81, 84, 87, 106, 124, 127, 129, 130, 144, 182, 259
objective tests, 45
obsessive-compulsive disorder (OCD), 164, 169, 170, 171, 172, 178, 179, 180
obstruction, 75, 76, 77, 80, 82, 109, 111, 142, 237, 259, 280
obstructive sleep apnea, 27, 40, 54, 56, 65, 68, 72, 76, 83, 91, 93, 107, 108, 109, 110, 111, 112, 113,

114, 115, 123, 125, 129, 131, 132, 133, 139, 140, 142, 156, 160, 235, 244, 254, 262, 268, 275, 287, 297, 298
Obstructive Sleep Apnea Syndrome, v, 77, 78, 123, 280, 289
occipital cortex, 187
occipital lobe, 279
occlusion, 139
occupational health, 44
oesophageal, 148, 149, 150
oil, 179
olanzapine, 167, 223, 228, 229, 320, 343
olfaction, 4
onset latency, 171, 204, 312
opiates, 234, 240
opioids, 337, 338, 348
opportunities, 45, 46, 167, 256
optic chiasm, 4
optic nerve, 326
oral cavity, 142
organic disease, ix, x, 158
organism, 193, 308
organs, 4, 193
orthostatic hypotension, 50, 324
oscillation, 3, 18, 201, 220
osteoarthritis, 104
osteotomy, 298
otolaryngologist, 43
outpatient(s), 116, 170, 175, 212, 213, 262
overlap, 49, 62, 65, 77, 105, 268
overweight, 124, 129, 130
oxidative stress, 87
oxygen, 44, 56, 77, 89, 90, 91, 115, 254, 259, 262, 280, 298
oxyhemoglobin, 40, 44, 125, 261

P

pain, 30, 35, 36, 40, 41, 69, 70, 95, 103, 106, 116, 121, 137, 138, 142, 147, 165, 276, 299, 311, 312, 314, 331, 337
pain tolerance, 311
palate, 83, 129, 133
palliative, 135, 138, 143
palpation, 137
palpitations, 174, 328, 329
panic attack, 49, 63, 70, 168, 169, 177, 178, 265
panic disorder, 163, 164, 165, 168, 169, 177, 178, 179
panic symptoms, 168
paradoxical sleep, 300
parallel, 40, 41, 47, 111, 235, 339
paralysis, 47, 50, 71, 165

paraneoplastic syndrome, 48
parents, 200
parietal cortex, 89, 92, 93, 282
parietal lobe, 92
parietal-occipital cortex, 92
parkinsonism, 71
paroxetine, 167, 171, 197, 331
paroxysmal nocturnal dyspnea, 78
participants, 30, 91, 105, 143, 211, 238, 324, 334
path analysis, 155
pathogenesis, 18, 98, 136, 139, 140, 188, 232, 284, 299
pathology, x, 39, 67, 69, 77, 98, 123, 124, 136, 137, 145, 204
pathophysiological, 17, 98, 139, 154, 181, 267, 273, 285
pathophysiology, 19, 21, 22, 23, 24, 28, 53, 57, 59, 68, 98, 99, 108, 117, 139, 171, 188, 191, 204, 205, 218, 219, 225, 258, 275, 283, 284, 285, 286, 346, 348
pathways, 5, 6, 41, 82, 98, 100, 155, 191, 214
peace, 312
pedigree, 118
peer group, 239
peer review, 90
peptide(s), 15, 57, 295, 332, 345
percentile, 88
perfectionism, 159
perforation, 245
perfusion, 279, 281, 285, 295, 296, 298, 300
periodicity, 50
periodontal, 138, 139
peristalsis, 142, 143
personal history, 31, 200
personality, 21, 31, 48, 66, 96, 141, 159, 162, 164, 175, 182, 259
personality characteristics, 31
personality disorder, 21, 162
personality factors, 21, 164
personality traits, 159, 162
pharmaceutical, 327
pharmacokinetics, 341
pharmacological treatment, 70, 172, 203, 204, 306, 320, 334
pharmacology, 59, 235, 342, 343, 344
pharmacotherapy, 167, 169, 170, 176, 179, 202, 206, 208, 240, 307, 316, 317, 341, 344, 345, 350
pharynx, 13, 75, 82, 108, 143
phase shifts, 211
phenomenology, 58, 99, 175
phenothiazines, 228
phenotypes, 94, 107, 190, 205

Philadelphia, 15, 16, 53, 54, 55, 59, 71, 109, 110, 115, 145, 146, 177, 345
phobia, 168, 172, 180
phosphocreatine, 279
phosphorylation, 183, 205
physical activity, 41, 118, 182, 308, 309
physical health, 104, 167, 175
physical therapy, 139
physicians, 96, 155, 217, 218, 315, 316
physiological, 13, 14, 42, 276
physiological arousal, 307
physiological mechanisms, 4
physiology, 3, 15, 136, 145, 146, 181, 182, 194, 228
physiopathology, 100
pilot study, 54, 121, 176, 214, 342, 347
pineal gland, x, 4, 207, 233
pineal hormone melatonin, 184
placebo, 25, 72, 90, 91, 112, 114, 115, 119, 180, 211, 214, 229, 298, 323, 324, 325, 327, 330, 335, 336, 337, 338, 339, 340, 341, 342, 345, 347, 348, 349, 350
plants, 237, 241
plasma levels, 335, 338
plasticity, 235, 245
playing, 287
plethysmography, 85, 111, 261, 271
polycystic ovarian syndrome, 80
polymorphism(s), 99, 157, 190, 214
pons, 9, 41, 185, 276, 282, 284, 285, 286, 290, 291
pools, 49
population control, 49
portability, 103
Portugal, 30
positive correlation, 47, 221, 325
positive reinforcement, 236
positive relationship, 221
positron, 33, 239, 293, 301, 344
positron emission tomography (PET), 33, 239, 276, 277, 279, 280, 286, 287, 288, 290, 291, 292, 293, 296, 299, 301, 344
post-hoc analysis, 347
posttraumatic stress, 63, 175, 176, 177
post-traumatic stress disorder (PTSD), 63, 66, 70, 71, 72, 156, 160, 163, 164, 165, 166, 167, 168, 169, 174, 175, 176, 177
prefrontal cortex, 9, 187, 239, 276, 279, 284, 290, 301
pregnancy, 31, 80, 94, 96, 116, 333
preparation, 179, 326
preschool, 42
preschoolers, 69
prescription drugs, 24
preservation, 3

preterm infants, 148
prevalence rate, 30
prevention, 145, 156, 159, 180, 210, 243, 244, 326
priapism, 324
principles, vii, 24, 272, 315
probability, 44, 84, 86, 101, 336
probands, 200, 213
probe, 86
prodromal symptoms, 208
prognosis, 158, 197
programming, 224, 315
pro-inflammatory, 193
project, 5, 8, 9, 12
prolactin, 179, 186
propranolol, 340, 349, 350
prosthesis, 135, 136, 137, 138
proteins, 183
proton pump inhibitors, 143
psychiatric diagnosis, 69, 154
psychiatric disorders, vi, vii, x, 30, 34, 35, 70, 151, 153, 154, 155, 159, 161, 166, 172, 174, 180, 200, 210, 211, 215, 231, 243, 244, 258, 275
psychiatric illness, 66, 154, 155, 163, 200, 232, 306, 314, 325
psychiatric patients, 219, 227, 343
psychiatry, vii, 57, 154, 243, 344
psychoactive drug, 56, 231, 234, 241
psychological distress, 153, 154
psychological problems, 166
psychological stress, 140, 147, 158
psychology, 226
psychopathology, 58, 66, 70, 177, 179, 193, 211, 232
psychopharmacology, 211, 214, 215
psychoses, 160, 226, 227, 301
psychosis, 49, 58, 157, 158, 159, 218, 219, 221, 226, 328, 329
psychosocial factors, 147
psychosocial stress, 32, 39
psychosomatic, 141
psychostimulants, 231, 237
psychotherapy, 199, 208, 212, 318
psychotic symptomatology, 218
psychotic symptoms, 157, 158, 224
psychotropic medications, 35
PTT, 86
puberty, 156
public health, 29, 76, 124, 154, 209, 238
pulmonary circulation, 87
pulmonary diseases, 35
pulmonary hypertension, 78, 87, 111, 280

Q

quality of life, 30, 42, 48, 53, 58, 91, 101, 104, 112, 115, 120, 121, 123, 124, 136, 154, 157, 159, 161, 175, 195, 200, 218, 225, 280, 297, 305, 320, 334, 337, 341
quantification, 102, 103
questionnaire, 30, 43, 84, 97, 101, 104, 105, 106, 110, 120, 132, 136, 264
quetiapine, 167, 172, 179, 207, 215, 229, 320, 325, 342, 343

R

race, 106, 108
racing, 168
rape, 241
rapid eye movement sleep, 63, 119, 162, 187, 211, 229, 236, 272, 293, 300, 301, 312
rapid eye movements, x, 11, 12, 252, 265
rating scale, 44, 120
reaction time, 88, 90
reactions, 49, 322, 336, 341
reactive oxygen, 87
reactivity, 95, 167, 195, 212
reading, 42, 43, 258, 308, 309, 320
reality, 49
reasoning, 192
recall, 66, 68, 71, 90, 178, 222, 270, 313, 322
recall information, 322
receptors, 4, 8, 9, 82, 98, 100, 142, 193, 197, 198, 206, 224, 228, 234, 235, 236, 237, 238, 239, 240, 279, 283, 284, 285, 290, 296, 299, 320, 321, 324, 326, 327, 330, 335, 336
recession, 138
reciprocal relationships, 49
recognition, 28, 75, 76, 160, 161, 213, 225, 243
recommendations, 21, 29, 44, 110, 111, 132, 256, 264, 271, 305, 307, 338, 348
recovery, 54, 63, 166, 187, 197, 198, 201, 208, 209, 277
recreational, 238, 241, 242, 245, 339
recurrence, 38, 154, 159, 187, 205, 326
reflexes, 12, 43
regression, 89, 97, 133
regression analysis, 97
reinforcement, 194, 240, 310
relapses, 157, 168, 204
relatives, 156, 187, 189, 200, 213
relaxation, 20, 142, 167, 208, 306, 307, 311, 312, 314, 315, 317, 320
relevance, 52, 202, 204, 205, 218, 220, 255, 338

reliability, 45
relief, 94, 194, 319, 331, 335
remediation, 218, 225
remission, 30, 38, 50, 52, 94, 154, 155, 160, 186, 195, 197, 200, 208, 209, 216
remorse, 238
renal dysfunction, 97
renal failure, 97
renin, 87
replication, 228
requirements, 75, 85, 267
RES, 116, 121, 349
researchers, x, 41, 88, 90, 138, 154, 219, 237, 238
resistance, 13, 14, 32, 44, 64, 76, 85, 87, 107, 111, 133, 140, 147, 156, 271, 334
resolution, 37, 51, 92, 94, 280
resources, 136
respiration, 14, 47, 76, 77, 81, 82, 137
respiratory arrest, 125, 127
respiratory disorders, 113, 125, 130
respiratory failure, 109
respiratory rate, 67, 77, 139, 169
responsiveness, 9, 14, 81, 109, 165
restless legs syndrome, 42, 96, 115, 116, 117, 118, 119, 120, 121, 185, 207, 255, 257, 262, 266, 272, 273, 275, 287, 299, 300, 320, 325, 333, 342, 346, 347, 348, 349, 350
restoration, 39, 184
restrictions, 206
restructuring, 198, 313, 315
retardation, 155
reticular activating system, 4, 33, 185, 277, 288, 292
retina, x, 4, 10
retino-hypothalamic tract (RHT), 18
rhythm, x, xi, 3, 4, 8, 9, 11, 12, 17, 18, 21, 24, 25, 57, 58, 82, 157, 163, 182, 183, 185, 190, 201, 203, 208, 213, 214, 215, 250, 257, 264, 272, 312
rhythmicity, 200
risk factors, 78, 80, 87, 95, 108, 109, 121, 123, 124, 128, 129, 130, 133, 155, 159, 209, 258, 259, 322
risperidone, 117, 167, 177, 223, 228
rodents, 205, 333
Rouleau, 112
routines, 31
rules, 71, 132, 219, 267, 270, 310

S

sadness, 42, 164
safety, 45, 256, 312, 319, 320, 323, 325, 327, 336, 343, 344, 347, 349
saliva, 140, 142, 148, 149
salts, 241

SANS, 218
SAPS, 218
SAS, 124, 268
saturation, 44, 56, 77, 125, 254, 261, 262
schizophrenia, vi, 48, 49, 58, 66, 157, 158, 160, 161,
    214, 217, 218, 219, 220, 221, 222, 223, 224, 225,
    226, 227, 228, 229, 287, 292, 301
schizophrenic patients, 49, 157, 161, 219, 220, 222,
    223, 226, 227, 228, 229
school, 21, 42, 77, 107, 332
school performance, 77
science, vii, 15, 229, 317
scope, 241
secretion, 4, 13, 16, 18, 100, 142, 149, 182, 184, 185,
    186, 188, 191, 207, 225, 228, 233, 237
sedative, 19, 203, 207, 231, 234, 235, 240, 243, 322,
    338, 341
sedatives, 63, 82, 222
segregation, 200
seizure, 63, 254, 255, 265
selective attention, 239
selective serotonin reuptake inhibitor, 66, 99, 140,
    167, 177, 199, 339, 341
self-assessment, 154
self-concept, 194, 211
self-control, 317
self-esteem, 42, 241
self-regulation, 312
self-reports, 324
sensation(s), ix, 83, 93, 94, 95, 104, 108, 139, 164,
    266, 268, 329
senses, 66, 68
sensitivity, 44, 46, 95, 102, 140, 147, 183, 189, 204,
    212, 235, 237, 257
sensitization, 182
sensors, 36, 44, 45, 85
sensory experience, 241
septum, 12, 43
serotonergic dysfunction, 210
serotonin, 6, 7, 8, 100, 167, 169, 170, 188, 196, 197,
    199, 208, 210, 214, 226, 233, 234, 238, 244, 245,
    319, 324, 327, 331, 349
sertraline, 72, 171, 197, 344
serum, 78, 98
serum ferritin, 98
sex, 22, 38, 49, 78, 87, 106, 126, 164, 170, 212, 214,
    244, 283
sexual abuse, 165
shame, 243
shape, 9
shortage, 315
shortness of breath, 174
short-term memory, 324

showing, 130, 155, 188, 232, 263, 265, 276, 281,
    286, 316, 324, 326
side effects, 197, 207, 208, 305, 306, 316, 323, 324,
    330, 331
signal transduction, 240
signals, 4, 41, 44, 161, 205, 225, 262, 282, 312
signs, 40, 66, 107, 147, 210, 267, 322, 338
simulation(s), 88, 113
Sinai, 161
single-nucleotide polymorphism (SNP), 140, 205
skeletal muscle, 62, 65, 185, 284
skeleton, 285
skin, 32, 64, 83, 254, 312
sleep apnea, 43, 56, 64, 65, 67, 72, 75, 77, 80, 81, 84,
    87, 92, 96, 107, 108, 109, 110, 111, 112, 113,
    114, 123, 124, 131, 132, 133, 140, 160, 164, 168,
    169, 236, 257, 259, 262, 266, 271, 280, 297, 298,
    328
Sleep Bruxism, vi, 135, 145, 146
sleep deprivation, 34, 39, 41, 42, 44, 46, 51, 54, 55,
    59, 62, 63, 66, 156, 158, 168, 174, 180, 188, 189,
    191, 192, 194, 201, 202, 203, 208, 209, 212, 213,
    215, 238, 277, 294, 306, 323, 328, 335
sleep Disorders, v, vi, x, xi, 1, 24, 27, 28, 51, 52, 55,
    61, 75, 76, 95, 102, 107, 126, 132, 133, 135, 136,
    231, 232, 249, 253, 267, 270, 271, 275, 306, 319,
    333, 349
sleep disturbances, vi, 153, 163, 186, 187, 200, 201,
    202, 204, 209
sleep fragmentation, 6, 23, 40, 43, 48, 86, 89, 130,
    166, 267, 332, 338
sleep habits, 30, 82, 105, 147, 153, 307, 328
sleep latency, 20, 32, 36, 38, 45, 46, 48, 51, 55, 56,
    83, 156, 157, 158, 166, 168, 170, 185, 186, 188,
    191, 197, 204, 209, 213, 219, 220, 221, 236, 249,
    255, 256, 257, 263, 270, 321, 324, 325, 326
sleep medicine, vii, x, 44, 71, 145, 146, 177, 258,
    275, 297, 301, 317
sleep paralysis, 47, 51, 62, 65, 66, 72, 164, 168, 175,
    262, 330
sleep physiology, 3, 59, 194
sleep propensity, 40, 41, 189
sleep spindle, 10, 11, 12, 184, 220, 312
sleep stage, 9, 10, 12, 15, 36, 64, 65, 101, 102, 126,
    139, 140, 143, 164, 192, 220, 249, 250, 252, 254,
    261, 262, 269, 276, 311, 337
sleep terrors, 62, 64, 65, 66, 70, 71, 169, 269
sleep walking, 269, 323
sleeping pills, 20
sleeping problems, 34
Sleep-Related Breathing Disorders, 76
Sleep-Related Movement Disorders, 93, 333

smoking, 87, 95, 106, 129, 140, 141, 142, 236, 237, 239, 244, 350
smoking cessation, 236
snacking, 310
snoring, 36, 42, 43, 67, 77, 79, 80, 83, 84, 85, 96, 107, 108, 109, 124, 125, 127, 130, 133, 140, 185, 253, 259, 262, 265, 271
social activities, 18, 23
social consequences, 20
social events, 20
social impairment, 168, 169
social interactions, 101, 182
social life, 22
social phobia, 49, 164, 165, 172, 180
social withdrawal, 42, 51
society, 27, 76, 234, 243
socioeconomic status, 200
sodium, 178, 319, 328, 329, 331, 345
software, 257, 271
somatization, 168
somatomotor, 252
somnolence, 20, 27, 39, 47, 50, 56, 57, 59, 88, 117, 197, 224, 326, 328, 331, 336, 337
Spain, 30, 79
spatial memory, 222
specialists, 79
species, 87, 182
specifications, 270
spectroscopy, 115, 295, 297, 300
speculation, 99
speech, 47, 63
spending, 307, 309
spinal cord, 12, 99, 101, 118, 119, 277
spinal cord injury, 99, 118
splint, 91, 139, 143
stability, 200
stabilization, 208, 240
stabilizers, 205, 206, 207, 332
standard deviation, 126
standardization, 44, 219
Stanford Sleepiness Scale (SSS), 43, 44, 56, 85
steroids, 35
stimulant, x, 49, 51, 237, 241, 256, 263, 280, 328, 329, 332, 333, 346
stimulation, 34, 55, 94, 135, 142, 145, 183, 197, 205, 206, 224, 280, 328, 335
stimulus, 31, 38, 47, 189, 208, 306, 307, 308, 309, 310, 314, 315, 316, 322
stomach, 142, 145, 241, 308, 309, 323
stratification, 104, 271
stress, 32, 35, 37, 66, 72, 95, 119, 139, 140, 141, 142, 147, 148, 149, 158, 161, 165, 175, 181, 182, 183, 191, 192, 193, 211, 212, 281, 313

stress response, 148, 313
stressful life events, 203
stressors, 208
stretching, 95
striatum, 4, 98, 239, 283, 288
stroke, 77, 79, 106, 107, 109
structural changes, 92, 114, 115, 297
structure, 109, 154, 193, 197, 266, 272, 283, 287
style, 182, 208
subdomains, 88
subjective experience, 32
substance abuse, 30, 39, 42, 66, 231, 264, 306
Substance Abuse and Mental Health Services Administration, 210
substance addiction, 243
substance use, 31, 34, 64, 69, 154, 231, 233, 243, 245, 263, 265, 267, 322
substitutes, 313
substitution, 90, 240
substrate(s), 41, 55, 343
succession, 252
sucrose, 205
suicidal behavior, 215
suicidal ideation, 155, 194, 209, 215
suicide, 209, 210, 215, 218
suicide attempts, 209, 215
Sun, 344
supplementation, 338
suppression, 46, 150, 192, 196, 197, 198, 212
suprachiasmatic nucleus, x, 4, 18, 21, 182, 183, 233, 326
surrogates, 86
surveillance, 261
survivors, 175, 216
susceptibility, 21, 99, 117, 118, 190, 217, 218, 306
synapse, 342
synaptic plasticity, 166, 192
synchronization, 18, 20, 183, 231
synthesis, x, 98, 116, 117, 197, 205, 284
systematic desensitization, 167
systolic blood pressure, 87, 106

T

tachycardia, 64, 70, 101, 169, 237, 331
tachypnea, 64
tardive dyskinesia, 157
target, 157, 198, 204, 206, 233, 306, 313, 315, 343
target response, 313
Task Force, 44, 56, 110, 111, 120, 132, 264
tau, 18, 201
T-cell receptor, 345
technetium, 279

technician, 254, 261

techniques, 15, 20, 99, 102, 103, 105, 110, 120, 132, 167, 273, 276, 287, 311, 312, 313, 314, 317

technological advances, 44

teeth, 69, 100, 103, 135, 136, 137, 138, 139, 268

telephone, 104, 105, 132, 315, 316

temperament, 154, 239, 245

temperature, 4, 13, 14, 18, 20, 32, 41, 46, 181, 182, 183, 184, 186, 190, 256

temporal lobe, 50, 89, 285, 291

temporomandibular disorders, 95, 135, 136

tendon, 12, 43

tension, 37, 86, 103, 128, 138, 168, 174, 311, 312

terminals, 286

testing, 49, 88, 91, 93, 110, 189, 203, 256

texture, 241

thalamocortical system, 41

thalamus, 5, 9, 14, 33, 42, 239, 276, 277, 281, 282, 283, 284, 286, 288, 289, 290, 291, 292, 293, 295

therapeutic agents, 157, 339

therapeutic approaches, 218, 275

therapeutic effects, 205, 211, 343

therapeutic interventions, 157, 332

therapeutic use, 333

therapeutics, 162, 244

therapist, 311, 314, 315

thermoregulation, 32

theta waves, 10, 11

thoughts, ix, 37, 164, 166, 168, 169, 306, 308, 309, 311, 313

threats, 165

threshold level, 100

thyroid, 13, 35, 183

tibialis anterior, 102, 267

time frame, 34

tissue, 75, 81, 133, 138, 193

tobacco, 82, 124, 236, 244, 339

tobacco smoking, 339

tonic, 72, 103, 104, 184, 235, 265, 268, 269

tonometry, 86, 111

tonsils, 80

tooth, 9, 95, 106, 138, 139, 143, 339

top-down, 100

torus, 138

total cholesterol, 106

toxin, 69, 139, 340, 350

trafficking, 344

training, 67, 208, 311, 312, 317, 334

traits, 159

tranquilizers, 63

transaminases, 327

transcription, 4, 183, 240

transcripts, 14

transferrin, 98, 117

translation, xi, 4

transmission, 5, 196, 205, 214, 233, 236, 238, 319, 329, 331

transport, 142, 344

trauma, 80, 138, 165, 166, 255

traumatic brain injury, 165, 175

traumatic events, 165

tremor, 174, 237

trial, 25, 46, 72, 91, 111, 112, 114, 119, 133, 146, 147, 176, 177, 211, 215, 225, 229, 256, 317, 318, 320, 325, 328, 330, 334, 336, 337, 340, 342, 343, 344, 345, 346, 347, 349, 350

tricyclic antidepressant(s), 66, 67, 169, 199, 214, 324, 327

triggers, 156, 168, 202, 319, 332

truck drivers, 46, 244

tryptophan, 196, 197

TSH, 186

tuberomammillary nucleus, 5, 7, 8, 12

tumor(s), 32, 48, 57

tumor necrosis factor (TNF), 32

turbinates, 43

turnover, 93, 197

twins, 141

tyramine, 330

tyrosine, 98, 118, 205, 284

tyrosine hydroxylase, 98, 205, 284

U

underlying mechanisms, 89

united, 30, 48, 80, 104, 132, 180, 239, 243

United Kingdom (UK), 30, 132, 239, 241, 244

United States (USA), 48, 79, 80, 104, 180, 243, 244

upper airways, 76

urban, 108, 133

urban population, 133

urinary retention, 324, 331

urinary tract, 67

urine, 13, 67

uvula, 83

V

Valencia, 114, 150

validation, 54, 111

valuation, 102

valve, 335, 346

valvular heart disease, 335

variables, 158, 161, 215, 216, 219, 220, 221, 222, 223, 227, 314, 322

variations, xi, 3, 12, 205, 257
varieties, 70
vascular dementia, 293
vasoconstriction, 32, 86, 87, 328
vasopressin, 67
vasovagal syncope, 172
venlafaxine, 66, 99, 169, 327, 332
ventilation, 81, 82, 166, 271
ventral periaqueductal gray matter, 5, 7, 9, 15, 55
ventricle, 287, 292
victims, 175, 176
video-recording, 103
videos, 43
Vietnam, 175
violence, 62, 175
violent behavior, 62, 323
vision, 4
visual environment, 21
vitamins, 24
vocalizations, 65, 70, 265
voiding, 67
vomiting, 329, 331, 336
vulnerability, 157, 166, 187, 200, 201, 204, 214

W

waking, vii, 6, 12, 13, 18, 19, 22, 27, 28, 32, 36, 37, 39, 40, 42, 55, 57, 58, 68, 81, 120, 135, 136, 140, 142, 166, 168, 186, 187, 204, 210, 211, 224, 250, 258, 266, 273, 276, 277, 278, 279, 287, 288, 292, 293, 294, 301, 308, 309
walking, 63, 83, 94, 102, 269, 284, 331
Washington, 15, 51, 72, 119, 174, 243, 317, 342
water, 49
weakness, 43, 95, 168, 262

wealth, 287
wear, 135, 136, 137, 138, 143, 257
web, 241
weight changes, 49
weight gain, 207, 320, 325, 331
weight loss, 331
well-being, 27, 28, 198
Western countries, 124, 236
Western Europe, 48
white matter, 89, 239, 281, 284, 285, 289, 290
windows, 64, 100
Wisconsin, 87, 105, 121
withdrawal, 87, 92, 202, 206, 232, 233, 234, 235, 236, 240, 243, 244, 320, 322, 329, 334, 345
withdrawal symptoms, 320
workers, 52, 76, 88, 89, 218, 220, 239
working memory, 92, 115, 218, 281, 298
World Health Organization, 236, 244
worldwide, 234, 236
worms, 93
worry, 31, 37, 141, 171, 306, 313

Y

Yemen, 241
yield, 266
young adults, 38, 89, 97, 159, 209, 228, 229, 241, 263
young people, 239
young women, 35, 238

Z

ziprasidone, 223, 229